# What Folks Have to Say

*"This book is a cornucopia of food and nutrition information! While it is a cookbook, it is also an educational piece packed with valuable tips and tools. The recipes are mouthwatering with something for everyone. Well-referenced and beautifully organized, Dr. Karr and her team have outdone themselves"!*

Nicole Hodson, NC, BCHN®, CDSP™
NANP Executive Director

~~~~~~~~~

*In the revised second edition of Our Journey with Food Cookery Book, Tammera Karr once again outshines herself with her unrelenting ability and dedicated passion to highlight just exactly why – and how – we ought to pay attention to anything related to food.*

*With contagious aplomb she takes the reader on a journey filled with encaptivating stories on often hilarious historical origins, traditional preparations and moving rituals but also modern, pragmatic tips so needed in a fast-paced and stress-pressured society that has lost touch with exactly how to, not laboriously but easily, prepare nutrient-dense food from scratch.*

*New chapters have been added while previous ones have been expanded. "Grains" as well as "Tubers and Roots" each have their own spotlight chapters now, so important in a time where trendy diets have demonized these two vitally nutritious food sources. Another new chapter "Umami" elevates the powerful mushrooms to the status they deserve, showcasing both their medicinal as well as they flavor power. "The Wild Side of Food" introduces the reader to mouthwatering recipes using edible plants that are often discarded as simply weeds to be destroyed. "Where's the Cheese" highlights the nutritional value of traditionally fermented dairy, reminding the reader how our industrialized, highly processed cheese is a far cry from the nutritional powerhouse of true cheese.*

*And of course, this would not be a Cookery Book without the addition of new scrumptious recipes, encouraging the reader to delve into often believed to be too cumbersome traditional food preparations by offering modern adaptations to allow the reader to, once again, connect to the unifying harmony that blends old and new, tradition and modernity, and serves but one purpose – to nourish Body and Soul, and became part of a universal Whole that transcends place and time.*

<div align="right">

Kirstin Nussgruber, CNC, EMB, BCHN®
Founder of Eat Holistic LLC
Vice President: National Association of Nutrition Professionals
Author of "Confessions of a Cancer Conqueror - My 5 Step Process to Transform Your Relationship with Cancer"

</div>

~~~~~~~~~

*No matter how much I think I know about food, Tammera Karr proves there is still so much more to learn. In-depth, well-researched, and filled with historical notes and quotes. I have to say, out of all the mouth-watering recipes shared within, the Recipe for Happiness is my favorite! A true gift of knowledge and wisdom. This book deserves a place in everyone's home!*

Susan Schiliro Guegan, NC, BCHN®, CHC
Author of *Don the Rooster and Me*

*Our Journey with Food*

# Cookery Book

*2nd edition*

Tammera J. Karr, PhD, BCHN®, CNW®, CGP

With

Chef Benjamin Qualls

Chef Christine Wokowsky, CN, CGP

Forewords by

Bill Schindler, PhD

Janet Ludwig, PhD

Editor & Content Advisor

Julie Thenell BS, MS, NC, BCHN®, CDSP™

Jacket Artwork by *JV Media Design*

Images/Illustrations
Waste Not Want Not WWI Canadian War Office Poster; Library of Congress
Oregon Historical Society
Vintage Advertising Archive
Adobe Stock Licensed
Authors Private Collection
Chetco, Crook, Wallowa and Grant County Museums, Oregon, USA

Copy Editor & Content Advisor
Julie Thenell, BS, MS, NC, BCHN®, CDSP™

1st edition ISBN: 978-0-9995562-8-3
2nd edition 2022-ISBN: 979-8-9864312-3-9

Library of Congress: 2018961169

All rights reserved ©2018, 2022 by Tammera J. Karr
and Holistic Nutrition for the Whole You

**SUMMERLAND PUBLISHING**
Summerland Publishing
Millcreek, UT

**Disclaimer:** Many of the recipes in this book originated from historical cookbooks still in use by the authors. As much as possible, the authors adhered to the original text and regional spelling of works for historical preservation. The authors of this cookery book do not endorse or subscribe to any set "dietary" approach. The emphasis is on locally produced, genetically, and culturally appropriate foodstuffs. This cookery book does not wholly represent the world's traditional /ancestral foods.

**If you have food allergies or sensitivities, you must modify recipes to fit your needs.** Consult with your healthcare provider before making broad dietary changes.

## *Dedication*

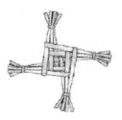

For all those who cook tasty food; past, present, and future. In remembrance of Betty Sitz, who flavored every meal with love and always had a recipe close at hand.

## *Acknowledgments*

This cookery book would not have been possible without help from many individuals. Thank you to all the students and colleagues who shared flavor and spice from their own cultures and histories.

A special thanks to Sherry Holub who created the notion, contributed, and designed the jacket.

Michael Karr who stood by taking notes in the kitchen, proofreading, formatting, and contributing research and quotes, is beyond compare. Michaels's continuous encouragement to create a legacy of traditional food knowledge for our son Brendan, grandson Michael, niece Neveah, and nephews Matt, Don, and Christian.

Countless dedicated hours from our editor, Julie Thenell. Gratitude to Chef Ben for proofing and adapting historic recipes, and Chef Christine who added a flair of exotic to the menus.

## *Advisors, Reviewers & Content Contributors*

Lorrie Amitrano, FNP-C
Sarica Cernohous, DACM, LAc
Nour Danno, Dietitian, PE
Mira Dessy, NE
Cynthia Edmunds, DACM, LAc
Jennifer Grafiada, MS
Sharena Graves
Stacy Gomes, EdD, MAEd
Leena Guptha, ND, DO, PhD
Soneil Guptha, MD, FACC
Nicole Hammond
Nicole Hodson, NC, BCHN,® CDSP™
Michael Karr
Karen Langston, CN, CHN, CNCP
Elizabeth Lipski, PhD, BCHN®

Janet Ludwig, PhD, MS
Denise Couturier Maitret
Mely Martinez
Medha Mujumdar Murtyy
Kirstin Nussgruber, CNC®, EMB, BCHN®
Benjamin & Cindy Qualls
Roseanne Romaine, BCHN®
Bill & Christina Schindler
Crystal Shephard, MS
BeeBee & Kelsi Sitz
Chris Smith
Anastasiya Terentyeva
Julie Thenell, BS, MS, BCHN®, CDSP™
Christine Wokowsky, CN, CGP
Miriam G. Zacharias, MS, NTC, BCHN®

# CELEBRATING 150 YEARS OF COOKERY MAGIC
# &
# CULTURAL CONNECTION!

Traditional, Cultural, Ancestral, Wild, or Just Plain Good Food has been provided by our contributors from:

Canada
Central America
Croatia
Cuba
Egypt
England
Euskadi Herria (*Basque Country*)
Finland
France
Germany
Greece
Hungary
India
Italy
Iran
Ireland
Korea
Lebanon
México
Scotland
Sicily
South Africa
South America
Turkey
Ukraine
United States
Wales

# Contents

| | | |
|---|---|---|
| 1) | ACKNOWLEDGMENTS | V |
| 2) | FOREWORD BY DR. BILL SCHINDLER | XI |
| 3) | FOREWORD BY DR. JANET LUDWIG | XV |
| 4) | INTRODUCTION ~ LET THE JOURNEY BEGIN | 1 |
| 5) | THE PANTRY | 11 |
| 6) | GIZMOS & GADGETS FOR THE KITCHEN | 51 |
| 7) | CULINARY HERBS & SPICES | 67 |
| 8) | VEGETABLES | 81 |
| 9) | TUBERS & ROOTS | 103 |
| 10) | BEANS & LENTILS | 119 |
| 11) | GRAINS | 135 |
| 12) | UMAMI ~ THE 5TH TASTE OF FUNGI | 169 |
| 13) | THE WILD SIDE OF FOOD | 181 |

| | | |
|---|---|---|
| 14) | BEEF, LAMB, PORK & POULTRY | *211* |
| 15) | CRUSTACEANS, FISH & MOLLUSK | *255* |
| 16) | FERMENTED FOODS | *269* |
| 17) | WHERE'S THE CHEESE? | *295* |
| 18) | DRESSINGS & SAUCES | *305* |
| 19) | BERRIES & FRUITS | *319* |
| 20) | DESSERTS FOR SPECIAL OCCASIONS | *331* |
| 21) | TRAVEL FOOD & SNACKS | *351* |
| 22) | BEVERAGES | *359* |
| 23) | WISDOM FROM THE PAST | *373* |
| 24) | FINAL THOUGHTS FROM CHEF CHRISTINE | *399* |
| 25) | LIST OF PRINCIPLES | *401* |
| 26) | MODERN & HISTORICAL COOKERY RESOURCES | *403* |
| 27) | INDEX | *409* |

## *Hidden Delights*

*I hold a perfect blackberry in my hand and reflect on all the hands that have done this before me.*

*The woman in skin garments, or gingham, the child with sun-bleached hair, or the work-hardened hands of a man. Wild animals have gingerly plucked or torn free the foods of the earth equally.*

*As I savor the sweet tartness of the berries, I'm scolded by the blue jay and gray squirrel for beating them to the last of summer's hidden delights.*

*Unlike those of olden days, hunger is not what stops me at the berry patch.*

*It is connection and preservation of knowledge.
Do not forget the bounty of the earth, a quiet voice on the breeze whispers to me.*

*Nor the pure joy in hidden delights.*

~ *Tammera J. Karr*
*2018*

x

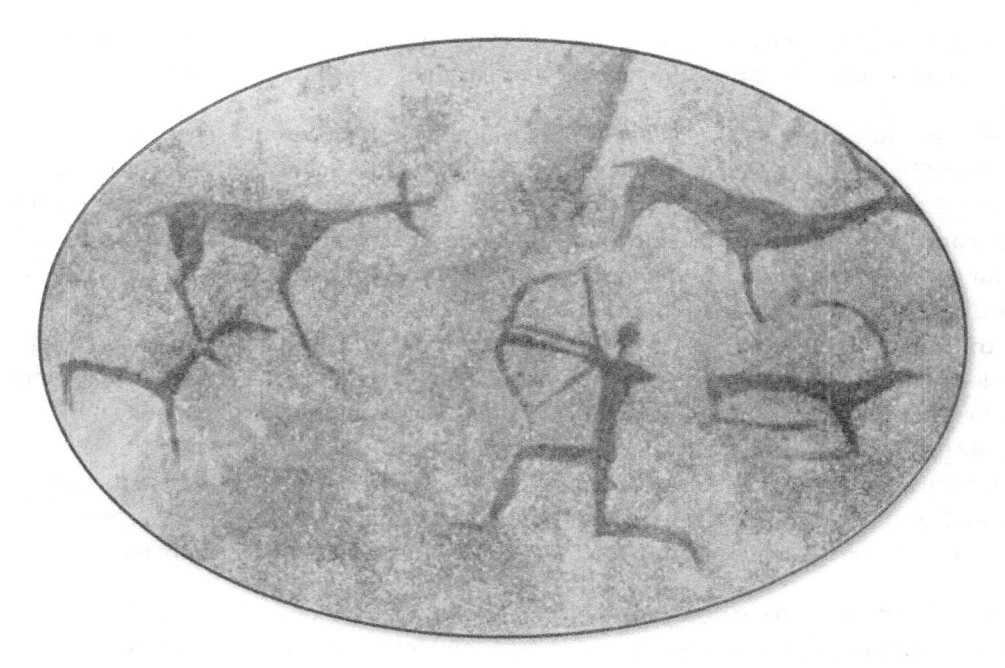

*"Food brings people together on many different levels.
It's nourishment of the soul and body; it's truly love."*

~ Chef Giada De Laurentiis

## Foreword by Bill Schindler, PhD

*2nd edition*

*I believe food can once again nourish us - and this book helps show us how.*

The way our ancestors approached food in the past provided life-sustaining and valuable nourishment that literally fueled our evolutionary growth of our bodies and brains, eventually resulting in us, the modern-day *Homo sapiens*. It also fueled our cultural, intellectual, and even geographic growth providing the nourishment necessary for populations to expand and inhabit the entire world.

This global expansion was all possible because we humans were viscerally connected to our entire food system. None of it was hidden from us - where our food came from, how it was prepared, eating together, and sharing food - all of it was a part of our lives in an intimate way - from the moment we woke until the time we retired at night each day. Every day.

Our relationship with food has changed — drastically. Beginning with the agricultural revolution and intensifying with the industrial revolution, resulting in the majority of present-day humans becoming increasingly separated from the food they consume day-to-day. The transition from hunting and gathering to food production resulted in some members working harder to raise food for everyone else within their community. While this allowed for specialization, it also opened the door to unintended disastrous consequences. One result came with the rise of industrialization in the 1760s which led to food production and preparation at home being regarded as an impediment to progress. With the birth of the industrial food system, the masses could be freed from the "burden" of growing, raising, harvesting, and cooking food and concentrate on the more important tasks of industrial expansion. Each of these steps, incremental at times and more dramatic at others, separated the population from their *daily bread* and, over generations, resulting in the loss of traditional food acquisition, preparation, and storage knowledge that once ensured food was nourishing, ethical, and sustainable.

In a world filled with a dizzying array of information regarding food, diet and health, we are starting to realize that so much of it is biased, false, and irrelevant. We are constantly bombarded with fad diets and false claims of health-inducing products. Today, most individuals are so far removed from their food that they don't know anything about what they are actually eating or the people and realities involved in the food chain. Our health and well-being are paying the price for the lost connection to the cycle of food that propelled us from the dawn of time to the modern age. The question is have we as humans lost the ability to include food in a meaningful and restorative way in our lives? Ancestral ways that nourish and connect us to the people and environment around us?

Traditional approaches to food are tried and true - put to the test through years, generations, and eons of trial and error. The most successful methods increased evolutionary fitness in populations, and unsuccessful approaches died out along with their practitioners. Natural selection extends to food and dietary practices. Without food, there would be no you or me.

What we need is to simply regain the power of real, genuine food made using time-honored traditions and high-quality ingredients, raised, and prepared in vitalizing ways. We need to return to our kitchens, take back control, and nourish our families. And that is precisely what makes this second edition of *Our Journey with Food Cookery Book*, from Tammera J. Karr, Benjamin Qualls, and Christine Wokowsky, so valuable. This comprehensive work is exactly what we need to begin to heal our broken relationship with food.

The foundational thread that runs through this book is tradition and is interwoven with personal stories, nutrition, history, science, and home economics. The authors share the powerful connections with food they enjoyed throughout their lives with the readers, and it is through those connections: connection to place, connection to the past, and connection to yourself, where true nourishment and enjoyment from food can be found.

This new inclusive edition contains over 395 adapted and historical recipes, representing cultural foods supported by citations and references — a true tome, chocked full of useful information needed to know in order to stock, maintain, and use your kitchen as a place that creates nourishing, meaningful food.

This book is also practical and accessible. Injected throughout the book are principles that make the massive amount of information provided both "digestible" and meaningful. The lessons and techniques come directly from the authors who actually cook and do everything they write about. For example, Tammera's Whole Chicken Routine illustrates how she breaks down a chicken and incorporates the different parts in various meals throughout the week, and it doesn't stop there. The practical information just keeps coming and includes tons of lists like what produce lends itself to cold storage, differences between various types of flour, and what tools and gadgets any well-stocked kitchen should have, and I wholeheartedly agree with the authors that a Vitamix® is a necessity!

Tammera Karr perfectly captured this book's essence in her poem *Hidden Delights* when she wrote, "*It is connection and preservation of knowledge.*" That is precisely what they have created with this practical, relevant, and powerful book. These authors have done something incredible and created a resource that entertains, informs, and empowers all of us to get back into our kitchens, dust off our aprons, and prepare truly nourishing food for our families.

~ Bill Schindler, PhD
Author of *Eat Like A Human*, Speaker and Educator
*Director of the Eastern Shore Food Lab and Executive Chef at Modern Stone Age Kitchen*

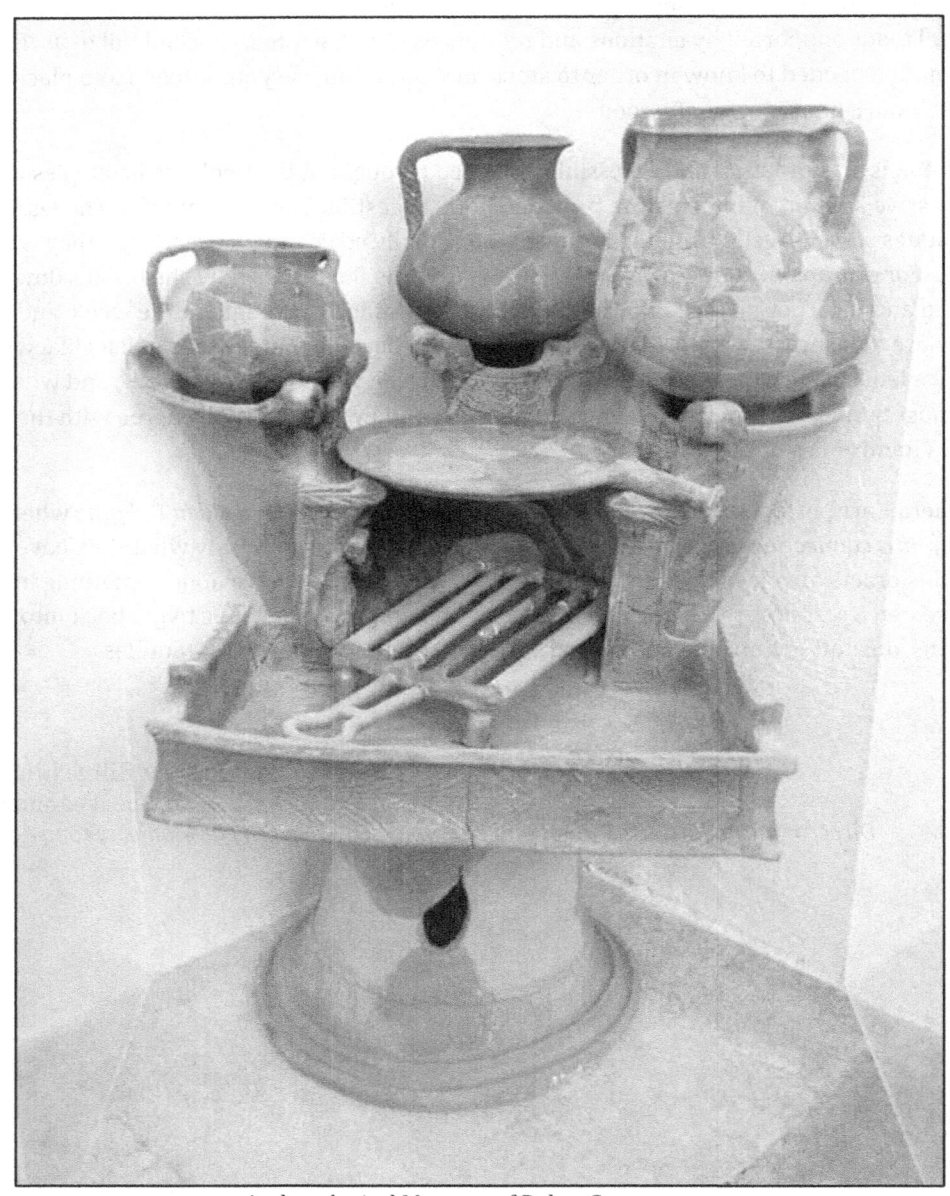

Archaeological Museum of Delos, Greece

A 2,500 year old stove (kitchen) made of clay with 3 burners, oven, grill and baking plate in Delos, Greece. This compact and practical design served the Greek household needs like todays electric or gas stove.

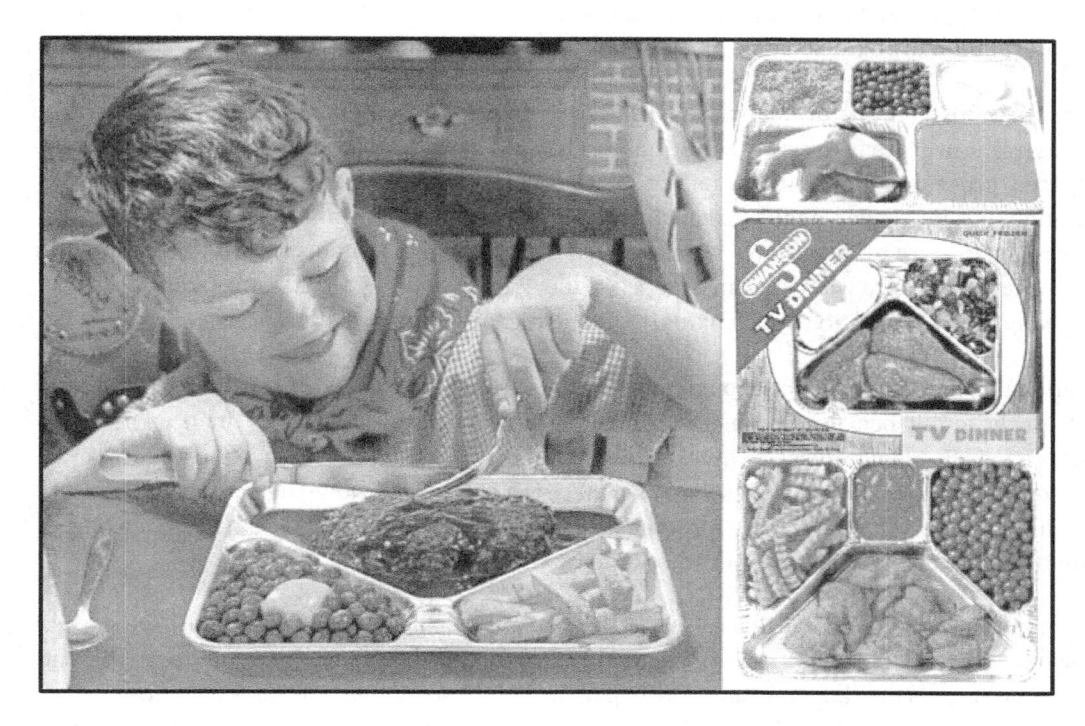

Trust Swanson ~ Meat loaf and gravy TV Dinner ad 1960s
Gerry Thomas conceived the company's frozen dinners in 1953 when he saw that the company had 260 tons of frozen turkey left over after Thanksgiving, sitting in ten refrigerated railroad cars. The refrigeration only worked when the train was moving. Betty Cronin, Swanson's bacteriologist, helped the meals succeed with her research into how to heat the meat and vegetables at the same time while killing food-borne germs. In 1954, the first full year of production, Swanson sold ten million trays.

# *Foreword by Janet Ludwig, PhD*

*1st edition 2018*

These are important times to be studying nutrition, food preparation, and the effect of eating on health. With the increasing prevalence of obesity and diabetes in adults and children, cardiovascular diseases, and cancer, there is a growing need for accurate and effective information to curb the prevalence of these diseases. Additionally, environmental toxins, epigenetics, and the microbiome are being identified as factors influencing diseases, all of which can be affected by nutrition. Thus, the evolution of how we eat and food preparation will provide insight into some of the associated risks and benefits to health conditions. As a nutrition educator and research scientist, the book *Our Journey with Food-Cookery Book* delivers this information in an informative, entertaining, and useful manner.

In the early 20th century, dramatic changes occurred when the population in the United States moved from rural areas to cities. Eating habits changed from farm foods to more corporate prepared, processed foods. Additionally, there has been increased exposure to air and water contaminants, pesticides, engine exhaust, and heavy metals. Eating habits, lifestyle, and increased exposure to toxins have resulted in changes in health. Concurrent with these changes was the fact that there was often an absence of the extended family to pass on traditions, especially food preparation and cooking, to the next generation.

Additionally, there is often not enough time for the caretaker of the family to shop, prepare and cook for the family because they are working long hours to meet the family's financial needs. Thus, eating has been reduced to quick meals, sometimes in the car on the way to and from work or picking up children from school. So, there is a gap in our knowledge of food that has been filled by food companies. The products from these companies that we eat are often based upon the company making a profit rather than its effect on our health.

Dr. Tammera Karr's book, *Our Journey with Food-Cookery Book*, fills this gap in our heritage and knowledge of food. This book is a unique blend of science, history, anecdotes, photographs, and wonderful recipes that begin to close the gap in our food knowledge. The book is logically arranged, beginning with explaining the benefits of staples in the kitchen and how to prepare and safely store many foods for later use. Measuring equivalencies and food substitutions are also provided to assist in cooking when it is difficult to obtain the specific ingredient at the time of cooking. Oils and how they should be safely used in cooking to preserve their benefits are explained based upon their chemistry. From there, herbs and spices, the staples of beans and grains, fermented foods, main dishes, and much more are provided with benefits explained as related to health and wellness.

Dr. Karr's insights into her upbringing in Oregon in a rural area provide a personal touch to the information many of us growing up in the cities or suburbs have never experienced. Her stories of her husband switching from buying fermented beverages to making them himself indicate the personal approach that she and her family have taken to ensure they are eating healthily. She personally explained tips on making many of these products, and the historical background with references that she brings to these recipes will make them easier to follow. The beverage recipes have more history and folklore than I could ever imagine being involved in something you drink. The historical references for these beverages bring it full circle to the image of sitting around a campfire drinking coffee and enjoying the camaraderie of fellow hikers as compared to the warriors drinking the wassail beverage in the 8th century. The "why" the food is important and the "how" are integrated throughout the book.

*Our Journey with Food-Cookery Book* is a sequel to her book *Our Journey with Food 2nd edition*, which traces the history of food and its relevance to health. The *Cookery Book* takes our knowledge one step closer to providing information on buying or growing good food, storing it, and preparing it with the best possible outcomes of preserving the essential nutrients needed for health. All of which will reduce the risk of nutrition-related diseases such as obesity, diabetes, stroke, auto-immunity, and many others. The book is carefully documented, in contrast to many books of this kind, done logically and without malice or fanaticism. It is not only a good read but an essential part of our history of food and the evolution of who we are.

~ Janet Ludwig, PhD, MS
*Biochemistry and Nutrition*
*Professor & Dean of Integrative Health and Nutrition, American College of Healthcare Science*

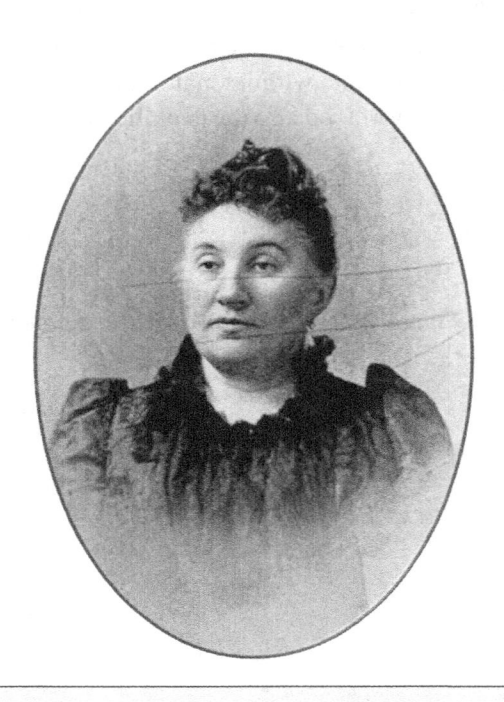

### European and American Cuisine
*1906*
Preface

    What science can boast of having done more for the happiness of humanity and the advance of the civilization of the world than the art of cooking?  It is strange that this, the most valuable, is so often left in the hands of the ignorant.  It should be the duty of every woman who expects to become a wife and mother to study the art and science of domestic affairs, for the destiny of the world depends upon the food we eat.
    Never is man more susceptible to kind and noble deeds than after partaking of a good meal. And I sincerely hope that this work may be of benefit, and give able assistance, to our many tired housekeepers in preparing healthy and nutritious food.

Gesine Lemcke<br>
Author

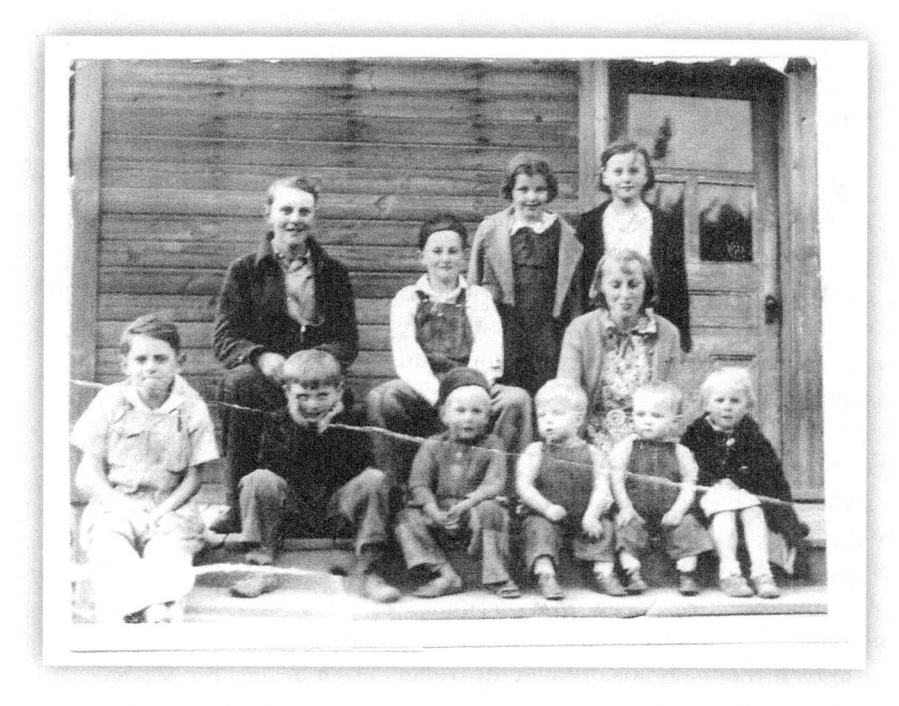

John Karr (back row left) with his siblings in Northern Idaho 1930s

## *Introduction ~ let the journey begin*

Like most, my husband and I have powerful memories stimulated by the smell or recollection of certain foods. For many individuals growing up in remote or rural areas, our childhoods were isolated from the advances and excitement of cities. My husband's grandmother came west in a covered wagon. My grandmother was a field laborer in the 1930s. She worked across the Southwest and eventually arrived in Idaho with her family. Our mothers made almost everything from basic ingredients once referred to as "staples" from which a wide selection of bread, cookies, cakes, and pies delighted us. The larder or pantry contained canned vegetables, fruits, and meats from which the nightly meal was made. Self-sufficiency and being stocked up was a way of life and still is.

When we reflect on favorite meals or foods, our brain chemistry changes and signals our hormones for digestion. The brain is so central to digestion that thinking about a favorite food can stimulate smell for some. The taste of Irish soda bread with currents cooked over an open wood fire in a *Folgers* coffee[1] can or the mouthwatering aromas from the Zabala kitchen that introduced me to Basque cookery are just a few.

I have always wanted a cellar like Mrs. Zabala who ran a boarding house in Burns, Oregon, and who I stayed with as a small child. The two-story white house had a cellar with walls lined with shelves filled with home-canned fruits, meats, vegetables, and jams. Ropes of chorizo and garlic, tied rosemary, sage, and oregano drying along with wooden boxes filled with potatoes and onions.

*Pure sensory heaven.*

In the 1960s, my mother tried different recipes from the *Trader Vics Pacific Island* cookbook, served hearty meals, and challenged herself with open fire cooking in a cast iron Dutch oven. Today when I smell the aroma of hot fried onion rings (a special treat shared with my older sister in the 1970s), for a moment, she is back. Almost everyone canned or bought food by the case for winter use. Trips to any store depended on the weather was an 8-15 hour day, and fresh produce was of poor quality or limited to those that didn't wilt and go bad.

By contrast, my husband, born in 1955, had a relatively bland midwestern-style diet. The highlight was fruit pie for breakfast and fresh bread with the foam off the new strawberry jam. The whole family would make the long trip to Warm Springs Ranch orchard at Penawawa, Washington, for canning fruit each summer. To this day, we still use his mother's pressure canner. A trip to St. Maries, Idaho, four times a year over remote roads brought the treat of drive-in hamburgers and fries. Home canned fruit, game meat, and thick slices of bread guaranteed someone wanted to buy his lunch in favor of their school lunch in later years after moving to Oregon.

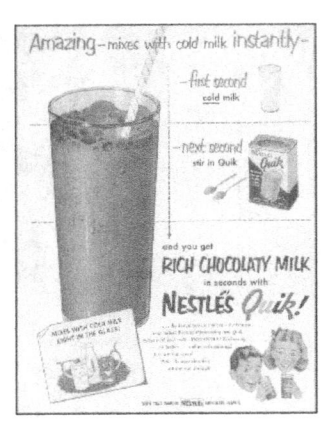

Good House Keeping Magazine 1950s

Availability of fresh vegetables in remote or rural areas depended on the family garden, orchard, berry patch, and foraging wild foods. Every type of food had a season when it was available. When abundant, if not home-preserved, individuals had to wait for the next year to taste a ripe peach or a succulent strawberry. While common in cities, refrigeration and electricity still had not reached remote areas of North America in the 1950s and 1960s.

Historical documents reveal that many rural North American families had safer and more food than their contemporaries in inner cities during the 1900s to 1940s.

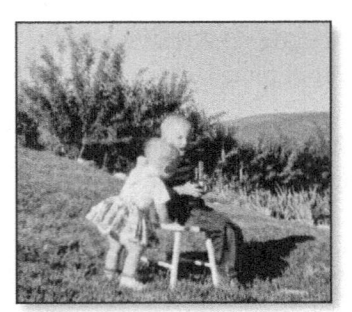

Fruit Orchard, Idaho 1960
Cindy and Vince Karr

Today, food insecurity for the elderly and low-income populations in cities is rampant, partly due to the vast quantities of food produced in factories and overseas. The second reason is the loss of knowledge on how to feed ourselves. We have lost our personal ability to gather and grow food and basic kitchen skills. From World War II to 1980, public schools and universities provided *Home Economics* education that taught students cooking, sewing, and personal accounting.[2] This provided basic knowledge that allowed individuals to enter the adult world with a measure of self-resiliency.

*Introduction*

## *Sharing What We Know*

A love of history and being exposed to Basque food as a kid have certainly influenced my gastronomy journey, especially regarding "ancestral foods." I'm not alone in this. Chefs Ben and Christine equally have family food stories. Since the 1st edition of *Our Journey with Food Cookery Book* in 2018, they have continued to recover and adapt recipes and seek and experiment with ancestral foods and cooking methods.

The people we have met through food are inspiring. Many of these individuals come from cultures like Persia, India, Italy, and Greece; all exotic and rich in food history. Our colleague and mentor, Dr. Bill Schindler, has encouraged many to return to traditional cooking by weaving his love of archaeology and anthropology with ancestral foods. Bill, a chef, and his family launched the *Modern Stone Age Kitchen* in 2020 and have continued educating and working to preserve ancestral cooking practices for communities and foodies far and wide. In my conversations with Bill, we invariably come back to modern-age individuals' disconnection from food. Dr. Schindler shares in *How to Eat Like a Human* that few people in today's modern society have the practical knowledge for acquiring, selecting, and preparing meals and understanding the life altering value of food. To paraphrase Bill, "Every technological advancement in human history resulted from harvesting, transporting, storing, cooking or preserving food."

## *The Research*

Research from Lancaster University, UK, in 2015 showed a startling decline in teens' views on food and their ability to prepare meals; something every home economics student could do at 15 in 1970. Researchers asked youth aged 16-20 about their attitudes toward food and how this can lead to obesity. One female first-year sports student told researchers she was "just not bothering" about what she ate as she was physically active. Another said, "I can't cook. I just can't be bothered …. I burn toast." What researchers found: The teenagers in the study utilize a microwave to heat up industrially manufactured pizza, chips or fries, ready meals, and cups of tea.

Thankfully virtual cooking classes in 2020-22 have improved children's nutrition knowledge, and school gardens are beginning to reconnect students with their food.[3, 4]

> ***Principle 1****: Food Knowledge and Culinary Skills must be taught to children and adults in order to improve health outcomes.*

## The Evidence

We learn more about *real* foods' vital and health-sustaining role every day through evidence-based science. Human and animal health depends on more than rudimentary chemistry, of calories in or out – to maintain or achieve longevity with vitality. The growing body of scientific and practical research, including that of Drs. Bill Schindler, Deanna Minich, and Terry Wahls, illuminates the wisdom of ancestral food knowledge in detail never dreamed of by our families.

Food preferences are shaped by environmental, cultural, and nutritional factors, including genetic ones. Rapid advances in molecular genetics have transformed the understanding of individual variances in aspects of human behavior. The heritability of food preferences has been described in twin studies of adults and children.[5, 6] While the world of nutrigenomics and nutrigenetics is complex and challenging, they provide fascinating information on food allergies, methylation, and disease prevalence.[7]

## Bio-Individuality

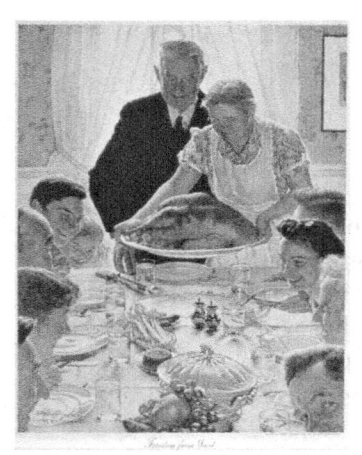

*Freedom From Want*
by Norman Rockwell Saturday Evening Post 1943
https://en.wikipedia.org/wiki/Freedom_from_Want

What is our idea of traditional or ancestral food? Is our image of food the 1940s Norman Rockwell picture of the family around the table at Thanksgiving? Our belief in a food tradition comes from a clever marketing campaign over cultural significance in today's modern North America. For example, the Hallmark image of Valentine's Day or Halloween, or how many Thanksgiving turkeys are sold based on the Norman Rockwell image, make up a modern myth of traditional food.

What is thought by one to be traditional or ancestral food may not be by another. Multiple factors come into play when we say traditional; family, history, location, time, and culture.

If we were to ask someone from Normandy and Paris what traditional French food was, you would get widely different answers, and both would be correct. If we were to ask individuals within our local community the same question, the responses would reflect a global collection of traditions from a wide range of countries and historical timelines.

Traditional foods are those prepared and consumed by a group of people for religious purposes, festivals, and daily life. These foods vary from household to household in preparation, technique, and economic status. They also vary within provinces, countries, and regions due to availability. <u>Ancestral foods have a story with them; by telling the story, we respect our culture and honor our ancestors.</u>

In today's world, there is a growing debate over ancestral diets. Some who are plant-based will say a vegan diet is the solution. Others following an animal-centered diet will say their eating habits have historical evidence supporting foods thought to be "hunter gather" in nature. These views are overly simplistic and generalized, with far more emotion than fact to support them. It is essential to distinguish the ideology of food from food history.

Foods intimately involved in religious belief systems are not the sum of ancestral foods. Food's place in religion is not always as finite as we think. Food choices are often mimicked due to respect, reverence, or adoration over actual availability and teaching. The practice of fasting is not a new idea. An aspect of early man's existence was at first due to food shortages, then later according to religious and cultural observances. By contrast, modern life's current abundance of calories and food availability is novel in humanity's dietary history.

Archaeologists are finding the availability of a food source does not mean a population consumed it. One such example comes from excavating a 6th century *Picts* village in Scotland. The *Picts,* a coastal culture, were skilled farmers who created elaborate stone carvings, often of the '*salmon of knowledge,*' believed to contain all the wisdom in the world. Forensic evidence found *Picts* avoided fish despite the community's seafaring prowess and proximity to the ocean. Fresh and saltwater fish were clearly missing from the diet. Scientists theorize the *Picts* may have intentionally avoided consuming fish for cultural and spiritual reasons. The current scientific data shows they primarily consumed barley, beef, lamb, pork, and venison.[8]

Think of it this way - ancestral foods are those our DNA responds to positively. The foods that make your DNA sing may be bone broth or mushrooms, broccoli or squash, salmon or lamb, and soy or corn. Our DNA has adapted to a wide range of natural and varied foods for over 200,000 years. But our DNA has not been able to adapt rapidly to all the human-made chemicals developed in the last 80 years. Genetic researchers now believe as we age, approximately 20% of health is determined by genes. The remaining 80% is influenced by lifestyle choices and how physical and social environments activate gene expression.[9]

> ***Principle 2****: Our cells carry information on Ancestral Foods.*

## What We Learn from History

In 2022, the largest of its kind study on ancient genomes homed in on the identity of the hunter gatherers who settled down to farm in the Middle East roughly 12,000 years ago. The blending of hunter-gatherers from Europe and the Middle East became the first communities to actively farm around 8,000 years ago in what is now the Balkans.[10, 11, 12]

In 2018, archaeologists discovered the charred remains of a flatbread baked by hunter-gatherers 14,400 years ago in northeastern Jordan. It is the oldest direct evidence of bread found to date, predating the advent of agriculture by at least 4,000 years.[13] Research technology can now determine what foods were present on ancient pottery and stone knives related to Paleolithic diets.

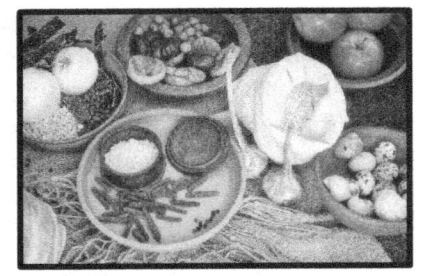

Anthropology and archaeology are gaining a greater understanding of ancient diets. Evidence shows a wide variety of foods, including insects and grass seeds, were consumed seasonally.[14] The keyword here is seasonal. Many of our clues on ancient diets come from detailed autopsies such as those on Ötzi, the 5,300 year old hunter "Iceman" found in the Ötztal Alps. Ötzi's preserved full stomach and colon illustrated ancient man's diet did include grains. Ötzi was an omnivore; he ate cereals, red deer, and goat meat the day before his death.[15]

However, the truth is that research will never fully answer what people ate in the past. Ancient humans scattered over vast areas and continents and consumed foods unique to the climate and terrain they lived in, many of which no longer exist. A lot has changed during our human journey with food; types of vegetation, animals, insects, and countless other aspects.

## *Romanticizing the Past*

As much as the authors value history, they are also honest regarding the facts about foods available to the masses following the civil war through the Great Depression. Food spoilage and contamination could arguably be the leading cause of death before the 20th century advances in food hygiene. When mass migrations of the population moved to cities (the great urbanization of America) following the civil war, it launched the Industrial Revolution. During this time, incredible advances in food production, including the automated assembly line developed by H.J. Heinz, predated Henry Ford by decades. These innovations went on to change the way consumers view everyday foods.[16] The efforts of early 20th century entrepreneurs altered the way food was marketed, made, stored, and transported. Innovations by Milton S. Hershey, W. K. Kellogg, J. L. Kraft and Marjorie M. Post make up 90% of the foods on the shelves of supermarkets today.

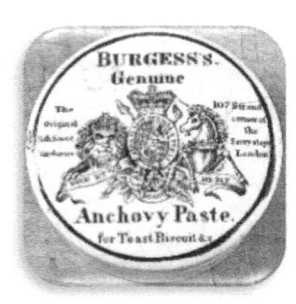

Burgess Essence of Anchovy paste was a top selling condiment used to camouflage spoiled meat. In the 1850s it was standard practice to adulterate with Armenian bole, an iron-rich clay, to imbue the sauce with a bright red color.

Inventions in food manufacturing in the 19th century came about when food was at its rottenest for urban consumers in North America. The earliest record of food adulteration has been traced to the Middle Ages.

The development of *analytic chemistry* allowed chemists to detect and describe the methods and effects of adulteration. Ironically, making *formulae for adulteration* available to unscrupulous hucksters. With the industrial revolution, the consumer market demand for *manufactured* food encouraged adulteration because of the prospects for improved profit. Food adulteration and outlandish claims in advertising led to suffering and death for countless Americans during the 19th and early 20th centuries. These events and recounts in the press increased awareness about food safety and resulted in federal legislation. The following are only a tiny sampling of North America's food state prior to the 1930s.

*17th century first food regulation*

- In 1641, Massachusetts introduced the first food adulteration law, which required inspection of beef, pork, and fish; followed in the 1650s with legislation regulating bread quality.

*19th century food adulteration*
In 1855, James F. W. Johnston published *The Chemistry of Common Life*, encouraging readers to understand their daily diet's chemical content and processes.[17]

- "Lie tea" was the dust of tea leaves—sometimes of other leaves—and sand, combined with starch into little cakes and painted to resemble black or green tea.
- Green tea was often covered with Prussian blue and sulphate of lime or gypsum or a yellow or orange-colored vegetable substance.
- Formaldehyde and boric acid were widely used by the dairy and meat-packing industries.
- Dairy producers thinned milk with water (and occasionally a little gelatin) and recolored the resulting bluish-gray liquid with dyes, chalk, or plaster dust.[18]
- Liquor, bread, cheese, pickled vegetables, and sugary confections were some of the items poisoned with copper, sulphuric acid, or lead.[19]

## *Convenience at a Cost*

A significant area of change during the last 150 years is human-made chemicals and plastics. Plastics contribute to the growing endocrine and chronic health challenges of the 21st century. No one would have believed in 1945 that plastics would be linked 80 years later to infertility, cognition decline, hypertension, and cancer. A return to earlier sustainable approaches to food storage and cooking with traditional tools is needed. While plastics are deeply entrenched in modern life, individuals can actively reduce waste and exposure through selective use.

Romanticized stories of food purity and quality from the past are far from honest. If one has never hunted, foraged, grown, or harvested food, it is unrealistic to understand the work involved in feeding one person.

The exertion of energy in growing, harvesting, and preparing food has been transformed by automation. Yet, is our food safer than that of the 19th century? A brief review of the USDA site for food safety is sufficient to support *No* as the answer. Moving forward brings challenges over food production's carbon footprint. One can find foods from all over the world in or out of season due to food inventors like Clarence Birdseye and global transportation. The modern convenience and trendy meatless food manufacturing carbon footprint far exceeds that of traditional and regenerative agriculture. The bottom line: the farther your food travels, the greater the risk to the health of individuals and the planet.

> ***Principle 3***: *Grow a garden, buy locally, know your farmer and rancher, and converse with the avatar and butcher.*

### *Return to Ancestral Food and Cooking*

Whether we call it plant or animal, fungi, or fish - food is everywhere and intimately involved in our lives. Without food, the human, animal, aquatic, or plant kingdoms would not exist. Without digestible nutrient rich foods, our bodies cannot achieve health or reproduce a viable next generation. Food is life and should bring energy, satisfaction, comfort, connection, and joy.

Not everyone can grow a garden or hunt down a deer. Still, the authors hope to provide the reader with solutions, resources, and knowledge fading from daily life. The sustainable and mindful option for human health and the earth is locally produced foods with minimal chemical exposure.

*The Goal of this Cookery Book is to Expand the Reader's Food Knowledge and Preserve Cultural Foods.*

*Let the Food Adventure Begin!*

*Introduction*

1 Folgers Coffee has been serving up great tasting coffee since 1850. While that was the year the company opened for business in San Francisco, the Folgers coffee story goes all the way back to the 1600s, when the Folger family left their home in Norwich, England and sailed for Massachusetts. Back in 1850, roasted coffee was something of a luxury for anyone living outside of large cities and ground coffee was virtually unheard of. Procter & Gamble, in early 1963 acquired Folgers Coffee and began to market it nationally under the Folgers coffee brand name.

2 Randolph, Elizabeth, "A Brief History of the Teaching of Home Economics in the Public Schools of the United States" (1942). Graduate Thesis Collection. 331. https://digitalcommons.butler.edu/grtheses/331

3 Elsevier. (2022, April 7). Virtual cooking class improves children's nutrition knowledge. www.sciencedaily.com/releases/2022/04/220407101056.htm

4 University of Texas at Austin. (2021, February 4). School gardens linked with kids eating more vegetables. www.sciencedaily.com/releases/2021/02/210204131408.htm

5 Robino, A., Concas, M. P., Catamo, E., & Gasparini, P. (2019). A Brief Review of Genetic Approaches to the Study of Food Preferences: Current Knowledge and Future Directions. Nutrients, 11(8), 1735. https://doi.org/10.3390/nu11081735

6 Precone V, Beccari T, Stuppia L, Baglivo M, Paolacci S, Manara E, Miggiano GAD, Falsini B, Trifirò A, Zanlari A, Herbst KL, Unfer V, Bertelli M; Geneob Project. Taste, olfactory and texture related genes and food choices: implications on health status. Eur Rev Med Pharmacol Sci. 2019 Feb;23(3):1305-1321. doi: 10.26355/eurrev_201902_17026. PMID: 30779105.

7 Marcum JA. Nutrigenetics/Nutrigenomics, Personalized Nutrition, and Precis on Healthcare. Curr Nutr Rep. 2020 Dec;9(4):338-345. doi: 10.1007/s13668-020-00327-z. PMID: 32578026.

8 Shirley Curtis-Summers, Jessica A. Pearson, Angela L. Lamb, From Picts to Parish: Stable isotope evidence of dietary change at medieval Portmahomack, Scotland, Journal of Archaeological Science: Reports, Volume 31, 2020, 102303, ISSN 2352-409X, https://doi.org/10.1016/j.jasrep.2020.102303.

9 Bland JS. Functional Medicine Past, Present, and Future. Integr Med (Encinitas). 2022 May;21(2):22-26. PMID: 35698609; PMCID: PMC9173848.

10 Marchi, N. et al. Cell https://doi.org/10.1016/j.cell.2022.04.008 (2022)

11 Allentoft, M. E. et al. Preprint at bioRxiv https://doi.org/10.1101/2022.05.04.490594 (2022).

12 Lazaridis, I. et al. Nature 536, 419–424 (2016).

13 14,400-year-old Bread Causes Major Re-think on the Birth of Agriculture; https://www.ancient-origins.net/news-history-archaeology/bread-production-0010388

14 The Sandal and the Cave: The Indians of Oregon by Luther S. Cressman 1962, Oregon State University Press, Corvallis

15 5,300 Years Ago, Ötzi the Iceman Died. Now We Know His Last Meal, by Maya Wei-hass National Geographic; https://ancientfoods.wordpress.com/page/3/

16 Rees, J.  Industrialization and Urbanization in the United States, 1880–1929. Oxford Research Encyclopedia of American History. Retrieved 15 Jun. 2022, from https://oxfordre.com/americanhistory/view/10.1093/acrefore/9780199329175.001.0001/acrefore-9780199329175-e-327.

17 Judith L. Fisher, "Tea and Food Adulteration, 1834-75": https://branchcollective.org/?ps_articles=judith-l-fisher-tea-and-food-adulteration-1834-75  Retrieved 6-15-2022

18 https://www.smithsonianmag.com/science-nature/19th-century-fight-bacteria-ridden-milk-embalminutesg-fluid-180970473/ Retrieved 6-14-2022

19 Victorian Era Dangers that People Faced; https://www.geriwalton.com/dangers-of-victorian-era/ Retrieved 6-14-2022

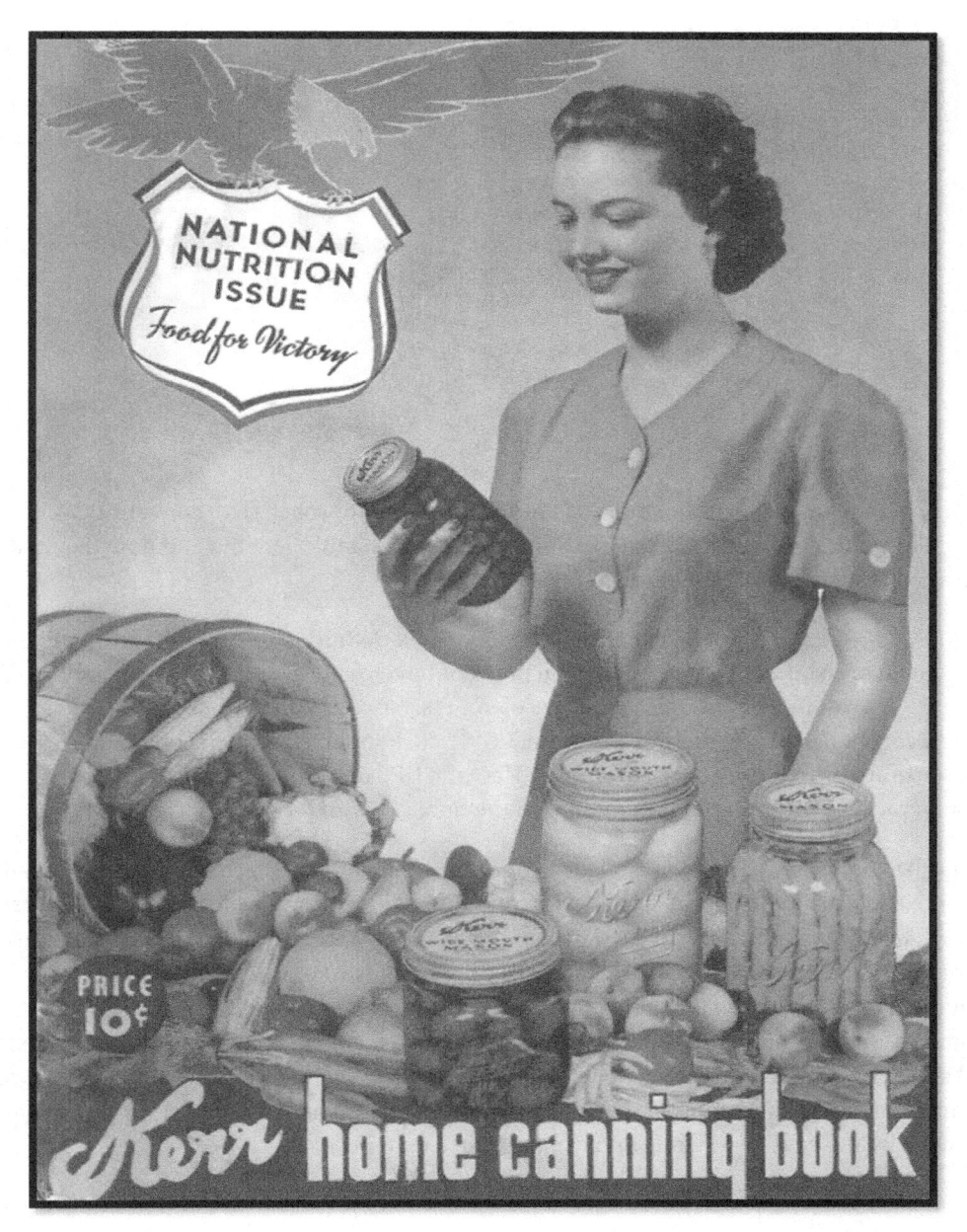

In 1943, American families bought 315,000 pressure cookers for canning vegetables, increasing from 66,000 in 1942. The National Center for Home Food Preservation was established in 2000 and developed a web-based home instruction program to improve food safety for children and adults.[20]

## *The Pantry*

> *"Good cookery means the knowledge of all fruits, herbs, balms, and spices, and of all that is healing and sweet in fields and groves, and savory in meats. It means carefulness, inventiveness, watchfulness, willingness, and readiness of appliance. It means the economy of your great-grandmothers and science of modern chemists. It means much tasting, and no wasting. It means English thoroughness, French art, and Arabian hospitality. It means, in fine, that you are to be perfectly and always ladies (loaf-givers)."* (1896 circ.)
>
> ~ John Ruskin
> *Elements of the Theory and Practice of Cookery*, 1900
> The Motto of the New York City Public School Kitchens, 1912

In considering the pantry, the authors take a slightly different approach than conventional cookbooks. The authors categorized this section according to health benefits and how the pantry contributes to balancing our wellbeing.

This cookery book section is not an exhaustive list nor is it a definitive one. Your pantry will be dependent on where you live. For example, you may not have ready access to sea vegetables, a unique source of protein, 56 minerals, and trace elements.[21, 22, 23] With the post COVID age, access to sea vegetables became easier to obtain. COVID lockdowns have changed how individuals acquire a wide range of food staples. Now the UPS or FedEx truck brings herbs, spices, flour, crackers, and even sea vegetables to the door.

From the earliest days of exploration and settlements, people had food caches, cellars, and well-stocked pantries to see them through the lean winter and *hunger* months of spring. The *Hidatsa*, *Mandan*, and *Arikara* people of the upper Missouri river developed farming tools, permaculture, and well-organized cellars (caches) in the banks of the Missouri river; for corn, squash, and beans hundreds of years before Europeans arrived.[24] While few people today are motivated to have a home pantry like those of the 1900s, having a well-stocked pantry of seasonally harvested foods and staple ingredients provides flexibility. The downside to dreaming of that pantry is room, so make sure you have thought through your storage space needs and location before you take up buying by the case or freezing and canning like a mad person.

> **Principle 4:** *An organized and stocked pantry allows for greater food security and dietary flexibility.*

**Keep it Simple**

Tammera likes humble food packed with health promoting nutrition. The uses become broader by having jars of fruits, vegetables, and meats without added seasoning, sugar, or salt. By keeping the preparation to basics, the risk of food waste decreases: that spaghetti sauce wasn't great; but the spaghetti sauce made with a quart of simple tomato sauce was a hit. Simple tomato sauce can be used for numerous recipes. Keeping home-canned, frozen, fermented, and dried foods in their natural flavor state make it easier to combine for nutrition gusto. The synergistic combination of the ingredients yields energy and enjoyment while feeding our DNA with culturally appropriate nutrition. Remember that *your cells carry the memories of your ancestors*. And our microbiome loves *real food*. To feed our unique genetics, we require an organized pantry stocked with staples that can be grabbed at a whim to create *recipes and meals our DNA sings for*.

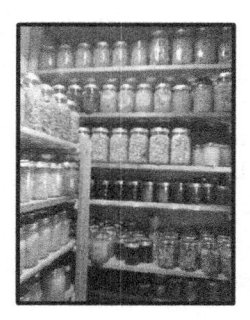

**Nonperishables**: Stocking up on nonperishable items from toilet paper, trash liners, foil, plastic wrap, paper towels, storage bags and other items used daily, including foods, frees resources for other things during the lean times of the year or when shortages occur. *Remember bread flour shortages and the run on parchment paper, Ball lids, and TP in 2021?*

These *mindfulness* practices save time, money, and energy while lowering stress and frustration. Taking advantage of sales, ordering in bulk, canning, drying, and freezing foods in season, along with canning or freezing meals ahead allows for convenience without compromising quality or nutrition. Individuals can spend less time cooking and prepping on weekends if they utilize leftovers from larger meals and pantry inventory for breakfast, lunch, and dinners during the week. The authors learned the value of seasonal availability and a flexible pantry from family members growing up.

Thousands of pre-packaged processed foods are waiting to fill your pantry shelves to the detriment of your health. These foods are devoid of real nutrition and can be wholly removed, saving you money and space once you learn to cook with whole foods and the tried and true staples. Here are a few of Tammera's: flour, coffee, organic sugar, tea, salt, lard, olive oil, butter, rice, beans, dried herbs, oatmeal, molasses, honey, and maple syrup.

Her pantry also includes room for cool storage and a freezer. Cool storage for potatoes, yams, onions, garlic, dried fruit, vegetables, spices, fermented foods, home-canned fruit, broth, beans, soups, salsa, jam, and pet food. The freezers for meats, berries, vegetables trimmings, butter, nuts, bread, and meals.

> **Principle 5**: *Make one or two larger meals so you have leftovers to turn into weekly meals in a hurry.*

Some of these items may be in ounces or pounds depending on the frequency of use and space. Example: Tammera bakes sourdough bread and uses a selection of flours. The all-purpose spelt flour is generally in 25 pound bags, whereas oat bran is in smaller packages along with tea and sugar. The meat selection in the freezer is determined by season and preference.

As you just read, we consider freezers part of the pantry. They allow for long term storage of foods like raw meat and reheatable meals.

*Here are some examples*:

- ❖ Tammera stocks up seasonally on lamb, beef, buffalo, fish, chicken, and pork. She includes venison, elk, halibut, wild salmon when the hunting and fishing seasons allow, and berries in her freezer.

- ❖ Ben may have more pork, poultry, beef, home-cured and smoked meats, and leftovers that heat efficiently on the stovetop, microwave, or oven in his freezer.

- ❖ And Christina, on the coast, will have more wild caught fish, broths, vegetables, fruits, and plant-based meals ready to heat.

*Note: Before you begin looking for the magic list, you should know we will not give you a regimented list of foods to have on hand; that would be assuming the foods available to us are the same for you. Because our food traditions are unique to our heritage, a list would miss the point of traditional/ancestral foods or bio-individual nutrition unique to you.*

> **Principle 6:** *Freezers allow for the seasonal rotation of plants and a complete protein profile of amino acids through the diet for balance, reducing the development of food sensitivities.*

### *Defining Processed Food*

Technically, a process is anything done in the preparation of food. That means washing, peeling, slicing, and cooking. Here are some accepted terms for types of processed foods.

**Ultra Highly Refined Processed**
- Chemicals are added to increase palatability (look for ingredients you don't recognize as food).
- Added salt, fat, and sugar create the desire to eat more.
- Flavor and color enhancers: CDG, MSG, MPG, and Inosinic acid.[25]

- Many steps are used to arrive at a final product.
- *<u>The processing can't be duplicated in your kitchen.</u>*

**Processed**
- Technically anything done to food but for these purposes, most or all the ingredients come from a factory.
- Generally packaged and branded.

**Traditional or Heritage Foods**
- Foods that have a process done to them but have long-standing origins.
- The original process might be done in a factory now, but it was developed by hand.
- Uses Real Food.

**Whole and Unprocessed**
- Origins are cultivated, slaughtered, harvested, or gathered.
- Your ancestors would recognize it as food; can be made or reproduced at home.
- Has the least possible modifications to be edible and safe for you.

## *Freezing versus Canning*

**A word on fresh produce**

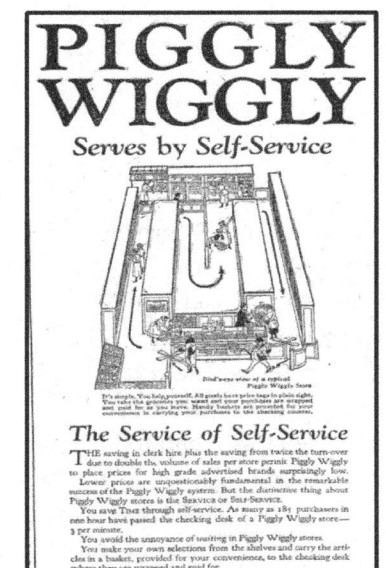

It is generally accepted that fresh fruits and vegetables contain the most nutrients. It is important to remember fresh produce in mega markets and chain stores is often radiated, transported over long distances, and left on store shelves with misters for prolonged periods. The misters, if not filtered, can be applying chemicals found in city water supplies. Additionally, if the misting system is not regularly cleaned, contamination of produce with bacteria and fungus can occur. The time lapse between picking and purchasing can cause fresh fruits and vegetables to lose nutritional value as they are exposed to light and air. Their taste and texture are also diminished. All the more reason to buy local and learn to garden.

Tammera remembers when she first began studying nutrition, an instructor insisted frozen was better than canned when it came to the nutritional content of food. She never completely agreed, living in an area with abundant fruit, vegetables, and fish that people have been canning for over 100 years. These local foods retain flavor, texture, convenience, and versatility better than frozen foods.[26]

Both methods allow for control over salt and sugar content and environmental chemicals if done mindfully. Fresh fruits and vegetables must be canned or frozen right after being harvested when nutrients are at their highest levels.

There does seem to be an exception to this rule when working with fruit. The Karrs often call ahead and order lugs (20 pound box) of fruit. Invariably, some are not fully ripe so they lay them out on old towels in the sun to ripen.

Peaches are another example. The Karrs bring home 4-6 lugs of peaches at a time and leave them covered in their boxes. Each day the peaches are checked for ripeness. They should peel easily and have a softness with a rich peach smell. Depending on room temperature, it may be two to seven days after picking before free-stone peaches are ready to can. <u>Be sure to ask the folks at the farm stand or market to recommend the best variety for home preserving – not all varieties are well suited to canning or freezing.</u>

**Added Resiliency**

When the refrigerator or freezer quits working and replacements won't arrive right away, or the power goes out for more than 24 hours, there is a mad scramble to save food from spoilage in freezers. Canning adds a measure of security to convenience and versatility. When traveling or living in an RV or tiny house, the refrigerator and freezer room is at a premium. Foods preserved in glass jars allow one to enjoy foods that can be quickly heated or consumed straight from the jar. *Each jar carries the intention of the cook on the day it was canned.* "I tell my family that every time you taste what you are cooking, you are seasoning it with love and a kiss," says Tammera.

**So, What Does Science Have to Say?**

Fresh vegetables can lose up to 75% of their vitamin C content after harvest. Spinach, greens, and green beans lose most of their vitamin C within seven days of harvest. A study by the University of Georgia and the Frozen Food Foundation showed that some frozen fruits and vegetables had higher folate, vitamins A, and vitamin C content than stored fresh fruits and vegetables. These findings also held true for carrots, green peas, and green beans. The study also suggested that nutrients degrade the longer fresh produce is stored in the refrigerator. Frozen broccoli, green beans, spinach, green peas, and carrots demonstrated less vitamin C loss than fresh produce stored longer than seven days.[27, 28, 29]

Research has shown that fruits and vegetables lose not only vitamins C but B vitamins when defrosted. Data supports that canning, like cooking, damages enzymes in foods; however, nutrients are otherwise retained.

A review published in the *Journal of the Science of Food and Agriculture* (2007) clarifies the nutrient loss conversation. Without refrigeration or processing, fresh fruits and vegetables have a shelf life of only days before they are unsafe or undesirable for consumption.

1) Refrigeration slows down the respiration of fruits and vegetables and allows for longer shelf life.
2) Freezing, canning, and drying transform perishable fruits and vegetables so they can be consumed year-round and transported to consumers worldwide.
3) As a result of processing, respiration is arrested, stopping *nutritious* components' consumption. The loss of moisture and the growth of micro-organisms are retarded by processing.
4) Washing, peeling, and blanching before processing are responsible for some loss of water-soluble nutrients.
5) The thermal processing associated with canning and pre-freezing is especially detrimental to vitamin C and thiamine. Blanching is an important preservation step in many vegetables' canning and freezing processes.
6) Since unprocessed and processed fruits and vegetables must undergo some transport and storage, degradation of nutrients before consumption is expected.
7) The degradation's extent depends on the cooking method, nutrients, and commodity. [30]

Dr. Deanna Minich and colleagues began research in 2022 on cooking through microwave, boiling, and autoclave (pressure cooker). The purpose was to determine which methods affected nutrients and inflammatory compounds in many plant-based foods.

**Excerpt from the Overall Conclusion Statement**

*Compounds are rarely ingested in their isolated format as we know from how these foods are traditionally consumed. Plant-based diets which contain these compounds also contain thousands of other compounds in the food matrix, many of which counteract the potential effects of the 'anti-nutrients.' Therefore, it remains questionable as to whether these compounds are as potentially harmful as they might seem to be in isolation, as they may act differently when taken in within whole foods that are properly prepared. Cooking and application of heat seems to be essential for the activation of some of these compounds.*

Following charts are from: Petroski, W, Minich, D.M, Is There Such a Thing as "Anti-Nutrients"? A Narrative Review of Perceived Problematic Plant Compounds. Nutrients 2020, 12, 2929. https://doi.org/10.3390/nu12102929

## *Food Preparation Determines Nutrient Content*

| 'Anti-nutrient' | Food Sources | Suggested Clinical Implications |
|---|---|---|
| Lectins | Legumes, cereal grains, seeds, nuts, fruits, vegetables | Altered gut function; inflammation |
| Oxalates | Spinach, Swiss chard, sorrel, beet greens, beet root, rhubarb, nuts, legumes, cereal grains, sweet potatoes, potatoes | May inhibit calcium absorption; May increase calcium kidney stone formation |
| Phytate (IP6) | Legumes, cereal grains, pseudocereals (amaranth, quinoa, millet), nuts, seeds | May inhibit absorption of iron, zinc and calcium; Acts as an antioxidant; Antineoplastic effects |
| Goitrogens | *Brassica* vegetables (kale, Brussels sprouts, cabbage, turnip greens, Chinese cabbage, broccoli), millet, cassava | Hypothyroidism and/or goiter; Inhibit iodine uptake |
| Phytoestrogens | Soy and soy products, flaxseeds, nuts (negligible amounts), fruits and vegetables (negligible amounts) | Endocrine disruption; Increased risk of estrogen-sensitive cancers |
| Tannins | Tea, cocoa, grapes, berries, apples, stone fruits, nuts, beans, whole grains | Inhibit iron absorption; Negatively impact iron stores |

| 'Anti-nutrient' | Food Preparation that Reduces | Food Preparation that Increase |
|---|---|---|
| Lectins | Soaking, boiling, autoclaving, germination, fermentation | Roasting, baking |
| Oxalate | Soaking, boiling, steaming, pairing with high calcium foods | Roasting, grilling, baking, low-calcium diet |
| Phytates | Soaking, boiling, germination, fermentation | n/a |
| Tannins | Cooking, peeling skins of fruits and nuts | n/a |
| Phytoestrogens | n/a | Boiling, steaming, fermenting (increases aglycone content) |
| Goitrogens | Steaming, boiling | |

**Principle 7:** The <u>How</u> of food preparation and processing is as important if not more so then the <u>What</u> when it comes to health and wellness.

**Cool Storage Top-Picks**

Root foods are perfect for stashing in an unheated garage or outbuilding if your winter temperatures go below 45°F. These crops will keep for two to six months at cool room temperature and require no processing, containers, or refrigeration.

| | | | | |
|---|---|---|---|---|
| Apples | Beets | Brussel sprouts | Cabbage | Carrots |
| Garlic | Parsnips | Pears | Potatoes | Onions |
| Rutabagas | Sunchokes | Sweet potatoes | Turnips | Unshelled nuts |
| Winter squash | | | | |

**Freezer Top Picks**

*What science is finding:* Time of day matters when harvesting broccoli.
Broccoli has a high content of *glucosinolates*, that promote specialized metabolism with anticarcinogenic activity. Harvesting at different times during the day changed broccoli heads' aging rate during post-harvest storage.[31]

**\*\*** *Glucosinolates are natural components of many pungent plants such as mustard, cabbage, and horseradish. The pungency of those plants is due to mustard oils produced from glucosinolates when the plant material is chewed, cut, or otherwise damaged.*

| | | | |
|---|---|---|---|
| Asparagus | Berries | Beans, snap | Bok choy |
| Broccoli | Cauliflower | Cantaloupe | Chard |
| Edamame | Eggplant | Kohlrabi | Peas |
| Peppers | Spinach | Summer squash | Sweet corn |

> **Principle 8:** *While the Industrial Revolution brought about many beneficial changes, it diminished our connection to local food and lore.*

## Home Canning

Food preservation history through canning begins in France in the middle of the Napoleonic Wars (1803-1815) followed by Bryan Donkin and John Hall, who developed the process of packaging food in sealed, airtight cans. Consumers rightfully didn't trust canned foods in the 18th and early 19th centuries. Food poisoning and spoilage, along with countless contaminants, meant eating canned food could and did result in death.

During the global depression of 1873, the U.S. exported canned foods led by the Campbell, Heinz, and Borden companies.[32] A game changing invention: Max Ams, in 1888, developed a can crimping machine. These folded seams of cans eliminated the need for solder (responsible for lead poisoning). The canned soup wars between Heinz and Campbell in 1904 forever changed how the world viewed canned foods.[33, 34, 35]

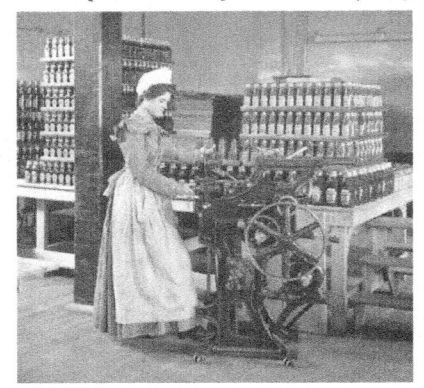

Women were the primary food industry workers in 1900. In 1904, the Max Ams Machine Company of New York patented the double-seam process used in most modern food cans. Today a double-seam machine can safely seal more than 2,000 cans a minute.

### Mason Jars

John L. Mason invented the mason jar. He created a machine that could cut threads into lids, making manufacturing a jar with a reusable, screw on lid practical. The difference between his design and his predecessors was the sealing mechanism: a glass container with a thread molded into its top and a zinc lid with a rubber ring. The rubber created the seal, and the threaded lid maintained it. The jar included his patent: "Mason's Patent November 30, 1858."

### Ball Jars

William Charles Ball and his brothers began manufacturing fruit jars in 1884 in Buffalo, New York. The Ball brand is the leading jar and lid used by home canners. Since 1993, the Alltrista Corporation has been manufacturing the Ball glass canning jars. They also make Kerr, Bernardin, and Golden Harvest canning jars.

### Kerr Jars

Alexander H. Kerr founded the Hermetic Fruit Jar Company in 1903. One of the first commercial products was the Economy and Self Sealing jars. The Economy jars were the first easy to fill wide mouth jars. They incorporated aspects from two 1903 patents held by another inventor, Julius Landsberger: a metal lid with a permanently attached gasket. This made the lids easy to use and inexpensive.

Mr. Kerr later (1915) invented a smaller, flat metal disk with the same permanent composition gasket. The lid was sealed on the top of a mason jar; a threaded metal ring held the lid down during the hot water processing. This allowed the re-use of old canning jars and inexpensive and easy to use disposable lids. The jar we know today was born! This two-part lid system transformed home canning safety.[36]

**Water Bath Processing Top Picks**

Pickles, acidic tomatoes, sweet jams and jellies, and fruit have a *pH* level of 4.6 or lower, which delays bacterial growth, allowing them to be canned in a traditional water bath canner or pot.

| | | | | |
|---|---|---|---|---|
| Berries | Chiles | Cucumbers | Fruits | Jams & jellies |
| Juice | Peppers | Rhubarb | Tomatoes | |

**Best Under Pressure**

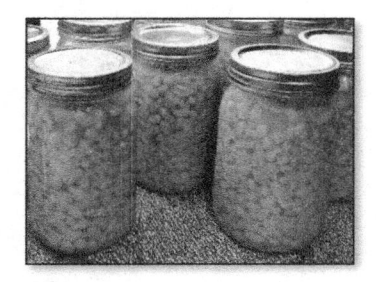

You will need a pressure canner to preserve foods with a *pH* above 4.6. The higher heat and pressure are necessary to kill bacteria that can spoil your hard work and potentially kill anyone who consumes the tainted food. Not to worry, using a pressure canner is perfectly safe when you carefully follow the directions. If you need more confidence, contact your local Extension service to inquire about joining a Master Food Preservers class.

| | | | |
|---|---|---|---|
| Black beans | Broth/ soup | Fruits /unsweetened | Garbanzo beans |
| Green beans | Lima beans | Meats /fish | |
| Pinto beans | Tomatoes | Vegetable mixtures | |

**Drying All-Stars**

| | | | | |
|---|---|---|---|---|
| Apples | Berries | Carrots | Cherries | Celery |
| Dry beans | Fruit leather | Grapes | Herbs | Peaches |
| Peppers | Plums | Mushrooms* | Sum. squash | Yams |

Dried peaches and citrus are fast in a food dryer. The citrus can be eaten with the rind, or the rind can be ground for adding zest to recipes. It makes a perfect digestive tea too!

*When drying mushrooms, use caution. As the fungi dry, they release spores that are vented by the dehydrator fan. It is wise to do this outdoors and clean equipment thoroughly when finished.*

**Home Food Preserving Resources**

Storing Food for Safety and Quality – ResearchGate
https://www.researchgate.net/profile/...to.../Frsh+food+longer+storage1.pdf

Current Food Safety Issues of Home-prepared Vegetables and Herbs
www.foodprotection.org/files/food-protection-trends/Jun-11-Nummer.pdf
SMART STORAGE — Keep Fruits and Vegetables Fresh
https://www.co.washington.or.us/hhs/swr/wasteprevention/smart-storage.cfm

National Center for Home Food Preservation https://nchfp.uga.edu/

Simply Canning: Canning Recipes, Equipment
https://www.simplycanning.com/home-canning-recipes-blog.html

Dry Canning:  https://www.grit.com/food/welcome-to-dry-canning-zb0z2103/

"Dry Canning" is Not Recommended: https://extension.psu.edu/dry-canning-is-not-recommended

**Print Resources**

***Ball Complete Book of Home Preserving***, 400 delicious and creative recipes for today.

***The Dehydrator Bible***: Includes over 400 recipes by Jennifer MacKenzie, Jay Nutt & Don Mercer

***Curing & Smoking Made at Home*** by Dick & James Strawbridge

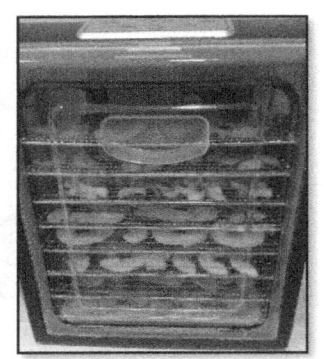

## *Beans & Grains*

From the Basque beans of the Oregon and Nevada High Desert to the frijoles of the Southwest and the cassoulets of southwest France, dry beans are a traditional food staple worldwide. Legumes (beans, peas, lentils) have been a staple of the diet in many parts of the world for more than 12,000 years.

Beans represented status in ancient Rome. "As remarkable and as yet unexplained sign of their status in the ancient world is the fact that each of the four major legumes known to Rome lent its name to a prominent Roman family: Fabius comes from fava bean, Lentulus from the lentil, Piso from the pea, and Cicero from the chickpea." [37, 38]

There are hundreds of dry bean varieties, each with its unique flavor, texture, cooking time, and culinary uses.[39]


**Bean Varieties**

**Adzuki:** Himalayan native, now grown throughout Asia. Small, nearly round red bean with a thread of white along part of the seam. Slightly sweet and starchy.

**Anasazi:** New World native (present-day junction of Arizona, New Mexico, Colorado, Utah). It is a white speckled bean with burgundy to rust-brown. Slightly sweet.

**Appaloosa:** New World native. Slightly elongated and curved, one end white and the other mottled with black and brown. It holds its shape well. Somewhat herbaceous and piney in flavor.

**Black:** New World native. Shiny, true black uncooked. Creamy texture when cooked. The flavor has an unusual, faintly sweet note reminiscent of chocolate.

**Cannellini or White Kidney:** New World (Argentina) native, now much loved and used in Italy. Creamy texture, slightly nutty.

**Cranberry:** New World (Colombia) native. Ivory or tan is beautifully mottled with red, burgundy, and bright pink striations. A melty, creamy texture, a little nutlike.

**Great Northern:** New World native. A white bean, slightly larger than the navy, meltingly textured.

**Kidney:** New World native. Kidney-shaped, shiny dark-red seed coat. Cooks up creamy with a little sweetness. Mild in flavor.

**Mung:** India and Pakistan native. Small, almost round, green with a small white stripe along part of its seam. Mild and starchy.

**Navy**: New World native. Smaller white bean. Soft but not creamily so.
A pleasant neutral flavor.

**Pinto:** New World native. Pink-puff bean mottled with a deeper brown-burgundy. It cooks up plump, creamy, a little sweet, and mild. These bean varieties and hundreds of others have been used to create extraordinary dishes representing a place in the world; locally grown ingredients, and traditional flavors that genuinely give a taste of a place.[40, 41]

## Health Benefits of Beans

What does "regular bean consumption" mean? The U.S. Dietary Guidelines recommend eating about 3 cups (cooked) of legumes per week, like pinto, kidney, or black beans. If you eat about a ½ cup of beans every day, you will meet the weekly Dietary Guidelines for beans.

Beans are part of the carbohydrate family. They are complex carbohydrates, slowing the release of glucose during digestion. Research supports the inclusion of beans in the diet to reduce the risks associated with diabetes, heart disease, hypertension, high cholesterol, and cancer. Complex carbohydrates also contain high levels of fiber, which is necessary for healthy bowel function and microbiome maintenance.[42, 43, 44]

## Whole Grains

Whole grains [45] contain vitamins, minerals, oils, and fiber. Like beans, whole grains are complex carbohydrates that have been part of traditional diets dating back over a millennium. Jared Diamond, PhD, identifies eight "founder crops" as the earliest cultivated. In this group are barley, flax, einkorn, and emmer wheat. Anthropologists believe these founder crops were grown over 9,000 years ago. Rice may have been developed in Thailand as far back as 4,000 years. Corn predates that, having been cultivated as early as 6,000 years ago in Central and South America. Teff and spelt are further examples of cereal grasses providing traditional food nourishment for countless generations.

Most grains must be processed to be edible. Ancient "processing" involved soaking and hand grinding between stones by a person. An additional bonus was grain flour. If kept dry and out of the reach of pests, the flour could be stored in caches providing food through the famine of winter and early spring.

Grain also provided an essential component for alcoholic beverages, notably ale or beer, a source of carbohydrates and calories for cultures prior to the 20th century and an additional means of preserving grain. This form of preserving grains played a central role in the Whiskey Rebellion of the newly formed United States in 1794. Following years of aggression with tax collectors, farmers feared for the loss of income if they could not malt and distill their excess grain for later use and sale. The region finally exploded and President Washington responded by sending troops to quell what some feared could become a full-blown revolution and collapse of the fledgling nation.[46, 47]

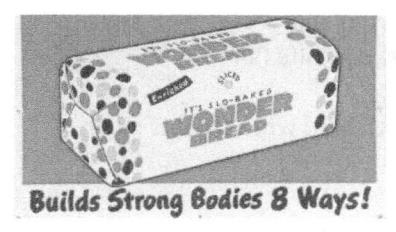

The world was first introduced to sliced bread in 1928. It was referred to as, "the greatest forward step in the baking industry since bread was wrapped."

A high intake of whole grains may increase the levels of betaine compounds, in the body. *Pipecolic acid betaine*, which is associated with improved glucose metabolism among other things.[48] Rye bread and whole grain foods also contain benzoxazinoids, a group of health-promoting substances. 5-aminovaleric acid betaine, seems to have the same action as some cardiovascular disease drugs. Scientists from Aarhus University in 2010 discovered their presence in whole grain.[49, 50]

The health benefits of whole grains are hotly contested in the modern functional nutrition field. GMO grains are a far cry from those produced worldwide before the 20th century. Bio-individual nutrition allows using non-GMO, traditional, and sustainably produced grains that are appropriate based on heritage, medical, family history, and availability.

## Types of Flour

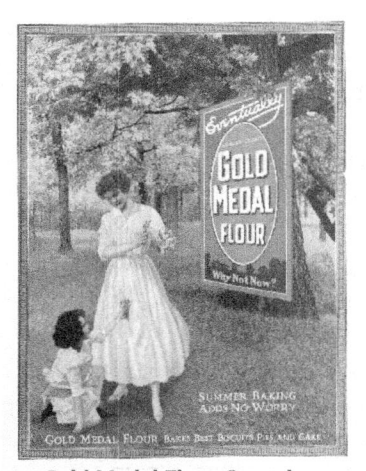

Gold Medal Flour Saturday Evening Post 1916

All flours are bleached, but unbleached flour is naturally bleached as it ages; exposure to oxygen causes it to whiten over time. It has a denser texture and duller color and provides more structure to baked goods. Bleached flour has been treated with bleaching agents (like *benzoyl peroxide*) to speed up the flour's aging process. The result is a paler color and lighter texture than unbleached flour. Baking with bleached flour yields softer results, but the two are interchangeable overall.

**All-Purpose**: This flour is likely already a staple in your kitchen, thanks to its versatility. It's milled from a combination of soft and hard wheat. It has a protein content of approximately 10%-12%, depending on the brand.

**Bread:** The texture of bread comes from the type of flour used. The bread flour is the strongest and has 12%-14% protein content. The extra protein is essential for yeasted bread that needs strong gluten to rise correctly.

**Whole Wheat:** All flours are made from wheat kernels separated into three components; the endosperm, germ, and bran, during the milling process. For white flour, only the endosperm is milled. Still, with whole wheat flour, some of the germ and bran is added back in, which gives it a nutty flavor and dense texture (plus fiber, minerals, and vitamins). Whole wheat flour has a protein content of around 14% but doesn't form gluten as readily as white flour.

**White:** Milled just like regular whole wheat flour, but it starts with hard wheat that is paler, called hard white wheat.

**Self-Rising**: Milled from soft wheat and has a protein content of approximately 9%. Self-rising flour yields lofty, light baked goods. Still, it can't be swapped as readily as other flours because the added ingredients can throw off other measurements in the recipe.

**Cake:** It generally has a protein content of 5%-8%, so it has less ability to form gluten bonds. Cake flour can absorb more liquid and sugar than other flours, so it keeps your cakes moist for longer.

**Pastry:** Pastry flour is between cake flour and all-purpose flour, with a protein content of around 9%. It can make extremely flaky, tender baked goods. It's often used for pastries, pie crusts, and cake.

**Double Zero**: An Italian flour milled from hard durum wheat with a protein content of 11%-12%.

**Semolina:** High in gluten and has about 12%-13% protein content, with a yellow color and nutty flavor.

**Instant:** Finely milled, low-protein flour pre-cooked and dried out.

**Rye**: Milled from rye kernels. Rye is closely related to wheat but has a lower gluten and protein content and more soluble fiber than wheat flour.

**Spelt:** A type of heritage whole wheat flour milled from the entire grain of spelt. It is lower in protein than regular whole wheat flour and behaves similarly to all-purpose flour.

**Einkorn:** The only wheat never hybridized and has only two sets of chromosomes. Low in gluten but higher in protein. Einkorn is unique and has gluten that is quite different than modern wheat. The same properties that make it easier to digest can make it a bit more challenging to bake than wheat with stretchier gluten. <u>For Best Results, Measure In Grams With A Baking Scale.</u>

**Khorasan:** This wheat, commercially known as Kamut, is a tetraploid wheat species. The grain is twice the size of modern day wheat and has a rich, nutty flavor. This ancient grain gives the dough a rich yellow color like durum but deeper and sweeter. Organic Khorasan also develops gluten better than durum, though their protein is typically similar. Protein 16%.

## Types of Yeast [51]

**Baker's yeast** is the common name for the strains of yeast used as an ingredient when baking bread. The earliest definite records come from Ancient Egypt.

Baking bread without yeast was done by mixing fresh and old dough that had risen. In the 19th century, bread bakers obtained their yeast from beer brewers who made sweet fermented breads. This was known as the Dutch process. By 1825 yeast was being sold in cream form, followed by a cake through the Viennese process. Charles Fleischmann brought the method of making yeast to the United States. He was trained as a young boy in a distillery and learned that yeast is a byproduct.

**Cream**: Cream yeast is used in industrial bakeries with professional dispensing and mixing equipment.

**Compressed**: This yeast is made from cream yeast for industrial and home use.

**Active dry**: Live yeast cells encapsulated in a thick jacket of dry, dead cells. It must first be rehydrated before use. Stored at room temperature, it can last for a year, while frozen can last 10 years or more. For home use.

**Instant**: Similar to dry yeasts but with a shorter life span, it does not have to be rehydrated. For home use.

**Rapid-rise**: Can be dissolved faster in the dough. It gives more carbon dioxide than other yeast types and raises the dough much quicker. Rapid-rise yeast is often used in bread machines.

## Carbohydrates, Fiber & Resistant Starch (Prebiotics)

One of the most significant nutrient deficiencies of Americans is fiber. The Standard American Diet is grossly void of fibrous foods. Nutritional fiber is essential for many biological functions. The digestive system and related organs, heart, skin, blood sugar control, and weight management need fiber to thrive.

Resistant starch and prebiotics play a significant role in gut health. Resistant starch feeds commensal gut bacteria, which is then broken down into short-chain fatty acids like butyrate, a substance with unique health benefits. A healthy microbiome controls the growth of pathogens and bacteria associated with chronic disease.

## Good Sources of Fiber

| | | | |
|---|---|---|---|
| Almonds | Avocados | Beans | Berries |
| Bok choy | Broccoli | Brussels sprouts | Cabbage |
| Cauliflower | Chia | Flax* | Hemp seed** |
| Kohlrabi | Onions | Peas | Pine nut |
| Pistachios | Psyllium | Pumpkin | Root vegetable/tubers |
| Sesame* | Squash | Sunflower seeds | |

*Flax and sesame seeds contain phytoestrogens and should be used cautiously if breast or prostate cancer is a concern.*

*\*\* Hemp and poppy seeds can cause false positive drug screening tests.*

## Best Sources of Resistant Starch

| | | | |
|---|---|---|---|
| Bananas, green | Black beans | Lentils | Plantain |
| Potatoes | Red beans | Rice | Sweet potato |
| White beans | White Great Northern beans | | |

## Best Sources of Prebiotics

The catch to this list is they need to be consumed raw to confer the prebiotic benefit. We have played around with dehydrating some raw, prebiotic vegetables in various ways, such as making Jerusalem artichoke chips and making onion and leek "flatbread."

| | | | |
|---|---|---|---|
| Asparagus | Apples | Apple cider vinegar, raw | Almonds |
| Artichoke | Bananas, green | Chestnut flour | Chicory root |
| Dandelion greens | Garlic | Jerusalem artichoke | Jicama |
| Leeks | Onions | Plantain | Radicchio |

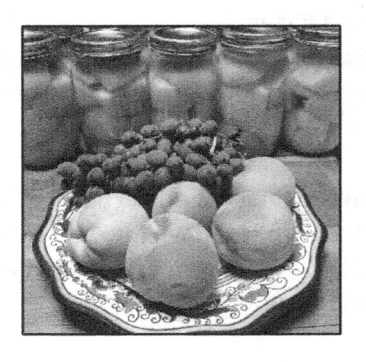

## Nuts & Seeds

Finely ground almonds have been used as a thickener in Mediterranean and Middle Eastern cookery since the 10th century. Raw nuts are a good source of healthy saturated fats that science and tradition support for daily consumption. Research supports the inclusion of nuts for heart, digestion, brain, bone, and healthy weight. Nuts are an excellent source of fiber, minerals, tocopherols, phytosterols, and phenolic compounds. Blood pressure, visceral adiposity, and metabolic syndrome are all positively influenced by nut consumption.

As often as possible, buy only organic raw nuts. Do not be fooled by packaging. Today, most nuts we think are raw in stores have been blanched to reduce *salmonella* contamination. Caution is advised for those with kidney disease or chronic inflammation.

**Should I sprout nuts and seeds?**

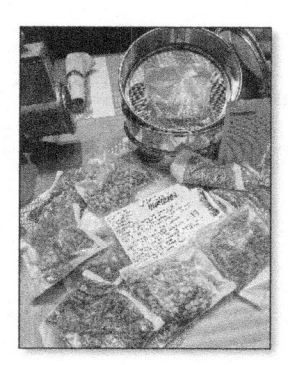

This traditional practice has regained popularity for breaking down phytic acid[52] and lectins. There is a reference to sprouting in the Old Testament[53] and Ayurvedic dietary writings.[54, 55] Current research supporting sprouting to reduce inflammation driven by phytic acid and lectin content is still in the early stages.[56] Time will tell if this is a benefit for everyone or for just those with elevated inflammation markers and autoimmune conditions. On the food security level, sprouting is a way to bring nutrient-dense fresh greens into the daily diet of humans and pet companions. Sprouting seeds come in different colors, sizes, and varieties. For $20.00, a selection of seeds can be purchased that will last one or two people for several months. Stainless steel sprouting trays can be purchased through natural food stores and the Internet. Basic glass jars can also be used.

The flavor of the sprouts varies based on the plant family: radish sprouts add a spicy zing, clover, and wheat a sweet grass taste, broccoli a sweet note, and beans all have their own distinctive flavor. The authors found sprouting time-efficient and easy in space-limited and mobile environments. Tammera believes sprouting is resilient enough it could have been done on ships, trains, and wagons for those who knew about sprouting.

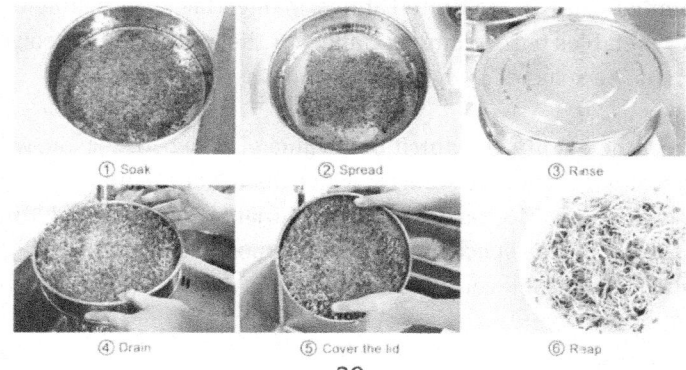

① Soak ② Spread ③ Rinse
④ Drain ⑤ Cover the lid ⑥ Reap

## Sprouting Seeds & Supplies

True Leaf Market: https://www.trueleafmarket.com/collections/sprouting-kits-and-supplies
Nature Jim's Sprouts: https://www.naturejims.com/seeds/
Johnny's Selected Seeds: https://www.johnnyseeds.com/vegetables/sprouts/
Stainless Steel Seed Sprouting Tray: www.amazon.com

## Top Picks

| | | | |
|---|---|---|---|
| Almond* | Brazil nut* | Chia seeds* | Hazelnut* |
| Macadamia nut | Pecan | Pine nut | Pistacho |
| Pumpkin seeds | Sesame seeds* | Walnuts | |

*Nuts and some seeds are high in potassium, phosphorus, and oxalate. These minerals are contraindicated for individuals with chronic or acute kidney disease.*

## Oxalate Low/Free Substitutions

| | | | |
|---|---|---|---|
| Cashew | Chile, seeds | Coconut | Hemp seeds |
| Macadamia | Nigella seeds* | Papaya seeds | Peanut |
| Pistachio | Pumpkin seeds | Sunflower seeds | Watermelon seeds |

*Kidney protective*

For more information on oxalate content: https://oxalate.org/

## *Sea Vegetables & Seaweeds*

Seaweed may be a staple in the pantries of many sea-bordering countries and is used daily in the diet. Seaweeds are not weeds but rather large marine algae that grow in coastal waters worldwide. They include thousands of species ranging from microscopic plants called phytoplankton to the large, floating, netted plants commonly seen washed up on shore. Sea vegetables rich in minerals are a vital addition to your pantry.[57] Thirty-five countries worldwide harvest seaweed commercially. In the United States, Maine, Hawaii, Washington, and Oregon are harvesting wild sea vegetables to sell commercially. For the most part, all sea vegetables are purchased dry and must be soaked in warm water and rinsed before use.

Many factors can affect the quality and nutritional value of seaweed. Season, water quality, salinity, water temperature, amount of sunlight, wave disturbance and large storms are only a few. All seaweed is high in salt. Most are high in antioxidants, minerals including trace minerals, melatonin, vitamin C and K. Some species, such as Irish moss, are incredibly high in iron, magnesium and zinc. The highest levels of melatonin in seaweed occur during the evening.

The phlorotannins in brown seaweed, responsible for many medicinal properties, are highly susceptible to oxidization, which is why seaweed must be stored in an airtight container. *Caution*: All sea vegetables can absorb toxins, heavy metals, and pollution.

> "There is no family of foods more protective against radiation and environmental pollutants than sea vegetables...sea vegetables can prevent assimilation of different radionucleotides, heavy metals such as mercury, and cadmium, and other environmental toxins."
>
> Steven Schecter, N.D.

## Types of Sea Vegetables

**Arame** - Perfect in salads as it has a firm texture even after soaking.

**Brown Algae** - Also known as bladderwrack, is rich in iodine. Use the young tips as a thickener for soup and stews. In addition to brown algae, additionally there are green and red algae varieties.

**Dulse:** Can be purchased as tiny flakes, which make a beautiful substitute for salt and can enhance any dish to give a nice salty flavor. It is sold whole in the form of stringy leaves and can be eaten like jerky or softened and added to soups.

**Hijiki:** The queen of sea vegetables, it is given credit for the lustrous hair and beautiful skin of Japanese women. Hijiki contains anti-inflammatory, antioxidant and anti-viral properties. This sea vegetable is typically found as flakes or powder.

**Kelp:** Available as noodles. Edible parts are the blades, leaves, stalks, and bulbs.

**Kombu:** The backbone for making Dashi, the Japanese stock that is a staple in their pantry. By adding a piece to the cooking liquid for soups, stews, beans, or rice, you are contributing alginic acid to your food. Alginic acid absorbs toxic heavy metals out of the body. Also, a strip of kombu added to beans will help reduce gas.

**Marine Grasses**: Best harvested in early spring and can be steamed or blanched. Eelgrass has a long history of use for fluid retention and in an alcohol, tincture provides antimicrobial benefits.

**Nori:** This is the ever-popular flat, thin sheets in sushi making. You can also buy it shredded, which is great to toss into salads, soups, etc.

**Wakame:** The fronds are the edible portion and work well in soups and salads and can be lightly fried and used as wraps for vegetables and meats.

## *Fruits & Vegetables*

When we consider the role vegetables and fruits play in our diet, we want to think of the rainbow according to nutrition expert Deanna Minich, PhD. Color, color, and more color: aim to consume five colors and portions of vegetables and fruits per day.[58]

**White and Brown** - Onions, garlic, leek, ginger, turnips, bok choi, and mushrooms. These colors signify immune-boosting compounds such as beta-glucans, EGCG, SDG, and lignans. They activate natural killer B and T cells.

**Yellow and Orange**: Apricots, peach, orange, grapefruit, butternut squash, carrots, butter cauliflower and pineapples. These are high in beta-carotene, zeaxanthin, flavonoids, lycopene, potassium, and vitamin C. These nutrients reduce age-related macular degeneration and the risk of prostate cancer, scavenging free radicals, and other supportive health benefits.

**Red:** Beets, cherries, blood oranges, radicchio, apples, and red peppers. The active compounds in red vegetables and fruits are *lycopene, ellagic acid, quercetin,* and *hesperidin*; to name a few. These nutrients can reduce the risk of prostate cancer, lower blood pressure, support heart health, reduce tumor growth, and support joint tissue in arthritis cases.

**Purple, Blue, and Black**: This is the family of fruits and vegetables the least eaten in the USA. It's considered to be a nutrient gap in our eating habits. Look to the berries, Concord grapes, purple figs, eggplant, black olives, purple cabbage, carrots, onions, broccoli, and asparagus to meet this vital nutrient need. These veggies and fruits are rich in *anthocyanin, resveratrol, zeaxanthin, vitamins C,* and *flavonoids.* They are essential for neuronal health, boosting immune system activity and digestive health, and improving mineral absorption.

**Green:** All the leafy greens, asparagus, Brussels sprouts, green beans, sprouts, green apples, green onions, snow peas, broccoli, cauliflower, and zucchini. They are rich in *chlorophyll, fiber, lutein, calcium, folate, vitamin C, vitamin K,* and *beta-carotene.* These nutrients help to reduce cancer risks, lower blood pressure and LDL cholesterol levels, normalize digestion, fight free radicals, and boost immune activity.

## *Proteins*

Consider protein as the heavyweight of health and vitality. Protein is an essential building block of bones, muscle, cartilage, skin, and blood. It is necessary for cell and mitochondrial health. Proteins are messengers that coordinate the biological processes of cell signaling, hormone communication, and tissue and organ integrity.

Proteins allow enzymes to carry out thousands of chemical reactions that take place. They are responsible for reading genetic information located in DNA and forming new molecules accordingly. Protein is a necessary macronutrient that includes fats and carbohydrates. Protein makes up about 15% of the mass of the average individual. [59]

**Sources of Protein**

| Beef | Bison/buffalo | Chicken | Crustaceans | Eggs |
|---|---|---|---|---|
| Dairy | Duck | Fish | Jerky, uncured | |
| Lamb | Organ meats | Shellfish | Turkey | Wild game |

*All animal products should be free-range, pastured, sustainably harvested, line caught and raw when possible: Organic if not.*

**Vegan and Vegetarian Protein Sources**

| Beans (legumes) | Edamame | Grains | Green peas | Lentils |
|---|---|---|---|---|
| Natto | Nuts & seeds | Nutr. yeast | Oyster mushrooms | |
| Rice protein | Seaweeds | Tempeh | Tofu | Vegetables |
| Whey | | | | |

## *Fats & Oils*

Fats are hydrophobic. In other words, fats repel water. Even oil based emulsions like mayonnaise rely on a third party to hold each tiny droplet of oil in suspension—egg yolk, mustard, or certain starches are common choices. Despite what some folks tell you, food fried at higher temperatures absorbs more oil than those fried at cooler temperatures.

Fats conduct heat and can do so at higher temperatures than water. When basting a roast with fatty pan drippings, the coating functions as a temperature buffer. This allows your food to heat evenly and prevents the exterior from drying out before the interior is fully cooked. Under normal conditions, water cannot be heated past its boiling point of 212°F at sea level. In contrast, fats can reach temperatures of 400-500°F. Fats lubricate food preventing it from sticking to cookware surfaces.

Fats add or boost flavor and enhance textural nuances of foods. This is vital for "mouth feel." Many of the flavor compounds that make herbs and aromatics such compelling seasonings are fat-soluble, meaning they will spread and coat your tongue better when immersed in lipids.

Using fat in anything from marinades to braises helps coax out, layer, and evenly distribute flavors.

Monounsaturated oils, specifically olive oil, increase the nutrients available through digestion. The tradition of tomatoes and olive oil is well supported by research; the antioxidant content of the tomatoes increases when combined with olive oil.[60, 61]

Natural oils and fats are traditional cooking mediums. Today's best options are cold-pressed, extra virgin oils and organic, humanely raised animal fats.

The more filtered the oil the lower the mineral and polyphenol content. Always buy solvent-free oils.

**Health Benefits of Traditional Fats**

Fats speak to the integral health of our whole body. Without healthy fats, we would not exist. [62]
- Fats give cells structure.
- They are a significant source of fuel for your body.
- Fats are required for absorbing vitamins A, D, E, K, and antioxidants lycopene and beta-carotene.
- You need healthy fats for optimum brain, nerve, and heart function.
- Fats make hormones and help to regulate them.
- Fats are essential for more youthful skin.
- Fats act as a cushion for your organs.

**Clarified butter** or **Ghee**[63] Cut butter into small pieces and melt over moderate heat. Skim off the foam, then pour the clear yellow liquid off the milky residue in the bottom of the pan. The clarified butter is now suitable for sautéing chicken breasts, vegetables, onions, fish, sauces, or anything you might choose.

It is the milky residue that turns black and bitter. Clarified butter will keep for weeks in a covered jar in the refrigerator.

**Washed Butter:** You will run into recipes, primarily vintage, that direct you to wash the butter and knead it until it is waxy. The process: Knead the butter in a damp towel until it is malleable. Place the butter towel in a cold water basin and continue kneading. Remove and knead on your work surface, still in the towel, mopping up moisture with paper towels. This method was used in the past to remove salt and moisture and to freshen the taste of butter if it had been kept too long.

**What is Smoke Point?**

Traditionally, oils are extracted from nuts and seeds through mechanical crushing and pressing. If bottled immediately, the oil is a cold-pressed (*raw* or *virgin*) oil, which tends to retain its natural flavor and color. In the case of olive oil, the "virgin" also signifies that only the perfect fruits were used. Unrefined oils are higher in minerals, enzymes, and compounds susceptible to heat and rancidity; these are the oils best suited to drizzling, dressings, and lower temperature cooking. The use of seed oils is controversial in some dietary models, and can be sources of mycotoxins.[64]

To produce oil with a high smoke point, manufacturers use industrial level refinement, bleaching, filtering, and high temperature heating to extract and eliminate extraneous compounds. This creates a neutral flavored oil with a long shelf life and a higher smoke point.

Clarified butter and ghee follow the same basic concept: a process designed to extract more heat-sensitive components; milk solids—from fat to raise its smoke point.[55] Fat breaks down when heated past its smoke point, releasing free radicals.

**Fat Smoke Point/Heat Reference Guide**

| | |
|---|---|
| Almond oil 520°F | Peanut oil 450°F |
| Clarified butter 450°F | Sesame seed oil 350-420°F |
| Walnut oil, semi-refined 406°F | Beef tallow 400°F |
| Coconut oil 400°F | Grapeseed oil 390°F |
| Avocado oil, virgin 375°F | Chicken fat 375°F |
| Duck fat 375°F | Olive oil, extra virgin 375°F |
| Lard 370°F | Butter 350°F |
| Unrefined olive oil 350°F | |

*Butter Substitutes.*
*There is no substitute for the taste of butter.*
Julia Child, 1912-2004

**Olive oil** is not only one of the oldest oils still in use for cooking, but it also has impressive science to support its use for health. Unrefined olive oil contains minerals, vitamins, and anti-inflammatory compounds. This is especially important when it comes to brain health.[66, 67, 68] The antioxidants in olive oil are essential for aiding the digestive system in absorbing nutrients found in vegetables. Especially those high in carotenoids, xanthine, and lycopene: winter squash, carrots, tomatoes, peppers, dark greens, cruciferous vegetables, and chard.

How you plan to use each type of olive oil matters because the flavor is affected by cooking. Olive oils, especially extra virgin, have varying smoke points. This depends on the type of olive, where it was grown, and how it was produced. For maximum flavor, reach for extra virgin olive oil.

Regular, pure, or classic olive oil provides many of the same health benefits as extra virgin olive oil. Pure, classic, light, and extra-light olive oils are authentic olive oils. All contain 100% olive oil and are not mixed with seed or vegetable oils unless explicitly stated on the package.[69]

Poor quality virgin olive oil with significant defects is called *Lampante* olive oil. Lampante olive oil is refined to remove bad flavors and odors, resulting in refined olive oil.

The International Olive Council (IOC) sets standards for a separate product category called olive pomace oil. Unlike olive oils, naturally extracted from olives, olive-pomace oil is a solvent removed from the leftover skins and pits after the olives are crushed and refined. The consumable grade olive-pomace oil is made by blending refined olive-pomace oil with virgin olive oil.

- The olive-pomace oil contains the same large proportion of monounsaturated fat, the "good fat," as olive oils but has few antioxidants.

- Olive-pomace oil can be used for high-heat cooking and manufacturing soaps and beauty products.

> **Principle 9**: *When it comes to fats and oils, read the label, consider the packaging, and look for country of origin to determines quality.*

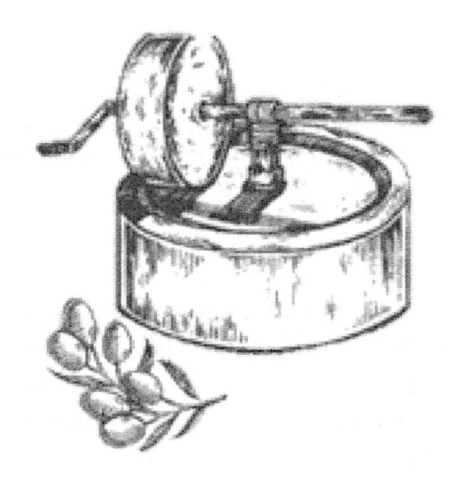

## *Olive Oil versus Canola Oil* [70]

The International Olive Council (IOC) in Madrid, Spain, sets the grades and standards for the world olive oil trade, including members of the North American Olive Oil Association.[71]

|  | **Olive Oil** | **Canola Oil** |
|---|---|---|
| Type | Fruit oil made from olives | Seed oil made from a variety of the rapeseed plant |
| Grades | The International Olive Council has established a grading system for olive oil that dictates how olive oil is graded and labeled. | No standards exist for Canola oil. While virgin canola oils exist, there is no consumer protection regarding the labeling. |
| Usage | Olive oil has been used for thousands of years. | Canola was developed in the 1970s. |
| Cost | Olive oil ranges in cost but is generally more expensive than canola. | Canola oil is less expensive than olive oil. |
| Production methods | Extra virgin olive oil is produced by pressing olives to extract the juice. Olive oil (often called classic or pure olive oil) may be extracted by applying heat. | Most canola is produced through a chemical extraction, refinement and bleaching process. |
| Solvents | No solvents are used to produce pure, classic, light or extra virgin olive oils. | Canola oil is generally extracted with chemical solvents such as hexane. |
| GMO | To date, there are no genetically modified olive oils. | Canola is a commonly genetically modified product. |
| Antioxidants | Olive oil of all grades contain antioxidants, which have powerful health benefits. | No antioxidants. |
| Rancidity | The antioxidants in olive oil help to protect the oil from rancidity and oxidation in storage and during cooking. | Canola should be used quickly after opening to prevent rancidity. |
| Flavor | Extra virgin olive oil has a fruity flavor. Pure and light olive oils have a neutral flavor. | Neutral flavor. |

## *Sweeteners*

*By including information on the varied forms of sweeteners, it is not the author's intention to support wholesale use. The following information is provided to aid cooks in selecting a suitable substitute for conventional recipes.*

**Sugar** was first introduced to cookery on the European continent by the Arabs. Cane sugar was not known before the 9th century when the Arabs filled the trade void after the collapse of the Roman Empire. It was called "white salt." The grains of sugar looked like those of salt, but unlike the grey color of salt, sugar was white. And, of course, it was sweet. Arabs had first learned how to take sugar from the cane from manufacturers in India. The process was time consuming, labor intensive, and expensive. Sugar was costly, and its exotic taste made it highly prized by wealthy Europeans. Apothecaries shaved flakes off sugar cones and sold them by the gram for toothaches.[72]

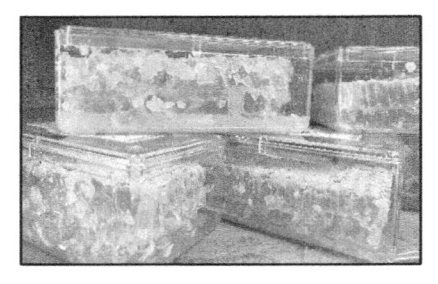

**Honey** has, by far, the oldest history when it comes to sweeteners. This would have been the *bee's knees* for the primitive hunter gatherer to find. By the time of the great Egyptian dynasties, honey was used as an antibiotic. Honey as a medicinal food is still in use today. Honey also became one of the world's first fermented alcoholic drinks, Mead. By medieval times, bees were so valuable for their honey, wax, and propolis that whenever one was seen to fly, a quick prayer to Saint Mary was said to keep the bees on the area of land spotted.[73]

**Sorghum** was carried west by pioneers and used as a substitute for molasses, honey, and maple syrup. This tall, broad-leaf plant resembles corn in the field and is best known for sweet syrup. Sorghum cane is typically harvested during September and October. Many sorghum syrup producers extract the juice from freshly cut plants in the field. The bright green juice then returns to the mill, where it is kept and heated in a holding tank. To avoid spoilage and produce the best syrup, it is cooked the next day into a light amber syrup and bottled. Ten gallons of raw sorghum juice yields about one gallon of syrup. Store sorghum as you would honey at room temperature. If it begins to crystallize, put it in a pan of warm water.[74]

**Molasses** is a byproduct of the sugar cane refining process. Sugar cane is mashed to create juice and then boiled once to make cane syrup. A second boiling creates molasses. After this syrup has been boiled a third time, a dark viscous liquid emerges known to Americans as blackstrap molasses. Blackstrap molasses contains vital vitamins and minerals, such as iron, calcium, magnesium, vitamins B6, and selenium.[75] It has the lowest sugar content of any sugar cane product.

**Maple Syrup and Sugar** are a traditional American Indian Nations sweetener. Maple sugar is made when the sap from the sugar maple trees is boiled for longer than it takes to make regular maple syrup. The remnants are solid sugar when nearly all the water has been boiled away.

In the United States, maple syrup is classified as grade A or B.

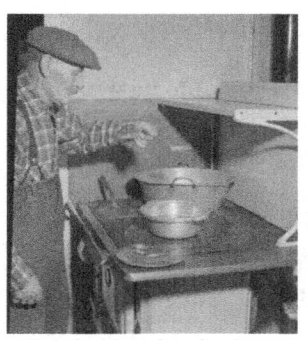

*Grade A* is further categorized into 3 groups: Light Amber, Medium Amber, and Dark Amber.

*Grade B* is the darkest of them all.

The main difference between Grade A and Grade B maple syrup is that the darker syrups are made from sap that is extracted later in the season. The dark syrups have a stronger maple flavor. They are used for baking, while the lighter ones are used as syrups. Pure maple syrup contains some minerals, especially manganese and zinc.

Reinhold Bieberdorf brewing maple syrup in his Scappoose kitchen, from sap gathered from local Oregon maple trees. February 24, 1952
*OHS photo. Scappoose 1952.*

Scientists from around the world shared research that expands the science of maple syrup's potential impact on health challenges affected by chronic inflammation. These include metabolic syndrome, brain health, liver disease, and the syrup's emerging link to a healthy gut microbiome.[76, 77]

**Agave** is a green, spikey looking succulent plant native to Mexico and the southwestern regions of the United States. It is primarily used to make tequila. The plant's sap is extracted to create what is popularly sold as agave nectar. For thousands of years, its anti-inflammatory and antiseptic properties have been used to treat burns, wounds, and insect bites. Most agave in the United States is adulterated with corn syrup.

Natural agave contains zinc, iron, calcium, and fiber as the prebiotic inulin. These nutritional benefits only come from agave in its raw, cooked, or dried states.[78] None of these benefits can be found in the sweet nectar commercially produced for grocery stores.[79]

**Coconut sugar** has been harvested and used throughout southern Asia for centuries. Some records state it has been used for as long as 6,000 years. The sugar is obtained from the sap of the coconut flower. The sap is boiled so that the water evaporates from it, which makes the sap become thick and concentrated, like molasses. Eventually, the sap is reduced to the point it crystallizes and becomes coconut sugar. This is the method used throughout history. Coconut sugar's nutritional profile is like ordinary white table sugar. It consists of 79% sucrose, with the rest being glucose and fructose.[80]

**Cane sugar** is what you typically find in your sugar bowl. It is the most common sugar in recipes when cooking and baking. "Regular" sugar granules are fine because small crystals are ideal for bulk handling and are not susceptible to caking. White sugar from beets is the most common form of sugar in North America. Unlike cane sugar is has a slightly bitter after taste.

**Demerara sugar** is light brown in color with large golden crystals, which are slightly sticky from the adhering molasses. This sugar can be made by dehydrating cane syrup after it is extracted from sugar cane. Popular in England, it is often used in tea, in coffee, or on top of hot cereals.

**Invert sugar** results from a process known as inversion, whereby sugar is split into its two components, glucose, and fructose. Because fructose is sweeter than sucrose or glucose, invert sugar is sweeter than white sugar. You can make it at home: when a recipe calls for sugar to be boiled gently in a mixture of water and lemon juice, the product is invert sugar.

**Liquid sugar** is white granulated sugar that has been dissolved in water. Simple syrup is liquid sugar with a 1:1 ratio of sugar and water. Liquid sugar is often used in drinks. Amber liquid sugar is darker in color and can be used when brown color is desired.

**Jaggery** is a traditional non-centrifugal cane sugar consumed in the Indian subcontinent, Southeast Asia, and Africa. It is a concentrated product of cane juice and often date or palm sap without separating the molasses and crystals. It can vary from golden brown to dark brown in color. Jaggery preserves some of the minerals and plant phytochemicals, providing a healthier option over refined sugar.

**Khus Shabat** is a fragrant, viscose sweetener made from the vetiver grass, found in south east Asia. Used medicinally and for beverages. Traditional vetiver syrup, is a dark amber color. Commercial versions are died dark green.

**Muscovado** is also known as Barbados sugar, is unrefined cane sugar in which the molasses has not been removed. It is very dark brown and has a robust molasses flavor. The crystals are slightly coarser and stickier than regular brown sugar, giving this sugar a sandy texture.

**Turbinado** is a partially processed sugar; only the surface molasses has been washed off. It has a blond color, mild brown sugar flavor, and larger crystals than brown sugars used in baking. Turbinado is the sugar in your packet of "raw sugar," but it is not unprocessed as the name may suggest.

## *Substitutions & Measurements*

1⅓ tbsp vinegar or 1½ tbsp lemon juice and sweet milk to equal 1 cup = 1 cup sour milk in place of buttermilk
½ cup evaporated milk and ½ cup cold water = 1 cup of milk
1 lemon = 3 to 4 tbsp juice
3½ tbsp cocoa and ½ tbsp butter = 1 oz or 1 square chocolate
1 tbsp cornstarch = 2 tbsp flour
1 tbsp almond flour = 1 tbsp cornstarch

1 tbsp potato starch = 1 tbsp cornstarch
4 tbsp quick-cooking tapioca = 1 tbsp cornstarch
1 cup granulated sugar with 1-2 tbsp blackstrap molasses = 1 cup brown sugar
1 cup honey = ¾ cup sugar plus ¼ cup liquid
1 cup sugar = 1 cup honey or maple syrup, and reduce the liquid in the recipe to ¼ cup
1 tablespoon potato or arrowroot powder = 1 egg

*Sorghum* as a substitute for honey (in recipes that do not use baking powder). When substituting sorghum in place of sugar, use ⅓ more sorghum than the amount of sugar called for in the recipe and decrease the amount of liquids by ⅓ When using sorghum instead of molasses, use an equal amount of sorghum, but cut the amount of sugar since sorghum is sweeter than molasses.

### How to Make Sweetened Condensed Milk

Yields 1¼ cup

Combine 1 cup whole milk, 1 cup cream, ¾ cup sugar or maple syrup, 4 tablespoons salted butter and 1 teaspoon vanilla extract.

Whisk together milk and sweetener in a medium sauce pan over medium-low heat. Whisking often, bring to a low simmer. Continue to simmer, whisking often, until milk has reduced by half, about 30 minutes. Once reduced, remove from heat, and stir in butter and vanilla. Allow to cool completely and store in a mason jar in the refrigerator for up to 1 week.

### *To Reduce Recipes*
To make half a recipe: Use exactly one-half the amount of each ingredient.

### *To Increase Recipes*
To double a recipe: use exactly twice the amount of each ingredient.

## *Size of Cans*

8 oz = 1 cup
No. 1 = 2 cups or 16 oz
No. 2½ = 3⅓ cups or 28 oz
No. 10 = 13 cups or 6 lbs 10 oz

Picnic = 1¼ cups or 10 oz
No. 2 = 1½ cups or 20 oz
No. 3 = 4 cups or 32 oz

## Measurement Equivalents

| CUP | FLUID OZ | TBSP | TSP | MILLILITER |
| --- | --- | --- | --- | --- |
| 1 C | 8 oz | 16 tbsp | 48 tsp | 237 ml |
| 3/4 C | 6 oz | 12 tbsp | 36 tsp | 177 ml |
| 2/3 C | 5 oz | 11 tbsp | 32 tsp | 158 ml |
| 1/2 C | 4 oz | 8 tbsp | 24 tsp | 118 ml |
| 1/3 C | 3 oz | 5 tbsp | 16 tsp | 79 ml |
| 1/4 C | 2 oz | 4 tbsp | 12 tsp | 59 ml |
| 1/8 C | 1 oz | 2 tbsp | 6 tsp | 30 ml |
| 1/16 C | .5 oz | 1 tbsp | 3 tsp | 15 ml |

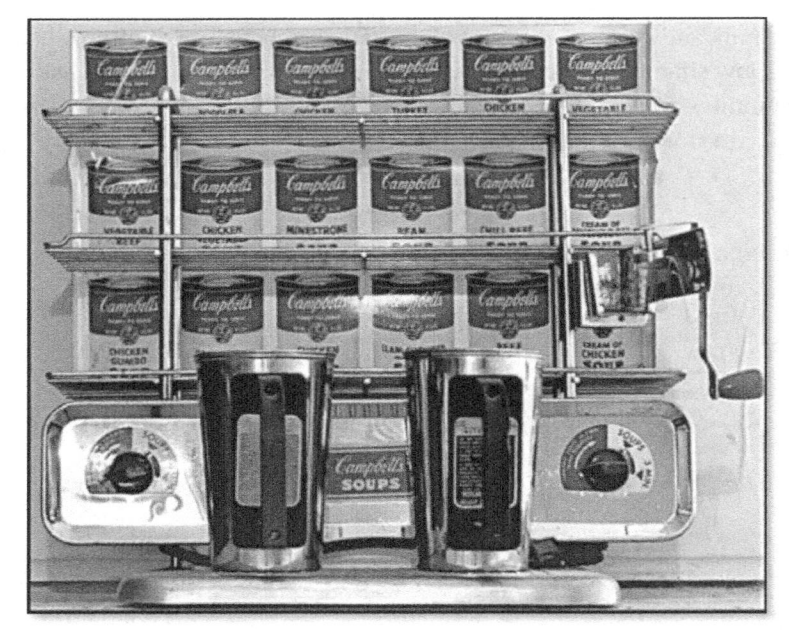

Commercial Campbell's soup warmer for restaurants and canteens. Two warming pitchers and a can opener made for a fast reheating circa 1960s. Wallowa County Museum, Joseph, Oregon

## Abbreviations Commonly Used

| | | | |
|---|---|---|---|
| tsp = teaspoon | tbsp = tablespoon | c = cup | oz = ounce |
| sq = square | lb = pound | pt = pint | qt = quart |
| doz = dozen | pk = peck | bu = bushel | g = gram |
| minutes = minute | hr = hour | mod = moderate | |
| DF = dairy free | EF = egg free | GF = gluten free | |
| P = paleo | V = vegetarían | VE = vegan | l = liter |
| WF = wheat free | | | |

## Vintage or Antique Measurement Conversions

When looking through cookbooks from the 1800s and handwritten recipes from distant family members – it isn't uncommon to encounter "period" measurements. Heritage and heirloom recipes reference measurements like "*dram, pinch, shake, knob, gill,* and my favorite *tad.*" Hopefully, this "*wee*" chart will help you recover an old family recipe.

1 drop or nip = 1/64 tsp     1 smidgen or shake = 1/32 tsp

½ pinch = what can be picked up between thumb and one finger

1 pinch or dash = what can be picked up between thumb and first two fingers; less than ⅛ tsp

2 fingers = less than ⅛ tsp     1 tad = ¼ tsp

1 salt spoon = ¼ tsp     1 kitchen spoon = 1 tsp

1 dessert spoon = 2 tsp or 1 soup spoon

1 tbsp = 3 tsp, ½ fluid oz     1 spoonful = 1 tbsp more or less

1 jigger = 1½ oz     1 wineglass = ¼ cup or ½ gill

4 large tbsp = half a gill     1 gill = ½ cup, 8 tbsp, 4 fluid oz [81]

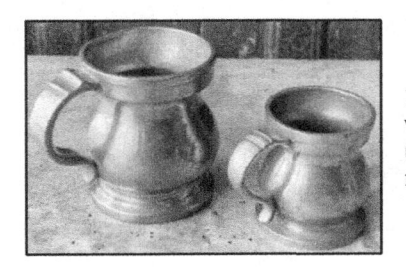

1 gill and ½ gill measure cups - volume equal to a quarter of a pint of alcoholic spirits. ¼ gill (35.5 ml) was also a common measure in Scotland and remains as the standard measure.

## *Elevation Adjustments for Baking and Cooking*

You may live in a coastal area or high in the mountains, but many do not realize that for every 1,000 feet of elevation, how foods bake and cook can change. This is especially true when home canning foods. The altitude to keep in mind is 3,500 feet above sea level. Not every recipe will have challenges, and most commercial mixes have ample leavening to compensate for elevation change. The higher a kitchen elevation is above sea level, whether camp or home, the less air pressure. The less air pressure, the more cooking and baking changes compared to most recipes' expectations. For example, at sea level, water boils at 212°F. At 7,500 feet above sea level, water boils at 198°F.

If you need to adjust recipes, here are a few suggestions.

- Increase oven temperature by 15-25°F.
- Decrease baking time by about 5 minutes (per every 30 minutes called for in a recipe).
- Egg whites should only be whipped to soft peaks.

**Reduce baking powder.** "Because of the decrease in barometric pressure at high altitudes, carbon dioxide gas expands more quickly and thus has greater leavening action." - *The Joy of Cooking*

**Reduce sugar.** Due to quicker evaporation, sugar becomes more concentrated in baked goods, so you won't need as much.

**Add liquid.** Foods such as flour dry more quickly at high altitudes. More liquid is needed to ensure the baked good doesn't turn out dry or crumbly.

**Increase oven temperature.** "Since leavening and evaporation proceed more quickly, the idea is to use a higher temperature to 'set' the structure of baked goods before they over-expand and dry out." - *King Arthur Baking*

| Feet above sea level | Baking powder or soda (reduce each teaspoon by) | Sugar (reduce each cup by) | Liquid (for each cup add) |
|---|---|---|---|
| 3,500 to 5,000 | ⅛ teaspoon | 0 to 1 tablespoon | 1 to 2 tablespoons |
| 5,000 to 7,000 | ⅛ to ¼ teaspoon | ½ to 2 tablespoons | 2 to 4 tablespoons |
| 7,000 to 9,000 | ¼ teaspoon | 1 to 3 tablespoons | 3 to 4 tablespoons |

## Sourdough Bread Adjustments

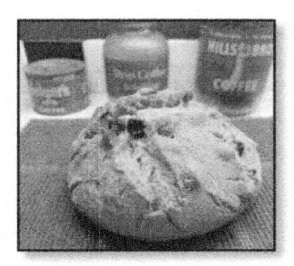

Living at high altitudes makes baking (and cooking) a little more complicated, especially when following recipes.

It takes bread (and other food) longer to reach a higher internal temperature at high altitudes.

### What to Change for High Altitude

| Oven temperature | Increase oven temperature by 25°F. |
|---|---|
| Bake time | Increase baking time unless oven temperature is increased. |
| Dough hydration | Generally, increase hydration. |
| Leavening | Sometimes a decrease, but not always. |

- ✓ The extra time needed depends on the bread; it is usually more for pan bread than free form loaves.

- ✓ Free-form loaves, on average, bake 10 minutes longer, depending on the style of bread and recipe.

- ✓ Loaves with higher hydration always require a longer bake time, whether this is a whole wheat loaf or a white loaf.

- ✓ Convection oven – Do Not reduce your oven by 25°F.

- ✓ Internal temperature should be near 200-205°F (93-96°C). However, at high altitudes (5,000 feet and higher above sea level), no matter how long the bread is baked, it never reaches the ideal temperature.

- ✓ With free-form loaves, a gentle squeeze should have a satisfying crunch (indicating the crust has sufficiently hardened off).

- ✓ There should be no pale colored areas on the crust.

- ✓ The loaf should feel light in hand, indicating sufficient water has baked away.

- ✓ Dough hydration is always relative to the flour used. Adjust as necessary.

- ✓ Humidity affects the amount of water your dough will ultimately handle. In many parts of the west and southwest, there can be a wide range of humidity levels, but generally, it's low, around 15-30%. To compensate, be prepared to add additional water to recipes.

- ✓ Performing an *autolyze* (mixing your flour and water and allowing it to rest) can improve sourdough bread at a high altitude, even if it's a short 15-20 minute rest.[82]

## *A Word on Dairy Substitutes*

The authors recognize there are individuals with food sensitivities, health conditions and preferences for not consuming animal milk. Over the last ten years dairy substitutes have become increasingly easy to buy or make. Nut milks are non-dairy milk alternatives derived from nuts soaked in water and blended into a creamy beverage. Commercial nut and seed milk typically contains preservatives, gums and added sugars that may not be suitable for dietary restrictions. Seed milks are lower in oxalates then nut milk and tolerated better by some. Oat milk is the easiest to make. Tools required for making nut and seed milks; blender and mesh strainer, or a home plant-based milk machine (Almond Cow Milk Maker Machine).

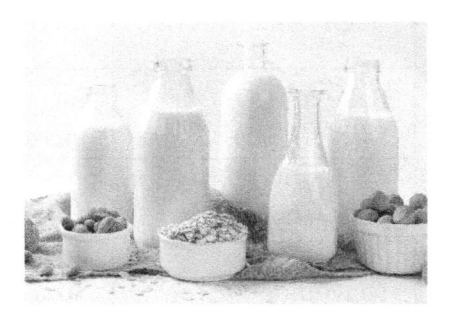

**Common non-dairy milk and cheese sources**: soy, almond, cashew, coconut, hazelnut hemp, macadamia, oat, peanuts, pecan, pistachio, potato, and walnut.

**Cautions:** Individuals with nut allergies, celiac disease, kidney disease, diabetes, and chronic inflammatory conditions are advised to avoid non-dairy milk products. Nuts contain aflatoxins, oxalates, potassium, and phosphorus which worsen kidney health. Diabetics with poor kidney function may be worsening their condition and elevating blood sugars. Other conditions that are worsened by anti-nutrients found in nuts and grains include auto-immune illnesses such as type 1 diabetes, rheumatoid arthritis, MS, crohns and lupus.

**How old is the use of plant milk?**
The answer to this question is hotly debated amongst foodies. So, acknowledging many plant milks have cultural histories and use, we will focus on commercial production.

Coconut milk largely unchanged from traditional forms
Almond milk 1880s, USA                              Soymilk 1917, USA
Oat milk 1990, Sweden                               Rice milk 1991, USA
Hemp milk 2015, Canada

20 National Center for Home Food Preservation; https://nchfp.uga.edu/how/store.html#gsc.tab=0

21 Seaweed: Nature's Secret for a Long and Healthy Life? Jane Philpott and Montse Bradford
https://www.semanticscholar.org/paper/Seaweed-%3A-Nature-%E2%80%99-s-Secret-for-a-Long-and-Healthy-Philpott-Bradford/3eeeca088571587f3f8c723ee90617c28d61a875?p2df

22 Algae as nutritional and functional food sources: revisiting our understanding;
https://www.ncbi.nlm.nih.gov/pmc/articles/PMC5387034/

23 https://www.thekitchn.com/sea-vegetables-22926349

24 *Buffalo Bird Woman's Garden* by Gilbs.ert L. Wilson 1917 and 1987; ISBN: 10:0-87530-219-7

25 Flavour enhancers are used in savoury foods to enhance the existing flavour in the food. Food flavour enhancers are commercially produced in the form of instant soups, frozen dinners and snackfoods etc. Monosodium glutamate is an example of a flavour enhancer. Salt is commonly used as a natural flavour enhancer for food and has been identified as one the basic tastes.
http://www.foodadditivesworld.com/flavor-enhancers.html

26 National Center for Home Food Preservation; https://nchfp.uga.edu/how/store.html#gsc.tab=0

27 Fresh versus Frozen Vegetables by Bertina Mcghee | 11/2/2017 3:58:06 PM;
https://www.lsuagcenter.com/articles/page1509638286014

28 https://foodandhealth.com/fresh-vs-frozen-whats-the-difference/

29 http://www.frozenfoodfacts.org/research/new-study-reinforces-nutritional-benefits-frozen-fruits-and-vegetables

30 Nutritional comparison of fresh, frozen and canned fruits and vegetables. Part 1. Vitamins C and B and phenolic comlbs.s, Joy C Rickman, Diane M Barrett and Christine M Bruhn* Department of Food Science and Technology, University of California – Davis, Davis, CA 95616, USA; J Sci Food Agric 87:930–944 (2007)

31 Casajús V, Demkura P, Civello P, Gómez Lobato M, Martínez G. Harvesting at different time-points of day affects glucosinolate metabolism during postharvest storage of broccoli. Food Res Int. 2020 Oct;136:109529. doi: 10.1016/j.foodres.2020.109529. Epub 2020 Jul 12. PMID: 32846593.

32 Early History of USDA Home Canning Recommendations -
https://nchfp.uga.edu/publications/usda/review/earlyhis.htm

33 The History of Canning and Can Making: https://www.acumence.com/the-history-of-canning-and-can-making/

34 How Canned Food Revolutionized The Way We Eat: https://www.history.com/news/what-it-says-on-the-tin-a-brief-history-of-canned-food

35 The Foods that Built America: https://play.history.com/shows/the-food-that-built-america

36 History of the Home Canning Jar and Collecting Antique Mason, Ball and Kerr Jars: https://www.pickyourown.org/canningjars.htm

37 On Food and Cooking by Harold McGee

38 Beans Around the World | Bean Institute. https://beaninstitute.com/beans-around-the-world/

39 Beans Around The World | Bean Institute. (n.d.). Retrieved from http://beaninstitute.com/beans-around-the-world/

40 Dragonwagon, C (2011). Bean by Bean – A Cookbook. More than 175 Recipes from Fresh Beans, Dried Beans, Cool Beans, Hot Beans, Savory Beans, Even Sweet Beans! New York: Workman Pub.

41 Beans Around The World | Bean Institute. (n.d.). Retrieved from http://beaninstitute.com/beans-around-the-world/

42 World Cancer Research Fund/American Institute for Cancer Research. Food, Nutrition, Physical Activity, and the Prevention of Cancer: a Global Perspective. Washington DC: AICR, 2007

43 Darmadi-Blackberry I, Wahqvist ML, Kouris-Blazos A, et al. Legumes: the most important dietary predictor of survival in older people of different ethnicities. Asia Pacific Journal Of Clinical Nutrition. 2004;13(2):217- 220.

44 Third Report of the National Cholesterol Education Program (NCEP) Expert Panel on Detection, Evaluation, and Treatment of High Blood Cholesterol in Adults (Adult Treatment Panel III), Final Report. Washington, D.C: National Heart, Lung and Blood Institute of the National Institutes of Health; September 2002. NIH Publication No. 02-5215.

45 The Mediterranean Diet between traditional foods and human health: The culinary example of Puglia (Southern Italy)MassimilianoRennaaVito, AntonioRinaldibMariaGonnellaahttps: www.sciencedirect.com/science/article/pii/S1878450X14000213

46 Guns, Germs, and Steel: The Fates of Human Societies Hardcover, by Jared Diamond Ph.D. 2005

47 http://www.thenibble.com/reviews/main/rice/whole-grains-cereals2.asp

48 University of Eastern Finland. (2018, October 3). Newly discovered comlbs shed fresh light on whole grain health benefits. ScienceDaily. Retrieved October 29, 2018 from www.sciencedaily.com/releases/2018/10/181003102720.htm

49 Aarhus University. (2016, February 8). Wholesome wholegrain. ScienceDaily. Retrieved October 25, 2018 from www.sciencedaily.com/releases/2016/02/160208124251.htm

50 https://www.semanticscholar.org/paper/Whole-grain-rye-breakfast-sustained-satiety-during-Isaksson Tillander/db0de1da9a2e43357e7f1415b2a45a5d9237d05f?utm_source=TrendMD&utm_medium=cpc&utm_campaign=TMD_50

51 History of Bread, retrieved August 2022. http://www.historyofbread.com/bread-history/history-of-bakers-yeast/?fbclid=IwAR3N-jeGc072IG72HC3WZ5yPatNcoDNhnWJ6PNX78d8qU3QsgCQGysgJELE/

52 Living With Phytic Acid by Ramiel Nagel, 2010

53 Ezekiel 4:9

54 A glimpse of Ayurveda – The forgotten history and principles of Indian traditional medicine; https://www.ncbi.nlm.nih.gov/pmc/articles/PMC5198827/

55 Traditional and ayurvedic foods of Indian origin; https://www.sciencedirect.com/science/article/pii/S2352618115000438#!

56 Are sprouted grains more nutritious than regular whole grains? 2017, by Heidi Godman Harvard Health Letter: https://www.health.harvard.edu/blog/sprouted-grains-nutritious-regular-whole-grains-2017110612692

57 https://www.researchgate.net/publication/261369332_Seaweed_and_human_health

58 Whole Detox by Deanna Minich

59 https://www.westonaprice.org/health-topics/abcs-of-nutrition/protein-building-blocks-of-the-body/

60 Lee, A., Thurnham, D. I., & Chopra, M. (2000). Consumption of tomato products with olive oil but not sunflower oil increases the antioxidant activity of plasma. Free radical biology & medicine, 29(10), 1051–1055. https://doi.org/10.1016/s0891-5849(00)00440-8

61 Lanza, B., & Ninfali, P. (2020). Antioxidants in Extra Virgin Olive Oil and Table Olives: Connections between Agriculture and Processing for Health Choices. Antioxidants (Basel, Switzerland), 9(1), 41. https://doi.org/10.3390/antiox9010041

62 https://www.euficorg/en/whats-in-food/article/facts-on-fats-dietary-fats-and-health

63 Is Ghee more Healthful than Butter?, Retrieved September 2022; https://www.medicalnewstoday.com/articles/321707

64 Bhat, R., & Reddy, K. R. (2017). Challenges and issues concerning mycotoxins contamination in oil seeds and their edible oils: Updates from last decade. Food chemistry, 215, 425–437. https://doi.org/10.1016/j.foodchem.2016.07.161

65 Cooking Fats 101: What's a Smoke Point and Why Does it Matter?; https://www.seriouseats.com/2014/05/cooking-fats-101-whats-a-smoke-point-and-why-does-it-matter.html

66 Extra-virgin olive oil preserves memory, protects brain against Alzheimer's; June 21, 2017, Temple University Health System: https://www.sciencedaily.com/releases/2017/06/170621103123.htm

67 Extra-virgin olive oil ameliorates cognition and neuropathology of the 3xTg mice: role of autophagy; https://www.ncbi.nlm.nih.gov/pmc/articles/PMC5553230/

68 Mediterranean-type diet and brain structural change from 73 to 76 years in a Scottish cohort; http://n.neurology.org/content/early/2017/01/04/WNL.0000000000003559.short?sid=f6a60041-6b89-41fe-827d-49a0f92359fa

69 North American Olive Oil Association; https://www.aboutoliveoil.org/what-is-pure-or-classic-olive-oil?utm_campaign=olive%20oil%20quality&utm_content=77894764&utm_medium=social&utm_source=facebook

70 North American Olive Oil Association; https://www.aboutoliveoil.org/oliveoil-vs-canolaoil?utm_campaign=olive%20oil%20health%20benefits&utm_content=77874684&utm_medium=social&utm_source=facebook

71 Grades of Olive Oil; https://www.aboutoliveoil.org/grades-of-olive-oil-video?utm_campaign=olive%20oil%20videos&utm_content=77894857&utm_medium=social&utm_source=facebook

72 Cuisine and Culture: A History of Food and People by Linda Civitello

73 Cuisine and Culture: A History of Food and People by Linda Civitello

74 What Is Sorghum? | The Difference Between Sorghum And ... (n.d.). Retrieved from https://www.farmflavor.com/at-home/seasonal-foods/what-is-sorghum/

75 Blackstrap Molasses Benefits - Healthline. (n.d.). Retrieved from https://www.healthline.com/health/food-nutrition/benefits-blackstrap-molasses

76 Can pure maple syrup help reduce chronic inflammation? https://www.eurekalert.org/pub_releases/2017-04/p-cpm033117.php

77 University of Rhode Island. (2010, March 25). Pure maple syrup contains medicinally beneficial compounds, pharmacy researcher finds. ScienceDaily. Retrieved September 19, 2022 from www.sciencedaily.com/releases/2010/03/100321182924.htm

78 Velázquez Ríos, I. O., González-García, G., Mellado-Mojica, E., Veloz García, R. A., Dzul Cauich, J. G., López, M. G., & García-Vieyra, M. I. (2018). Phytochemical profiles and classification of Agave syrups using 1H-NMR and chemometrics. Food science & nutrition, 7(1), 3–13. https://doi.org/10.1002/fsn3.755

79 What's Wrong with Agave Nectar? By Andrew Weil, MD: https://www.drweil.com/diet-nutrition/nutrition/whats-wrong-with-agave-nectar/

80 Coconut Sugar: The Sustainable Sweetener - Spiceography. (n.d.). Retrieved from https://www.spiceography.com/coconut-sugar/

81 1938 Qt.er gill measure pot: https://www.bbcco.uk/ahistoryoftheworld/objects/dCVOH-rrQ_udb-MJIK9ixg

82 The Perfect Loaf: https://www.theperfectloaf.com/guides/how-to-bake-sourdough-bread-at-high-altitude/

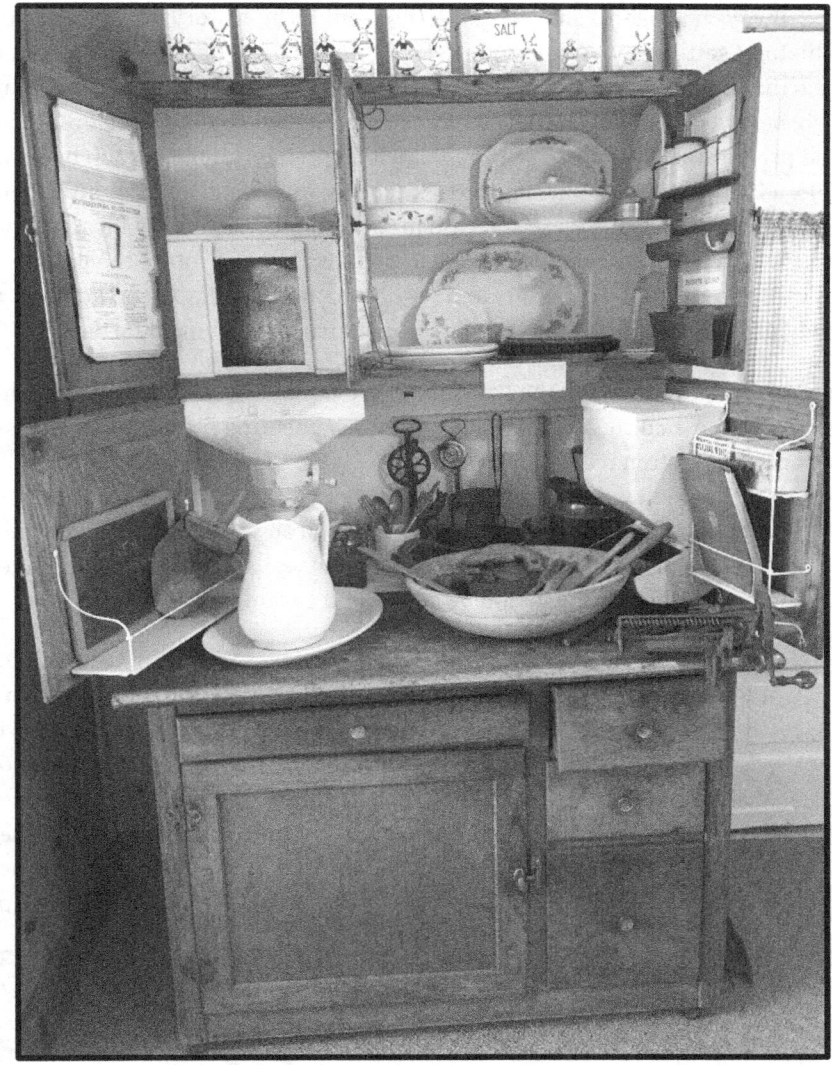

Chetco County Museum, Harbor, OR.

A Hoosier is a kitchen all-in-one cupboard and work center. The Hoosier Manufacturing Co. began in Indiana in 1898. The factory made 600 a day; by 1920, the company had sold nearly 2 million. The cabinet featured drawers for utensils, shelves, a spice rack, pie safe, cookbook stand, a breadboard, flour bin, a sifter, and a pullout porcelain worktop. In some models, the bin could be lowered for easy filling. Cabinets came equipped with fitted glass coffee and tea jars. Another feature of the Hoosier Kitchen Cabinet was measurement conversion cards inside the doors. These also included sample menus, cooking times, and household hints.

# *Gizmos & Gadgets for the Kitchen*

The kitchen is and always has been a shared space, by people. The history of our modern kitchen goes back to prehistoric settlements worldwide.[83, 84] In the *Choukowtien* cave system in northern China, ancient hearths contain traces of cooking attributed to "Peking Man" from an estimated 780,000 years ago, believed to be the earliest evidence of a central cooking area or kitchen.[85] Using fire for food preparation was a breakthrough. Just like today, kitchens soon became the repository of tools; a 2,600 year old fully equipped kitchen was unearthed in Anatolia, Turkey, in 2016.[86] In the past, kitchen locations were selected for accessibility, centrally located, and ventilation; Moroccan kitchens placed cook pots in a "roofless kitchen" off of the pantry. Bulgarian homes utilize summer kitchens located outdoors. In India, the Mogul kitchens were frequently located outdoors to remove the smells and heat from the living quarters.

The kitchen was also the focal point for the transmission of culture and teaching, from origin stories to homework. In most cultures, the kitchen became a meeting place between classes; long time family cooks were often treated with the respect due to family members. In segregated societies, the kitchen was a connection between whites and blacks. The invention and mass distribution of the large cast iron stove, called the "iron sow" in early Sweden, radically changed the design of the kitchen.[87] Now, this room was filled with heat, cleaner air, and the temperatures needed for baking could be controlled easier.

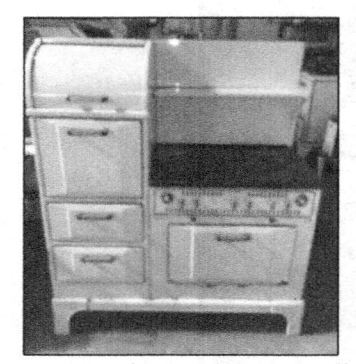

Even with the addition of cookstoves in the 1800s, the kitchen was an afterthought in America's homes. It had little to no cabinetry or storage space, sparse counter space and was ill-equipped for meal preparation. By the 1890s, incomes had increased and individuals had more money to spend on convenience; cooks began using standalone baker's cabinets which provided storage and some much-needed workspace. The Hoosier cabinet promised to save time, work, and *do away with all kitchen drudgery*.

Hoosier advertisements presented a woman as an *efficiency expert* using a stopwatch and a pedometer to measure steps used while preparing three meals. Ads read: *By combining the storage functions of the pantry and the work table, 1,592 steps could be saved using the cabinet.* The Hoosier Manufacturing Co. was the first in the nation to provide a time-payment plan with its *Hoosier Club* membership.

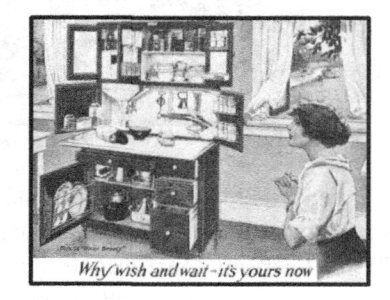

While uniform kitchen cabinets were standard by the mid-1900s in populated areas, rural kitchens depended on standalone cabinets until 1950. Other versions appeared during this same time. One was the Possum Belly baker's table. The Holistic Nutrition for the Whole You kitchen centerpiece is a baker's table made by M. FrudRick Furniture CO., San Francisco, CA, circa 1880- circa 1900. The tin-clad rounded deep drawers give the table its unique possum belly.

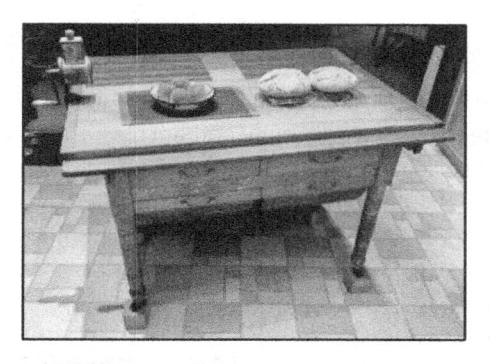

The table surface expands for use as an eating surface or a smaller work surface with drawers easily accessible. The Pie Safe and Kitchen Hutch joined the Hoosier and Possum Belly in safeguarding food staples from vermin.

By 1944, 85% of American homes had refrigerators and ranges; some even came with built-in radios. Every piece of cabinetry was sleek and had a purpose; by the 1950s, some refrigerators came with ice makers, and the kitchen was filled with chrome and color.

### The Knife

In its many forms, the knife is the oldest and most prevalent of cookery tools. Early humans would have been challenged to chew and tear meat or fibrous tubers without the aid of a sharp edged stone tool. The development of knives combined with cooking made it possible for culture and complex communities to develop. The advent of knives and cooking, some assert, is what led to the superior brains of humans. Now, foods once uneatable due to their fibrous nature could become staples during the famine, adding more nutrition and calories to the human diet.

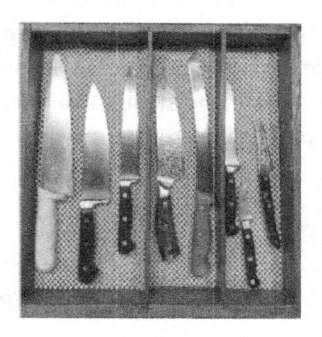

Over the centuries, cultures have developed knives more than all other utensils. Materials used included bone, granite, obsidian, jade, copper, bronze, and steel. Some are works of art or ceremony, while others have coveted places in the kitchens of master chefs.

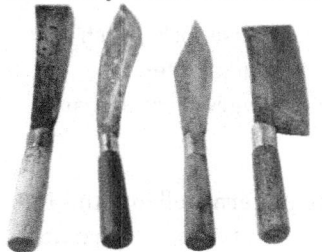

In Asian culture, it is a knife that holds the position of honor; it is the *Tous*. This knife is responsible for the artful blending of flavors. It is used for slivering vegetables and chopping meat, fish, poultry, and vegetables into perfect bite sized pieces. This perfect balance in flavors ranks Chinese cookery second only to French fare in popularity.

Ingredient Guru Mira Dessy has this to share about knives. *"Everyone needs a good chef's knife. A chef's knife is my favorite with an eight-inch blade and a perfect balance. I use it all the time. When Hurricane Harvey displaced me for a few months, the one thing I missed the most was my knife."* The size of the knife really depends on the cook, they range in size from 8 inches to 12 inches.

As a rule, the most dangerous knives in or out of the kitchen are dull ones made from inferior quality steel. Individuals may not know how to properly use a steel or whetstone to smooth out the work roughened edge of a favorite knife; take heart, with the Internet at hand you can find a video or blog that will tell you how to keep this important tool tuned and safe for use.

## The Spoon's Early Technology

Once we moved from using our hands and knapped stone implements for food preparation, the materials easiest to mold to our needs was wood, bone and horn. Archaeologists can point to evidence around 1000 BC of spoons from Ancient Egypt. Spoons in Egypt and Britain carried significance in ceremonies as a sign of wealth and power. The spoon became a symbol of love in Wales and Norway. Carved elk antler spoons represented wealth to members of the Confederated Tribes of Cow Creek Indians in Southern Oregon; a man with 250 spoons was considered rich. [88, 89]

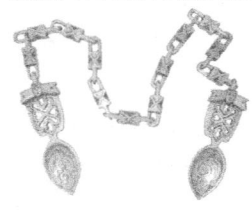

*Norwegian wedding spoons (Vladimir Alexiev/ CC BY SA 4.0 )*

Our current "*cookery*" would be harder without the technological breakthrough of the spoon; long handles, short, oval, round, big, or small. The simple spoon is a marvel; tiny spoons for measuring critical ingredients to mega spoons used in industrial work. A kitchen would not be complete without a jug or jar stuffed with wooden spoons. Their safe and straightforward efficiency when mixing or stirring a hot pot or pan is hard to surpass.[90]

> **Principle 10**: *Quality cooking utensils and cookware last a lifetime and are a measure of safety from unknown chemical contaminants.*

## Enter the Fork

The fork is a relative newcomer to the table. Many parts of the world do not use forks, such as the Orient, Outback, and the jungles. The Orient adopted the fork for some functions after colonization and the influence of Europeans. In the western world, almost every meal we eat involves the use of a fork in preparation, serving, and eating.

Anthropological information suggests humans had an *edge-to-edge* bite pattern well into the 18th century. Professor Charles Loring Brace realized in the 1960s that the overbite of modern man was not a result of the age of agriculture, but instead the result of a change in dining utensils in the late 18th century.[91] This marked the timeline when upper middle class circles embraced eating with a fork and dull table knife for cutting food into small bites before eating.

Initially, the fork attracted laughter and scorn. The resemblance to Poseidon's Trident or the devil's pitchfork led many to shun its use. Historians believe the first fork used had two prongs, was made of gold, and had an ornate handle. It was believed to belong to a Byzantine princess married to the Doge of Venice in the 11th century. She was damned by saints and ridiculed by clerics for her "excessiveness" for using her little gold fork. It is said the princess felt she was too "delicate" to use her hands to eat. It could be she was very sensitive to heat or cold, didn't like the messiness, or in the minds of her contemporaries, thought she was superior to everyone else. For over 200 years, the story of her extravagance was recounted in church sermons warning of the gratuitous natures and evils to all who would listen.

The Italians embraced the fork before any other European group in the Middle Ages. Why? The love of pasta proved the undoing of their reticence to embrace the fork for everything placed on the table that was not a soup or sauce. The rest of Europe would shun its use until the 17th century.

The new kid on the block by some belief is the spork. The term spork was first recorded in a dictionary in 1909. However, the first patent for a spork was not issued until 1970. Some myths attribute the development of the spork to General MacArthur during World War II. However, the actual utensil, if you can call it that, was used earlier. The Pixar character *Wall-E's* reaction to the spork is a classic for many of us; it invokes frustration, confusion, and humor. Even former President Bill Clinton made jokes about the confused utensil and called the spork a symbol of his administration. In 2008, a man in Anchorage, Alaska, attempted to rob someone with a spork from a fast-food chicken restaurant. The arrest records recount parallel scratches and shock over how much damage was done before the spork shattered.

Today the spork has had an image makeover and is deemed the perfect utensil for backcountry campers, hikers, and others.

## *Innovation Brings Convenience*

World War II did not just launch us into the modern era of space and flight, it changed the types of tools we use in our kitchens, how we cook, where we eat, and our perception of food. In the eight decades following World War II, we have gone from a meal based on what was available that day at the local market to exotic meals delivered to your door, pre-measured to assure perfection at the table.

Before the development of orange juice concentrate, the juice was either freshly squeezed or pasteurized to be sold in cans. The former was inconvenient and the latter not pleasing to the taste. Pasteurization killed most of the flavor and left a bland, watery beverage. Frozen concentrate juice was developed by a U.S. Department of Agriculture scientist named Cedric Atkins while working at the University of Florida. Concentrating the juice allowed for volatile oils and other essences, which produced flavor to be added back in, enhancing the appearance of the beverage in addition to taste.

California Fruit Growers Exchange Saturday Evening Post 1915

According to the Smithsonian, Michael J. Cullen, founder of King Kullen in 1930, launched the supermarket of the same name. Cullen was a former employee of the Kroger Co. The early days of the Great Depression had most grocers wary of risk as prices rose and jobs vanished. It wasn't long before chain stores found they could reduce costs and offer lower prices. Although meat could be purchased under the same roof as fresh vegetables, it still required the assistance of a meat clerk or butcher. Before using plastics and polystyrene, natural items such as leaves, bark, newspaper, cheesecloth, or wax paper were used to wrap meat.[92] Research data in 2021 revealed plastic wrap used for meat and vegetables directly contributes to hypertension.[93, 94]

> ***Principle 11***: Lower dependence on plastics by using bees wax coated papers, cotton, and parchment paper bags.

Americans think they invented barbecue, particularly in Texas and Tennessee, famous for slow cooked brisket and dry rubbed ribs. Slow cooking by fire and smoke is among the oldest ways of preparing food. Nearly every culture has its own take on slow cooked meats, and the earliest recording of barbecue comes from the *Tainos*, people that lived in Puerto Rico, the Dominican Republic, and much of the Caribbean in the 16th century. The word *barbacoa* (barbecue) was a wooden platform set over a fire, allowing smoke to billow up and preserve and season the ingredients above (in essence, an ancient smoker).[95] The gas grill strategically positioned on the porch or outside an RV looks nothing like the wooden platform or heavy iron grate used over wood fires from antiquity. In the 1950s a dim view was taken on those who did not entertain executives, clients, and important personages at home, and the brick fireplace barbecues became popular. *I Love Lucy,* one of the most popular television shows of all time, featured the building of a barbecue (episode 23) in 1957.

The faithful portable Weber® Kettle Grill came on the scene in 1952 developed by George Stephen. The 70th anniversary of the Weber line in 2022 covers twenty two models and a price range from $57.00-$4,500.00, a far cry from a free wooden rack over a fire.

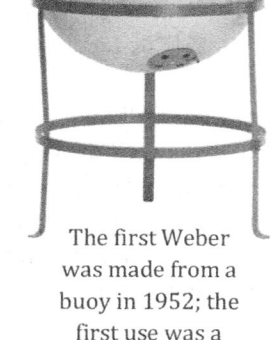

The first Weber was made from a buoy in 1952; the first use was a disaster.

## Cookware

**Stainless steel** is a terrific alternative to a non-stick cooking surface. Most chefs agree that stainless steel browns foods better than non-stick surfaces. When purchasing stainless steel cookware, be sure it is of the highest quality to prevent the leaching of toxins into foods.

## Aluminum

Many are under the impression aluminum cookware is a product of the 1940s and 1950s; hence the connection to Alzheimer's, which has been put into question with newer research. Aluminum cookware dates to 1807 in Germany. Aluminite cookware was shaped into bake and sauté pans, gratin and soufflé dishes, vegetable steamers, plates, coffee and tea pots, ramekins and shells. Alcoa began marketing the Ware-Ever brand in 1903, and West Bend Company began distributing cookware through Sears, Roebuck and Company. In the 1940s, Wear-Ever and EKCO courted homemakers with the latest in pressure cookers. A full-color ad in *Woman's Home Companion* in February 1947 promised lima beans in one minute, rice in five, and fried chicken in fourteen. [96]

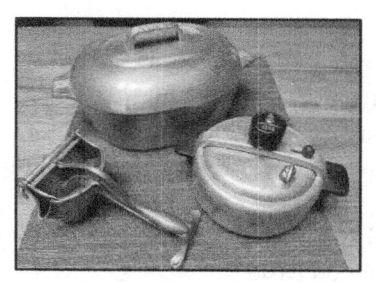

Wagner Magnalite roaster 1930, Ekco Pressure pan 1940s and Ware-Ever Juicer 1950

## Cast Iron

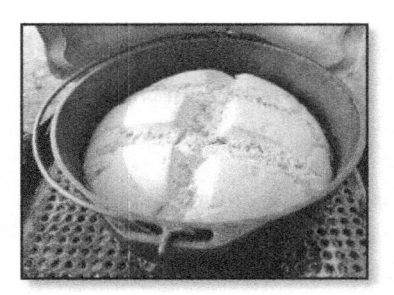

Cast iron has been used since the appropriately named "Iron Age" roughly 2,500 years ago. Aside from stone, iron is the oldest cooking surface still in use.[97] Today it remains an alternative to cheap non-stick cookware. Lodge®, America's oldest family-owned cast iron manufacturer, refers to its cookware as "natural non-stick." Cast iron is durable and can be preheated to temperatures that will brown meat and withstand oven temperatures well above what is considered safe for other pans.

Seasoning is not just recommended for cast iron pans; it is a requirement. The seasoning layer is comprised of broken down, then polymerized unsaturated fatty acids. Multiple thin layers of seasoning built up over time are a sign of a well-seasoned pan. The pros of the seasoning process are that eggs cook without sticking, you don't have to re-season as often, and the pan will not rust.

The cons are harder to quantify. Bits of the seasoning will come off over time and be replaced by more seasoning. Nobody knows exactly how much seasoning comes off over time, nor do they know what health effects there may be if any. Do not be overly alarmed. The oil seasoning on your cast iron pan may be oxidized, but it is not rancid. Daily, the authors use cast iron that is three generations old. The pans work just as well now as when they were bought at the turn of the 19th century.

### *How to Clean a Cast Iron Skillet*
NEVER RUN cast iron through the dishwasher.

Even though many DO NOT USE soap on cast iron, it is often the most efficient way to remove strong-smelling foods and rancid oils. Rancid oil is never a good thing to consume. Tammera uses cast iron that is three generations old; all of it has had dish soap used by more than one family member over the decades. But it has never been subjected to the horrors of a dishwasher.

1) Wipe the pan clean with a paper towel, preferably while it's still warm, making removing bits of food easier.

2) Using a non-metal brush or non-abrasive scrubber, rinse the pan under hot water and give it a good scrub.

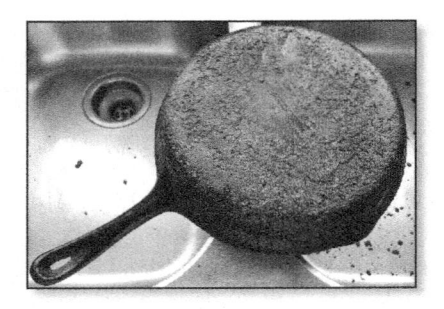

3) Dry the skillet thoroughly with a cloth or paper towel, then heat it on a medium-low burner to evaporate any remaining moisture. Rust will accumulate if water is allowed to sit on the pan's surface. If your pan develops rust, use a paper towel, and wipe the "inside only" with olive oil. The paper towel and oil will remove the rust.

4) Add a half teaspoon of olive oil to the pan when it's cooled down but is still warm to the touch.

5) Using paper towels, spread the oil around so that the interior is coated. Continue to wipe down the pan with the oiled towels until the entire surface is smooth and there are no pools. Select oils that do not turn rancid at room temperature: olive oil, grapeseed oil and avocado oil.

6) To remove heavy crusting from the cast iron outside – DO NOT USE OVEN CLEANER!!! Cast iron is porous and these toxic chemicals can enter your food.

Place cast iron in a gas barbecue on 500°F for 30-45 minutes. Let cool, then using a small metal scraper work any large chunks free. You may need to repeat this process several times. The traditional method also works. Place the skillet or pan directly into hot coals as the wood fire is dying low (not flaming and not red hot). After the pan has cooled with the fire, check the outside, and wipe off ash and any carbon.

**_NOTE_**: *Overheating the cast iron will damage it or even crack it, so error on the side of caution.*

**What About Toxins and Iron Overload?**

When you buy and properly care for quality cast iron, many of our concerns over toxins vanish.[98] Clinically, Tammera has had far more clients who needed iron than those with excess iron. Even when we consider anemia a digestion issue, deficiencies will persist until intrinsic factors and the microbiome are optimized. [99, 100, 101] Based on a bio-individual model, there will continue to be individuals who, no matter what, always come up short on iron.[102]

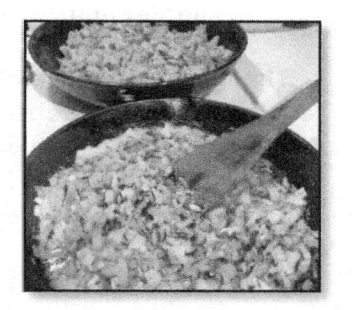

For individuals with elevated risks of hemochromatosis, hepatitis C, liver, or kidney disease, cast iron or copper cookware is counter indicated.

"New" cast iron releases more iron into food until it is fully cured. When tests are done on older cast iron, the iron release is a fraction of a new skillet or Dutch oven. Additionally, the foods you cook in cast iron affect the level of iron released.[103] For example, tomato based dishes should be made in stainless steel, glass, or toxin-free ceramic pans. Lead poisoning from glazing for ceramic and porcelain can be dangerous for children. Be sure you are buying quality over marketing hype.[104]

**Carbon steel**

Many of the concerns or challenges of cast iron apply to carbon steel pans apart from price. Depending on your area and the age of the cast iron (vintage Griswold can be worth hundreds of dollars), new modern carbon steel pans may come with a hefty price tag.

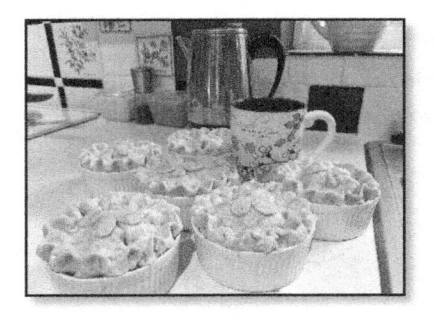

**Heat-resistant glass** pans and baking dishes conduct heat efficiently and are easy to clean. The oldest manufacturer of glass cookware in America is Pyrex® by Corning Inc. The authors use several different sizes of baking dishes that also double for storage in the refrigerator and freezer. DO NOT place a cold dish in a hot oven; it will break. DO NOT place a glass dish or pan in the oven, microwave, or stovetop with a plastic lid on. Plastic will melt and expose food to hormone disrupting chemicals, especially foods containing oil or fat.

**Inventions of Heat-resistant Cookware**

The story of Pyrex® glass began in 1914. Bessie Littleton's earthenware casserole dish had cracked. Her husband, Jesse Littleton, was a physicist at Corning Glass Works in Corning, New York. He evaluated the company's formula for temperature-resistant glass for use in railroad lanterns and battery jars. Mrs. Littleton asked if the glass might work for baking. Mr. Littleton sawed off part of a battery jar for his wife to try. With this makeshift dish, America's first cake was baked in heat-resistant glass, and Corning launched Pyrex® in 1915.[105]

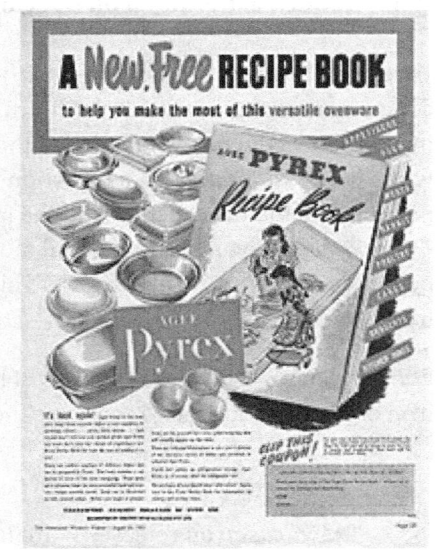

American Woman Weekly 1952

**Stone bakeware** is made from stone fired at a very high temperature. The firing of the stone produces a nonporous surface on the bakeware, which does not need glazing. The stone bakeware absorbs the heat from the oven and distributes it evenly. It retains the heat well and keeps food warm long after it is removed from the oven. Because the stone bakeware distributes heat so evenly, there is less chance of burning or overcooking the food. It does take a little longer to initially heat up, so if you are baking something that requires a short baking time, you may have to extend the time by a couple of minutes. Most stone bakeware must be seasoned before using for the first time. To season, rub the surface with oil. To care for stone bakeware, do not use soap to clean. Scrap off excess food and wash with warm water.

Stoneware is also available with an enamel glazed surface. The glazing provides for an easier cleaning surface, which is scratch resistant; however, the glaze may contain heavy metals.[106]

***Principle 12***: *Reduce lead exposure by verifying the heavy metal content of stoneware, ceramic, and China dishware. Dishware manufacturers still utilize heavy metal in the glazing process.*

## Kitchen Appliances for a Lifetime

**KitchenAid®** makes a stand mixer with grating and shredding attachment. Over the years, we have used this workhorse for grinding our own meat, milling wild berries for juice, grating cheese, making bread, whipping cream into herb butter, and so much more. I cannot imagine going through a busy canning season here in the Pacific Northwest without my KitchenAid® to help.

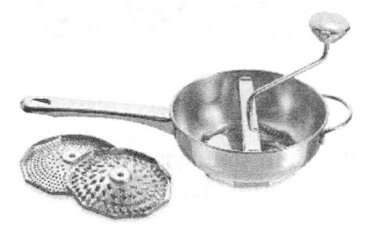

**Food mills or ricers** are old-fashioned kitchen tools viewed as the pureeing implement of choice dating back to 1932. They are part strainer and part masher or saucer in that a *food mill* crushes foods by forcing them through a perforated disk that separates any seeds, core, or skin. They are often used to make applesauce, tomato sauce, pureed soups, and rice (or mashed) potatoes. Foley Manufacturing Company is my brand of choice.

**Vitamix®** is the most used appliance in the author's kitchen next to their KitchenAid® stand mixer with attachments. We make simple cream of vegetable soups in the winter, chop nuts for holiday cooking, and make coconut milk ice cream and sorbet in the summer.

**Food drying** has been a way to preserve food forever. Man had to find ways to retain unused foods to survive. In eastern Oregon, ancient food storage caches were uncovered by Luther Cressman, the father of modern anthropology and archaeology in the 1930s. Ancient settlement sites near Silver Lake, Oregon dating back 5,600 years[107] contained dried foods in various forms; whole, sliced, and ground foods. Fermenting may be the only food preservation method dating back as far as drying.

We use a small food dryer to preserve grated carrots, chili peppers, celery, tomatoes, bell peppers, onions, garlic, herbs, and in a pinch, it acts as our Kombucha warmer.

**Pressure Canning/Cooking**

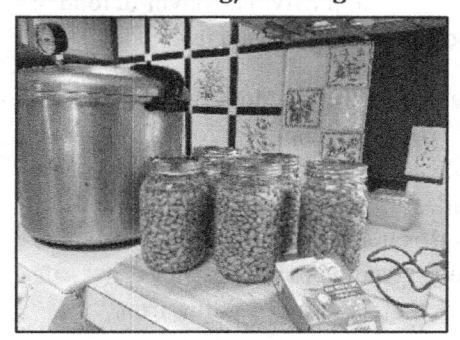

A lot has changed for home food canners since the 1917 Kerr® canning book was published that sits on Tammera's shelf. Gone are the glass lids with rubber gaskets and bear-trap wire bungs to hold the pressure.[108, 109] For the Karr family, the 1966 Presto® canner makes it possible to take advantage of seasonal foods for winter enjoyment. Reusable glass jars reduce waste and eliminate worries over plastic and petroleum contamination.

The **Instant Pot**® hit the market in 2016. Clients and colleagues alike were all talking about how much easier this tool made meal preparation. Tammera recommends using an electric pressure cooker to make broth, soups, stews, pot roasts, beans, and lentils. Consider buying an additional insert to have on hand when one is in the wash. Is the Instant Pot® faster? It depends; some foods are, and others take the same amount of time as on a range. Compared to a Crockpot®, the authors find the food quality and convenience of the auto program function on the Instant Pot® preferable. This appliance allows for ease of use in RVs, apartment kitchens, busy homes and at work.

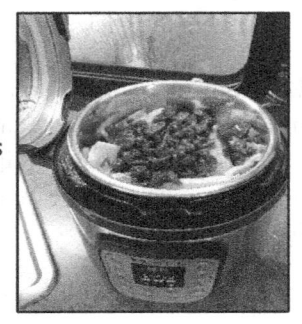

**Farber ware**® *stainless steel coffee pot* is my choice for brewing tea and coffee. Gone are the plastic coffee makers from Tammera's counter. The Vianté electric glass and stainless tea pots are perfect for herbs and French press use. Stainless steel is tried and true old school and helps keep plastic contamination to a minimum.

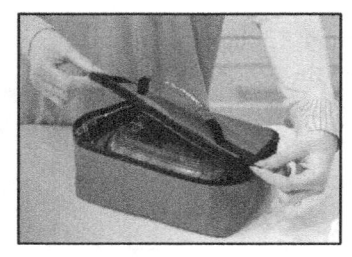

**Hotlogic**®, without a doubt, is my husband's favorite appliance. This handy portable heating unit has allowed for hot meals on the go. The Hotlogic® Mini plugs into a cigarette lighter port in heavy equipment or vehicles. In 90 to 120 minutes, he has chili, stew, soup, and more hot and ready to eat. The glass container doubles as a bowl and worries about microwaves and plastic are gone.

## *Word on Water Filters*

Traditional foods go hand in hand with water. We use words like sweet, pure, artesian, glacial, ancient aquifer, and mountain spring to describe water's quality and purity. The flavor of food or the ability to ferment foods depends on water. Water is a primary medium used in cooking.

In today's world of chemicals and pollutants, it is necessary to filter water. Modern municipal water treatment is designed to remove only the largest of particulates and treat for common pathogens. It is not geared to remove countless pharmaceutical medications and industrial chemicals. Well water may not be any better. Over the decades, Tammera has seen rivers and aquifers in the Pacific Northwest go from pristine to polluted as industrial and agricultural chemicals use increased. Even without those challenges, some ground or runoff water is not safe to drink. The unique geology of an area will contribute heavy metals, arsenic, sulfur, iron, alkaloids, viruses, parasites, and bacteria.

Areas under construction or left vacant for long periods of time allow for other water contamination to occur. Old water lines are perfect breeding grounds for bacteria, and most of our cities have more than a few old lines.

Modern appliances, like refrigerators and coffee makers, may come with water filters. However, just like the pitcher type, these filters contain a simple carbon filter that primarily removes chlorine and fluoride. Some high-tech personal water bottle filters will remove parasitic ameba and some heavy metals. We use these when traveling.[110]

Most used is the reverse osmosis under-the-counter filter. The upside to this type of filter is its ability to remove all but prescription medications. The downside is that the filtration is only at one location, can be expensive, and waste water. Reverse osmosis filters may, however, be the only option available to you if you live in an apartment or condominium. They can be removed easily and relocated to a new residence.

Our preference is a whole house filtration system that can be installed at the water main, well, or in the garage. This multi-stage system can include UV light for bacteria in addition to filters capable of removing containments down to very small microns.

When you do some looking on the Internet, you will find countless countertop water filters that claim to do everything from changing the energetic flow to preventing cancer. Bottom line; do your research and do not believe everything you read. The alkalinity or acidity of water may be the least of your concerns.

> ***Principle 13***: *Filter all the water used in drinking and cooking. Filtered water reduces toxic chemicals, solvents, and pathogens from contaminating food. Fermenting requires filtered water.*

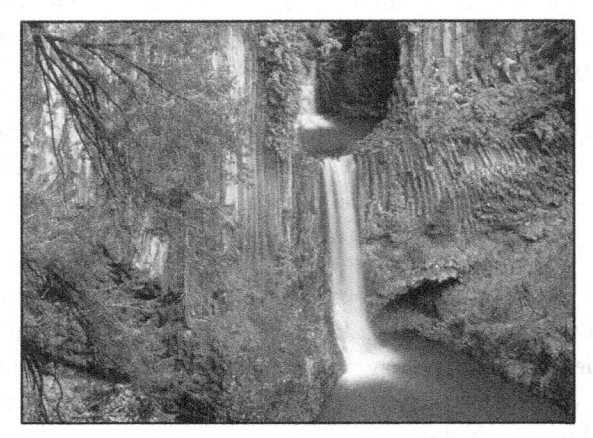

Toketee Falls, North Umpqua River, Umpqua National Forest, Oregon

---

83 University of Leiden. (2016, March 16). How people prepared food in prehistoric times. ScienceDaily. Retrieved August 22, 2022 from www.sciencedaily.com/releases/2016/03/160316105806.htm

84 Integrating Lipid and Starch Grain Analyses From Pottery Vessels to Explore Prehistoric Foodways in Northern Gujarat, India; Front. Ecol. Evol., 16 March 2022, Sec. Paleontology
https://doi.org/10.3389/fevo.2022.840199

85 BLACK, D. Recent Discoveries at Choukoutien*. Nature 133, 89–90 (1934).
https://doi.org/10.1038/133089a0

86 Ancient Kitchens Unearthed in Western Turkey, Archaeology Dec 2016:
https://www.archaeology.org/news/5140-161215-turkey-anatolia-kitchens

87 The Ancient Kitchen; https://www.encyclopedia.com/food/encyclopedias-almanacs-transcripts-and-maps/ancient-kitchen

88 The Sweet Symbolism of a Welsh Love Spoon; Retrieved September 1, 2022, https://www.ancient-origins.net/history-ancient-traditions/welsh-love-spoon-009894

89 Confederated Tribe Cow Creek Indiand display, Canyonville Historical Society, Canyoneville Oregon

90 Consider the Fork – A History of How We Cook and Eat, by Bee Wilson

91 C. Loring Brace, https://anthropology.iresearchnet.com/c-loring-brace/

92 Environmental Health Perspective 2012; https://www.ncbi.nlm.nih.gov/pmc/articles/PMC3385451/

93 Plastics Softeners Tied to Spike in BP During, After Pregnancy:
https://www.medscape.com/viewarticle/965549

94 Phthalates: 'Safer' replacements for harmful chemical in plastics may be as risky to human health;
https://www.sciencedaily.com/releases/2015/07/150708160531.htm

95 A Guide to Barbecue Around the World—in All Its Tangy, Spicy, and Charred Glory July 2022, Conde Nast Traveler: https://www.cntraveler.com/story/a-guide-to-barbecue-around-the-world?utm_source=join1440&utm_medium=email&utm_placement=newsletter

96 Encyclopedia of Kitchen History by Mary Ellen Snodgrass page 9-10

97 Are cast iron pans unsafe? By Kamal Patel - https://examinutese.com/nutrition/are-cast-iron-pans-unsafe/

98 The Truth About Cast Iron by Americas Test Kitchen; https://www.americastestkitchen.com/guides/cook-it-in-cast-iron/busting-cast-iron-myths

99 Use Cast Iron Cookware as an Iron Deficiency Treatment by Chelsea Clark, 2018 University Daily Health News: ;https://universityhealthnews.com/daily/energy/use-cast-iron-cookware-as-an-iron-deficiency-treatment/

100 Food prepared in iron cooking pots as an intervention for reducing iron deficiency anemia in developing countries: a systematic review.; https://www.ncbi.nlm.nih.gov/pubmed/12359709

101 Heavy Metal: the Science of Cast Iron Cooking; http://www.cookingissues.com/2010/02/16/heavy-metal-the-science-of-cast-iron-cooking/index.html

102 The Health Benefits of Cooking with a Cast-Iron Skillet by Janet Rausa Fuller; https://www.epicurious.com/expert-advice/the-health-benefits-of-cooking-with-a-cast-iron-skillet-article

103 Are cast irin pans unsafe? By Kamal Patel - https://examinutese.com/nutrition/are-cast-iron-pans-unsafe/

104 Release of Iron into Foods Cooked in an Iron Pot: Effect of pH, Salt, and Organic Acids; Journal of Food Science 2006; https://onlinelibrary.wiley.com/doi/abs/10.1111/j.1365-2621.2002.tb09582.x

105 How Pyrex Reinvented Glass For a New Age by Liz Logan 2017; https://www.smithsonianmag.com/innovation/how-pyrex-reinvented-glass-new-age-180955513/#H4TRxcD7Ol0OodgT.99

106 Recipe Tips.com; https://www.recipetips.com/glossary-term/t--37441/stoneware-baking-dish.asp

107 Sandal and the Cave by Luther Cressman page xxii

108 Who Made That Mason Jar? - https://www.nytimes.com/2012/04/29/magazine/who-made-that-mason-jar.html

109 Encyclopedia of Kitchen History by Mary Ellen Snodgrass 2004

110 Oko water filter: https://okoh2o.com/

*"If more of us valued Food and Cheer and Song above hoarded gold, it would be a Merrier World."*

~Thorin Oakenshield, The Hobbit

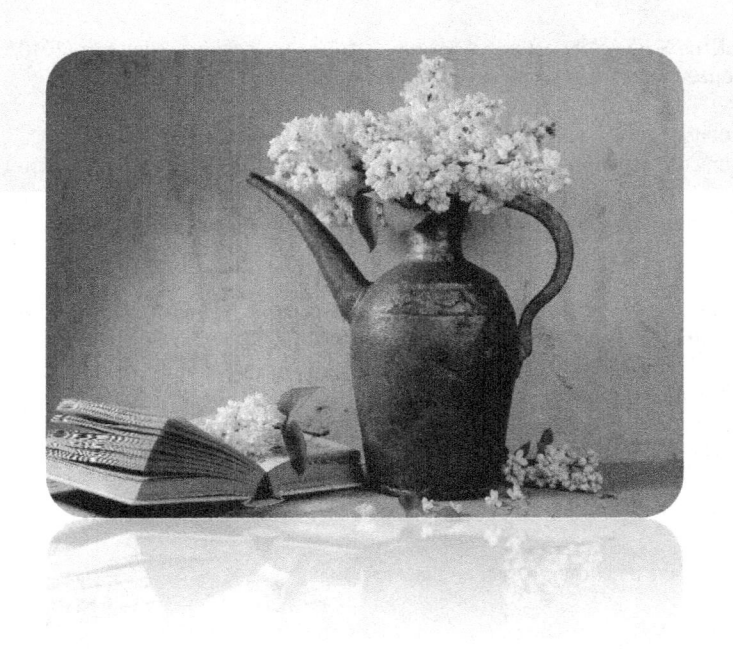

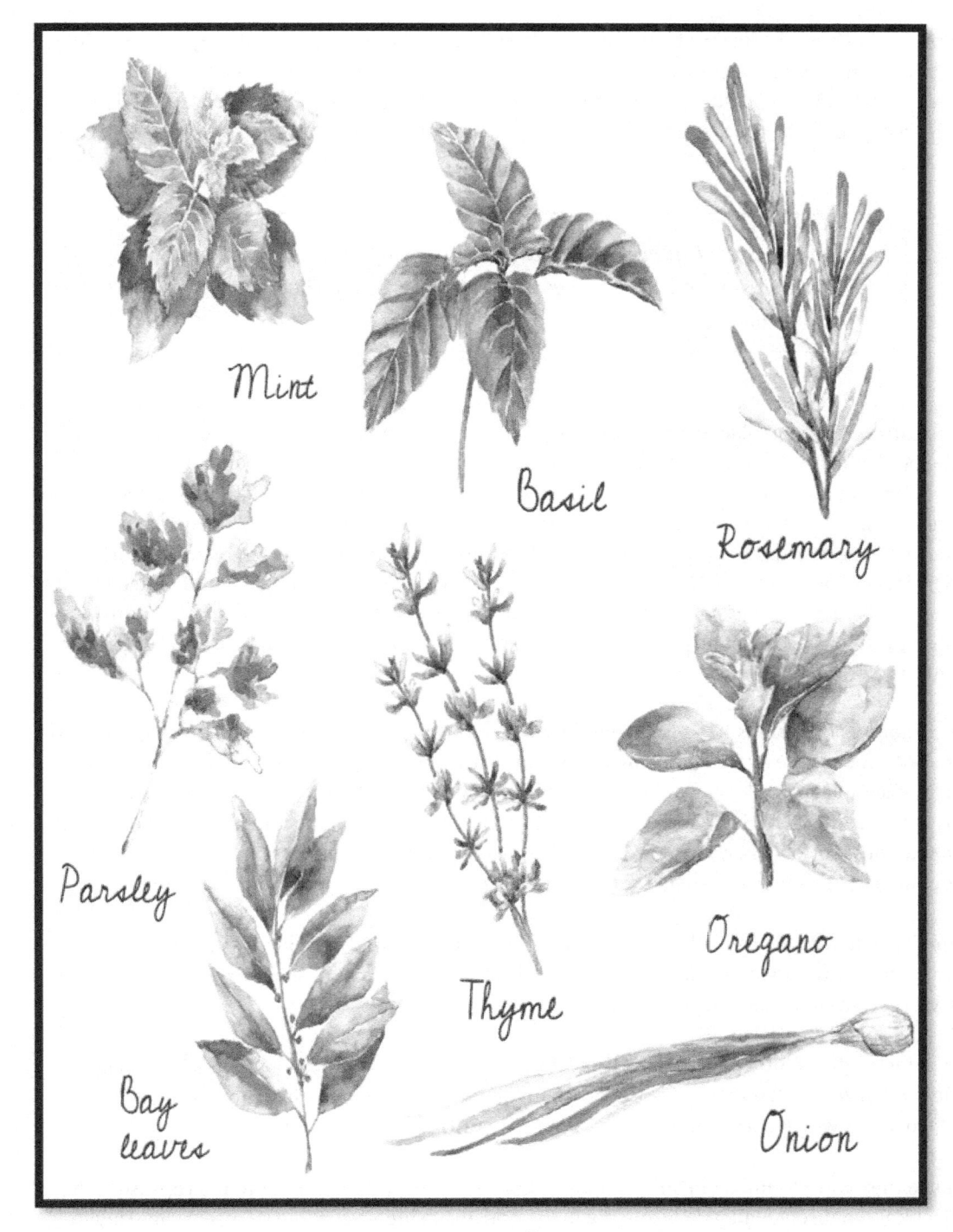

**Culinary Herbs & Spices**

The role of herbs and spices in traditional cookery is more than flavor; herbs played a vital role in nutrition and health for past generations.[111] The daily use of herbs in cookery supplied minerals, vitamins, and volatile compounds effective at killing pathogens and parasites. They provided expectorant, glucose-regulating, diuretic, and anti-inflammatory properties.[112, 113]

> **Principle 14**: *Understanding the healing properties of herbs and their inclusion in cookery is essential to fully grasp the concept of "food as medicine."*

For centuries, the food placed before humanity was nourishment and the sole source of medicine. A *goodwife*[114] during medieval times was the mistress of the household and was known for keeping order. *Housewife* later became the accepted term and further denoted a married woman in charge of the home. Additionally, the *lady of the house* was judged on how well provisioned the pantry, how well the kitchen garden was tended, which included herbs for food preservation and medicine, and how flavorful the foods were coming from the kitchen. All of these were considered before beauty. The medieval *goodwife's* skill reflected on her family and the prosperity of her husband and his charges, making the place of *goodwife* an elevated and essential role.

This all sounds ridiculous to us in the modern age, but remember, these were different times, and these skills meant life or death during famines or war. A skilled *goodwife* would be called on to care for the injured or ill. She could find herself in chains or on the fire for being a witch if her ability was lacking. This is historically the earliest beginning of holistic nutrition for those of European descent. The Persians and Asians extensively used culinary herbs, predating the European *goodwife* by more than a century.[115, 116, 117]

When did individuals begin adding flavor to their food? Food anthropologists cannot give us a definite answer because the plant remains rarely last, so researchers seldom speculate on how they were used thousands of years ago.[118]

That being said, in 6,000-year-old pottery from Denmark and Germany, a team of researchers found *phytoliths* small bits of silica that form in the tissues of some plants, most notably garlic mustard seeds which carry robust and peppery flavor but little nutritional value.

Because they were found alongside residues of meat and fish, the seed remnants represent the earliest known direct evidence of spicing in European cuisine. According to researcher Hayley Saul of the University of York, *"It certainly contributes important information about the prehistoric roots of this practice, which eventually culminated in globally significant processes and events."*[119]

The flavors associated with Europe, Mediterranean and Asian traditional foods are primarily due to the influence of the Arabian Agriculture Revolution. After the fall of the Roman Empire, the Muslim ships and caravans carried their cuisine rich in spices and fruits across three continents. The Muslims brought melons, pomegranates, grapes, raisins, peaches, almonds, pistachios, cherries, pears, and apricots to the Persian Empire.

Muslims introduced to Europe spinach, melons, eggplant, and artichokes. They planted orchards of stone fruits; peaches, cherries, and apricots. In Spain, the introduction of sugar, saffron, rice, and the bitter orange became the foundation of the British marmalade. All this happened before 700 A.D. By the 10th century, the Muslim influence on the world's flavor of food was firmly in place.

The earliest Muslim recipes dated from Baghdad in 1226. They were recorded by al-Baghdadi, who *"loved eating above all pleasures."* Many recipes are for *tagines* – meat and fruit stews simmered for hours over a low flame until the meat is falling apart melt-in-your-mouth tender. The inclusion of spices in almond stuffed meatballs called *mishmishiya* consisted of cumin, coriander, cinnamon, ginger, and black pepper. Saffron added color, and ground almonds were added to thicken. Stews were also perfumed with waters distilled from rose and orange blossoms.

According to *Le Viandier*, cooking with spices was considered a new cookery style and was written by Frenchman Gillaume Tirel circa 1312- circa 1395. This became the first European cookery book. Le Viandier reflects the influence of the Middle East on the cooking of the Middle Ages of Europe, especially the use of spices such as cinnamon, ginger, cumin, coriander, and cardamom. These spices can be found in the traditional Christmas drink known as *wassail*.

The fall of the Christian Eastern Roman Empire to the Turks in 1453 sent the European world and its now addicted sweet tooth and love of spices into a tailspin. All roads east were closed, and the need for food explorers brought us Cristoforo Colombo (Christopher Columbus) and a whole "new world" of flavors.

> *"In general, mankind, since the improvement of cookery, eats twice as much as nature requires."*
>
> ~ Benjamin Franklin (1706-1790)

## *Western Culinary Herbs* & medicinal properties

**Basil** leaves are best when used fresh. They are often used on pasta, soups, salads, chicken, fish, pesto, sauces, dressings, teas, and rice. This herb has digestive properties, benefits the nervous system, and has positive effects on controlling diabetes and asthma.

**Bay** (*wax myrtle, waxberry, candleberry, vegetable tallow bush*) is used to season meat, fish, poultry, soups, and broths.

**Blackberry** (*bramble, dewberry*) leaves are used in teas to aid digestion. The fruit is used in jam, jellies, juices, and syrups. Brandy, wine, and cordials are also made from the fruit for culinary and medicinal uses.

**Carrot seed** (*Queen Anne's Lace, bird's nest, bee's nest*) is used to season soups, sauces, dressings, stuffing, and roasted meats. Carrot seed should be used with care, especially if pregnant. Consumption benefits the bladder and kidneys, reduces edema, and stimulates digestion.

**Celery seed** (*smallage*) is the dried fruit of the *Apium graveolens*, which is closely related to the vegetable celery. They are tiny light-brown seeds that give the flavor and aroma of celery. In culinary use, the seeds provide the taste of celery taste without using the celery stalk. They are used in soups, salad dressings, tomato dishes, and pickling. Celery seed has been used as medicine for thousands of years in the Eastern world. During ancient times, Indian Ayurvedic medicine used celery seed to treat colds, flu, water retention, poor digestion, different types of arthritis, and certain liver and spleen diseases. Beneficial as a diuretic and for arthritis, gout, reducing muscle spasms, calming nerves, reducing inflammation, and lowering blood pressure.

**Chicory** (*wild succory*) has a long history as a pioneer coffee in America. The roots are roasted and ground. Leaves are added to salads or cooked. Good for digestion.

**Dill seed or herb** is used with fish, potatoes eggs, salads, pickled vegetables, soups, and dressings. Beneficial for colic, gas, and indigestion. The name "dill" originates from the Old Norse word *dilla*, which means "to soothe."

**Elder** (*black elder, European elder, boretree, devil's wood*) is found wild and domesticated in America and Europe. The flowers and berries of this tree are used to make jam, jelly, juice, syrups, and drops. Used to build the immune system.

**Fennel** (*sweet fennel, large fennel*) has been used in many cuisines worldwide. It grows wild in many vacant areas in the Pacific Northwest. This sweet aromatic herb is used in teas, soups roasting, salads, and stir-fries. It is known for eliminating colic in babies and digestive spasms in adults with IBS. Fennel is good for digestion.

**Ginger**, both wild and domesticated, is used in soups, sauces, teas, drops, and ferments. It is an effective digestive aid.

**Hops** (*cannabacea*) are most associated with beer. Still, they have a long history of being used in teas for digestion and as a relaxing herb for the central nervous system.

**Juniper** (*ginepro, enebro*) berries and leaves have been used to flavor meat, soups, and distilled beverages. Juniper should be used with caution. This plant benefits the stomach, bladder, and kidneys.

**Lemon balm** (*bee balm, sweet balm*) is in the mint family. It is best suited to container gardens to prevent spreading. The lemon balm provides a beautiful citrus flavor to dressings, sauces, fermented beverages, and teas. This plant is mentioned in the Bible and in writings from Homer. It is calming to the nervous system.

**Licorice** *(lick weed, sweet wood)* adds sweetness to teas, dressings, sauces, candies, and fermented beverages. Used for digestion and adrenal support. Contraindicated in individuals with high blood pressure.

**Lovage** (*old English lovage, Italian lovage, pioneer celery*) is perfect for soups, sauces, roasted meat, cordials, and teas. Tastes like celery and grows easily in gardens. Used for digestion, the lymphatic system, heart, and kidneys.

**Mint** comes in many varieties—spearmint, peppermint, chocolate mint, apple mint, pineapple mint, orange mint, and lemon balm. Mint is used in teas, sauces, dressings, jellies, and fermented beverages. It benefits the respiratory and digestive systems.

**Nettle** (*stinging nettle*) has a long history in traditional Irish dishes, soups, and teas. Nettle benefits the kidneys, liver, and respiratory system.

**Parsley** (*Italian parsley, curly leaf, flat leaf*) is used in soups, egg and potato dishes, sauces, dressings, salads, and roasted meats. Beneficial to the digestive system, bladder, kidneys, and stomach. Reduces garlic odor on the breath.

**Plantain** (*snakeweed, ribble grass, broadleaf plantain, white-mans-foot-print, yard weed*) leaves are used in salads, cooked greens, and soup. The seeds can be roasted or parched. They have been used for centuries for treating sore throats, coughs, bronchitis, and mouth sores.

**Oregano** is a traditional Mediterranean herb used dry in dishes containing tomato, chile, garlic, and onions. Used in salads, soups, broth, dressings, dips, and sauces. Oregano oil and tea contain antibacterial properties. Benefits cough, bronchitis, asthma, and the immune system.

**Oregon grape** (*mountain grape, California Barberry, berberis, holly-leaf, marberry*) contains cambium. This herb has a long history in regional native diets. They harvested the berries for drying. Teas, jellies, juices, and cordials were made by pioneers. Oregon grape benefits the digestive and elimination systems, purifies the blood, and improves skin health primarily through helping the digestive system and liver.

**Rose** (*rosehip*) collection for teas and dishes is thought to predate any medieval cookery mention. This herb provided cultures with a valuable vitamin C source before modern international transport and nutraceuticals.

**Rosemary** (*compass weed, poplar plant, old man*) is considered a Mediterranean herb; however, it also has a long history in colder climates. Rosemary is used in soups, gravies, the roasting of meat, and teas. This herb can thrive in damp, cooler climates making it useful for illnesses associated with such environments. Beneficial for the brain, heart, digestive and respiratory systems, for blood sugar balance, and as a nerve tonic, Strong anti-inflammatory properties.

**Sage** (*garden sage, meadow sage*) is used in dressings, the roasting of meat, stuffing, soups, sauces, and teas. Sage is beneficial to the digestive and respiratory systems and reproductive organs. It supports oral health, breaks down blood clots, has a calming effect, and is an astringent for use on the skin.

**Thyme** (*garden thyme, whooping cough herb*) is used as tea, seasoning on poultry, dressings, stuffings, and soups. This herb contains antibacterial properties, soothes the respiratory tract, and supports singers' vocal cords.

**Watercress** (*Nasturtium officinale*) is the source of Saint Brendan's health and longevity in Ireland. This green plant can be found under ancient Roman bridges and along streams in Great Britain. Plato and Homer wrote about watercress as a source of healing; Plato is said to have selected his hospital location based on proximity to watercress. This slightly spicy, crisp green can be used fresh in salads or added to soups. Beneficial for anemia, heart health, and cancer prevention, it is high in vitamin C.

## *Herbs & Spices of Mexico*

**Ancho chile powder** differs from traditional chile powder due to its sweet, rich flavor, mildly fruity with hints of plum, raisin, and tobacco.[120] Most "chile powders" in the store are blends of various spices, not Ancho. Mexican chile spice is 100% a dried version of the Poblano chile.

**Anise seeds** are used in savory dishes comparable to Mole, paired with vanilla and cinnamon. Anise is used in sweet dishes like desserts, cakes, cookies, and sweetbreads.

**Avocado leaves** are edible with a flavor that can be compared to anise and hazelnut. The leaves are often used in Central and Southern Mexico for tamales, roasting meats, steaming, or grilling fish. The dried powder is aromatic when used in sauces, stews, and salad dressing.

**Achiote** paste is made from an obscure spice common in the Yucatan peninsula. Mildly spicy and earthy, achiote adds complexity to any dish. Used most often as a paste like a bouillon cube. Achiote is known for giving color to Cochinita, a famous pit-oven pulled pork, pastor meat, brightening chorizo sausages, and providing cheese with an orange hue.

**Cilantro** was brought by Chinese workers to the Spanish silver mines in southern Mexico and South America during the 1500s. This herb comes from the leaf of a small plant in the same family as parsley and carrots. Cilantro is added to tacos, salsas, Moles, cheeses, broth-based soups, rice, and beans.

**Coriander** is the whole dried seeds of the leafy cilantro plant. A native to southern Europe, northern Africa, and southwestern Asia, coriander is a versatile spice with lemony, floral undertones and a hint of sweet spiciness. Coriander is often paired with cumin, thyme, and black pepper.

**Cumin** is popular in Tex-Mex dishes more than traditional Mexican food and is mainly used in sauces and stews. Use cumin to balance the flavor of chiles, but be careful; too much cumin can easily overwhelm a dish.

**Garlic powder** has advantages over fresh garlic as it is less prone to burning. Mixing a 1:1 ratio of water to garlic powder and letting it rehydrate for a few minutes will bring out the flavor before cooking.

**Hoja Santa, the holly leaf** is grown in the Oaxacan highlands, where the most celebrated Mexican dishes come from (Mole). Hoja santa leaves are used to wrap fish and tamales to infuse them with the most delicate, floral, citrusy, anise aromas. Used in sauces or Moles to give them a distinct feature.

**Mexican allspice** is native to Latin America and the Caribbean. Allspice is confused as a blend of spices with the fragrant aroma and flavors of cinnamon, ginger, clove, and nutmeg. It compliments all of those spices. You can use it in cakes, cookies, stews, and meats.

**Mexican Oregano** is more aromatic and citrus scented than its European cousin and almost tastes sweet. Oregano is ubiquitous in pozole pork stew and is often added to pickled onions or tacos.

**Mexican vanilla** is amongst the best in the world. Vanilla is native to Mexico and is still the best source for the highest quality vanilla beans.

**Onion Powder** adds a sweet and savory flavor to dishes and robustness difficult to get from fresh onions.

**Mexican smoked paprika** originated in central Mexico, where it has been seasoning dishes for generations. Christopher Columbus introduced it to Europe. Smoked paprika brings a hint of barbecue flavor or subtle smokiness to a dish. Paprika's versatility adds flavor to meat rubs, vegetables, or garnish on guacamole.

**Common Western Herbs** *(*additional information in text)*

| | | | | |
|---|---|---|---|---|
| Basil* | Bay* | Celery seed* | Chives* | Chocolate mint |
| Dill* | Fennel* | Garlic* | Lemon balm* | Lovage* |
| Oregano* | Parsley* | Rosemary* | Shallots* | Thyme |
| Watercress* | | | | |

## *Garlic, Onions, Shallots & Chives*

This group of herbs holds a special place in almost any traditional kitchen. They play a pivotal role in French cookery for soups, sauces, and by themselves. In Spain and Portugal, garlic is king, along with red onions and shallots. Asian, Basque, Greek, Italian, and Persian food utilizes these herbs from the Lily family.

**Garlic** is high in allicin, which is responsible for this herb's aroma. The highest concentration of allicin is found in the Siberian variety. Garlic benefits the heart, lungs, and immune and digestive systems.

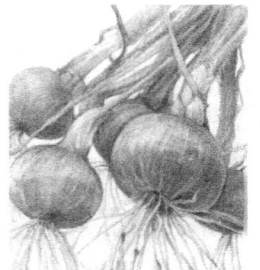

**Onions**, like garlic, can be mild or hot. Yellow onions are also known as winter keepers. They contain the highest levels of bioflavonoids used for immune support and the prevention of viruses. Yellow and Spanish red onions add a robust, rich flavor to hearty stews, broths, and gravies. Walla Walla and vidalia are sweet onion varieties. They are used in light summer cooking and salads.

**Shallots** contain higher levels of bioflavonoids, sulfur compounds, and active ingredients than onions. The rich pungency of shallots lends a rich flavor to soups, and chutneys.

**Chives** bring a bright green onion or garlic flavor to salads, dips, and dressings. They make a flavorful garnish to cream soups, potatoes, parsnips, and rutabaga dishes.

## *Culinary Spices* & medicinal properties.

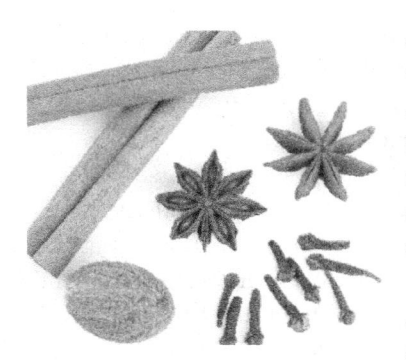

**Allspice** (*Jamaica pepper, myrtle pepper, clove pepper*) is the only spice grown exclusively in the Western Hemisphere. Allspice is used as a seasoning for desserts, sausages, pork, poultry, pate, terrines, smoked and canned meats, liqueurs, marinades, mulling, and pickling. Benefits digestion and circulation and is antimicrobial, warming, and a mild anesthetic

**Anise** (*Pimpinella anisum, aniseed*) is one of the spices written about in the Bible and Tora. Anise was so highly prized it was used for tithes and paying taxes in Palestine. Anise leaves can be used as an herb, mainly the seeds used in cooking. Aniseed is used in baked goods, desserts, sausage, and charcuterie. Benefits digestion and helps prevent intestinal gas and flatulence.

**Cardamom** (*capalaga, Ilachi, green cardamom, true cardamom, Ceylon cardamom*) comes from the seeds of various ginger plants. Native to southern India and grown in Guatemala. Cardamom is considered one of the world's oldest spices, dating back at least 4,000 years. Cardamom pods were chewed to help keep breath minty and to help clean teeth.[121] Used in Indian and Middle Eastern cuisines, curries, teas, Scandinavian mulled wine and glogg, sweet pastries, and bread. Benefits indigestion, asthma, and bad breath.

**Cayenne** (*pimenten picante, cayenne pepper*) is prepared from various seeds and pods of different types of chile. Cayenne is hot chile pepper used to flavor food. It is known as "the king of spices" for its incredible healing power. The capsicums used are small-fruited varieties. Culinary uses include spice, garnish, tea, pickling, sauces, seafood, meat, poultry, stews, soups, pizza, and baked foods. Benefits include relief of cramps, stomach pain, indigestion, nerve and joint pain, headaches, asthma, the immune system, and weight loss.

**Cinnamon** (*true cinnamon, yook gway, Dal-chini*) used in North America is from the cassia tree, which is grown in Vietnam, China, Indonesia, and Central America. Cinnamon is used in baked goods, milk and rice puddings, chocolate, fruit dishes, lamb tagines, stuffed aubergines (eggplant), hot beverages, pickling, curries, pilaus, garam masala, wines, creams, syrups, and tea. Cinnamon benefits blood sugar regulation, cholesterol, triglycerides, digestion, poor circulation, blood pressure, and infantile diarrhea. It is considered stimulating, antiseptic, and astringent.

**Cloves** (*Ding xiang*) are unopened flower buds of a tropical tree native to India and Indonesia. The spice is most often paired with cumin and cardamom. The ancient Romans highly valued cloves, pepper, and nutmeg. Culinary uses include tea and Indian and Mexican cuisines. Used medicinally in traditional Chinese medicine and Ayurveda to relieve indigestion, diarrhea, hernia, fungal infections, colds, cough, and toothache.

**Cumin** (*Machin, kammun, jeera*) is native to the shores of the Mediterranean Sea and Upper Egypt. Originally cultivated in Iran and the Mediterranean region, cumin seeds are used as a spice in North Africa, Middle Eastern, western Chinese, Indian, and Mexican cuisines. It typically flavors sauces, fish, vegetables, cheese, sausages, soups, stews, grilled lamb, chicken, curry, stuffing, bean dishes, and rice. It is used as a fragrance. Beneficial as a stimulant, antispasmodic, sedative, and antibacterial agent. Aids digestion, colic, and headaches.

**Ginger** [122] (*Zingiber officinale*) is commonly found in Asia, Africa, and tropical areas in the Americas. It is an underground rhizome, also known as ginger root or ginger. Color varieties are red, yellow, and white, but the genetic variation is not limited to colors. The distinctness depends on where the ginger grows or is cultivated. Ginger is used as a spice or food, and beverage condiment. Ginger is also an ingredient for fragrances and cosmetics. Benefits digestion, circulation, and those with diabetes. Known for its anti-inflammatory and anti-cancer properties.

**Grains of Paradise** (*melegueta pepper*) is the seed of *Aframomum melegueta*, a species of plant in the ginger family, and native to coastal regions of West Africa. It was commonly combined with three other spices: anise, ginger and cinnamon in medieval recipes.

**Nutmeg** residue was found on ceramic potsherds and is estimated to be 3,500 years old; about 2,000 years older than the previously known use of the spice.[123] The nutmeg fruit, seed, and mace for thousands of years have been highly prized as food and medicine. Europeans became so obsessed with this plant that blood was shed to obtain it. Two spices come from the nutmeg tree: mace and nutmeg.

**Mace** is a beautiful and bright red skin located around the nutmeg seed. It is used in cooking and as a medicinal spice. Nutmeg is the brown seed inside the mace. The health benefits of nutmeg include reduced anxiety, sound sleep, better digestion, and help for colds and the flu.[124]

*If a person eats nutmeg, it will open up his heart, make his judgment free from obstruction, and give him a good disposition.*

Hildegard of Bingen
12th century Benedictine Abbess

**Paprika** (*bell pepper, sweet pepper*) to the Hungarians is like cheese to the French. There are hundreds of flavored and regional paprikas used in traditional Hungarian foods. Ground paprika is used in sauces, chickens, potatoes, stews, soups, meats, sausages, rice, and other dishes. Benefits digestion, skin and hair health, cardiovascular health, is anti-inflammatory and induces sleep.

**Saffron** (*za'farân, zang hong hua, saffron crocus*) is an expensive spice produced from crocus flowers. The saffron is derived from the Arabic word zafaran, which means yellow. Saffron is mainly used in Mediterranean and Asian cuisines.[125] It is primarily added to give color and fragrance. Saffron is also used in cakes, chocolate, liqueurs, and fabric dye. Benefits the respiratory system, digestion, fever, asthma, and is anti-spasmodic

**Turmeric** (*Indian, saffron, turmeric, yellow ginger, wong geung fun*) is native to tropical South Asia. It is known as Indian saffron in Europe since it is widely used as an alternative to the far more expensive saffron. It has a distinctly earthy, bitter, slightly peppery, hot flavor and a mustardy smell. Widely used in Malaysian cuisines and non-south Asian recipes, canned beverages, baked products, dairy products like ice creams and yogurt, yellow cakes, orange juice, biscuits, popcorn, sweets, cereals, sauces, and gelatins. Benefits digestion, circulation, cognition, skin health, the microbiome, and is anti-inflammatory.

**Common Spices** (*additional information*)

| | | | | |
|---|---|---|---|---|
| Allspice* | Anise | Black pepper | Cardamon | Chile* |
| Cinnamon* | Clove* | Cumin* | Ginger* | Nutmeg* |
| Paprika* | Saffron* | Turmeric* | | |

The more, the better! The broader the diversity and globe trotting additions, the tastier the food, and a vast spectrum of positive health-incurring benefits.

> **Principle 15:** *Herbs, spices and seasonings are shared and interconnect worldwide cultures.*

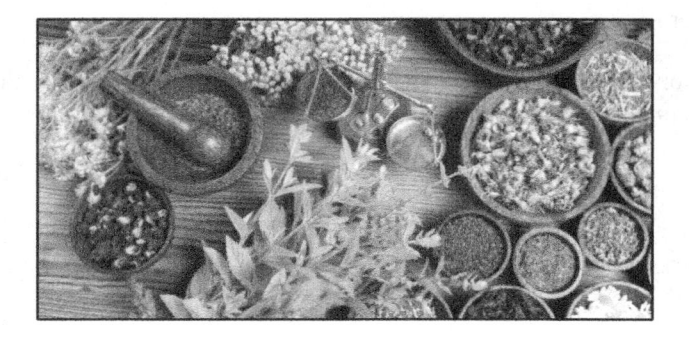

## Seasonings

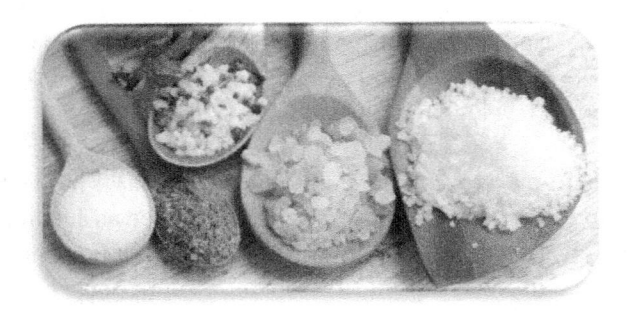

### Salt

*"For thousands of years, we have been making salt from the sea or finding it in the land, and the worlds thousands of regional cuisines have evolved in concert with the availability and character of locally made salts. For most of human existence, salt has been scarce in the extreme, difficult to transport, and of dramatically varying quality. Salt was, literally, a treasure, and everyone everywhere who could make it would. Yet salt making was a challenging, physically demanding, risky job requiring the participation of an entire community. The salts were unique, each bearing a mineral and crystalline imprint of the elemental and human forces that wrought it. Salt was a natural, whole food, intimately tied to a place and a way of life."*[126]

When Tammera read this passage in *Salted* by Mark Bitterman, she pondered how our current view of salt has changed dramatically. This one seasoning, above all others, is a requirement for life. Without salt, maintaining homeostasis and electrolyte balance would be impossible. When observing nature, invariably, a game trail frequented by large and small animals will involve a "mineral or salt" lick; a source for supplementing essential minerals necessary for health, reproduction, and vegetation.

The mantra "salt is bad for you" is based mainly on a poorly designed study from 1905. However, the artisanal salts described in *Salted* are nothing like the white stuff in the Morton® salt container. Industrial salt produced in North America contains a wide array of solvents, fillers (including sugar), chemicals, and contaminants. These aspects of industrial table salt do nothing to promote health or to connect us with the ancestral cultivation and harvesting of this essential element for life.

The salt you select for dishes will reflect care, intention, and creativity. The authors keep several different artisanal salts in the pantry.

## Pepper

An ancient trading commodity, black pepper dates back over 4,000 years. The black peppercorns you use in your grinder originated from the Western Ghats of Kerala State in India. The green berries produced by the *Piper nigrum* flowering vine are left to ferment and dry in the sun. *Piper nigrum* still grows in the wild in Kerala.

Pepper is an essential spice in Indian cooking; this spice was mentioned in the early Tamil literature. The Mahabharata, written in the 4th century BC, describes feasts that included meats flavored with black pepper. The spice was valued equal to precious pearls, and the peppercorns were used as a form of money along the trading routes.

Tellicherry black peppercorn refers to the size, not a place. Tellicherry peppercorns are bigger than regular black peppercorns, both from the same vine. The pepper fruit is picked from the vine and allowed to shrivel and dry. Then the peppercorns are sorted by size. The smaller peppercorns are considered whole black pepper, while the larger peppercorns become the Tellicherry. The Tellicherry peppercorns are more pungent and provide an increased complex flavor with added citrus notes.[127]

Black pepper factored into Indian medicine as a prescription to cure constipation, earache, gangrene, and heart disease. Hippocrates used pepper as part of his healing arsenal. The benefits are that it aids digestion, increases hydrochloric acid, and possesses antioxidant and antibacterial properties. Another use includes keeping ants from walking across your counter. Sprinkle a line of black pepper wherever ants enter the home.

*"What science demands more study than Cookery? You have not only, as in other arts, to satisfy the general eye, but also the individual taste of the persons who employ you; you have to attend to economy, which every one demands; to suit the taste of different persons at the same table; to surmount the difficulty of procuring things which are necessary to your work; to undergo the want of unanimity among the servants of the house; and the mortification of seeing unlimited confidence sometimes reposed in persons who are unqualified to give orders in the kitchen, without assuming consequence, and giving themselves airs which are almost out of reason, and which frequently discourage the Cook."*

~ Louis Eustache Ude (1813)

111 Health-promoting properties of common herbs
Winston J Craig: https://academicoup.com/ajcn/article/70/3/491s/4714940

112 Opara, E. I., & Chohan, M. (2014). Culinary herbs and spices: their bioactive properties, the contribution of polyphenols and the challenges in deducing their true health benefits. International journal of molecular sciences, 15(10), 19183–19202. https://doi.org/10.3390/ijms151019183

113 Williams A (2021) Historical Uses of Herbs and Spices in different Cultures. J Nutraceuticals Food Sci Vol.6 No.3:12.

114 Oxford Dictionairy of English, Seconed Edition, Revised: good wife, goodwives, chiefly Scottish, the female head of a household.

115 Eight Essential Foods in Iranian Traditional Medicine; https://www.ncbi.nlm.nih.gov/pmc/articles/PMC5288958/

116 Ancient Persian Nutrition; https://healthandfitnesshistory.com/ancient-nutrition/ancient-persian-nutrition/

117 Perian Cuisine, a Brief History by Massoume Price, 2009; http://www.cultureofiran.com/persian_cuisine.html

118 Snezana Agatonovic-Kustrin, Ethan Doyle, Vladimir Gegechkori, David W. Morton,

Journal of Pharmaceutical and Biomedical Analysis, Volume 184,2020,113208, ISSN 0731-7085, https://doi.org/10.1016/j.jpba.2020.113208.

119 Europes Historical Hunger, by Samir S. Patel, Ancientfoods; https://ancientfoods.wordpress.com/

120 Retrieved July 2022: https://nerdyfoodies.com/traditional-mexican-spices-1130.html

121 The History Of Cardamom | Myspicer.com | Spices, Herbs ... (n.d.). Retrieved from https://www.myspicer.com/history-cardamom/

122 Chapter 7The Amazing and Mighty Ginger; https://www.ncbi.nlm.nih.gov/books/NBK92775/

123 3,500-year-old pumpkin spice? Archaeologists find earliest use of nutmeg as a food ; http://www.southeastasianarchaeology.com/2018/10/04/3500-year-old-pumpkin-spice-archaeologists-find-earliest-use-of-nutmeg-as-a-food/

124 Nutmeg Benefits - Herbalremediesadvice.org. (n.d.). Retrieved from https://www.herbalremediesadvice.org/nutmeg-benefits.html

125 Saffron, Saffron Spices,crocus Sativus Spice. (n.d.). Retrieved from http://www.spicesmedicinalherbs.com/saffron-crocus-sativus.html

126 Salted by Mark Bitterman page 5

127 The Difference Between Tellicherry Peppercorns And Black ... (n.d.). Retrieved from https://www.myspicer.com/difference-between-tellicherry-peppercorns-and-black-pe

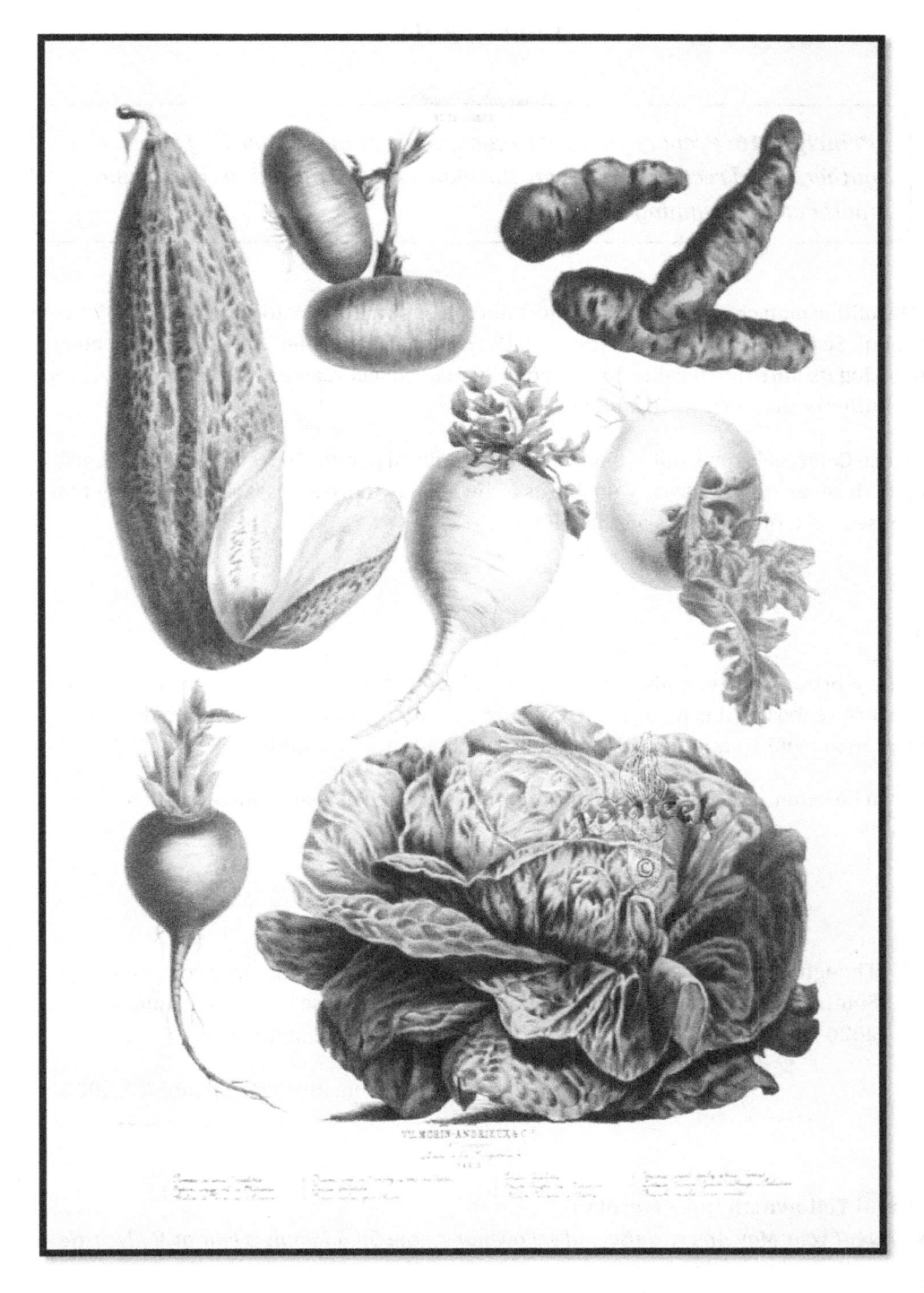

**Vegetables**

## Sea Vegetables

> ***Principle 16:*** *Prepare yourself to cook. Mise en place = putting in place or gather. Read recipes all the way through, and assemble ingredients and tools before beginning.*

The Mesolithic man chewed weed, but most notably, its written history began in the 7th century. Irish monk St. Columba, freshly relocated to the island of Iona, refers to *'dulsing'* in a poem.[128] Recognizing its nutritional value, Ionan monks would collect seaweed to feed the poor, softening it with butter or mixing it with oatmeal.[129]

Ever since Columba's time, dulse held value for medieval people. In Ireland, it was recorded that a crop of dulse on a rock was as valuable as a cow. Today there is research suggesting that cows who eat seaweed produce less methane.[130]

### Dulse

This winey-brown seaweed, also called *dillisk*, is found all around the Irish coast, particularly on the western seaboard. It is mentioned in the 8th century by *Brehon Laws,* which describes a penalty for consuming another person's dulse without their permission.

Dulse can be eaten raw or added to fish soups or stews. It can also be mixed with potatoes; Dulse Champ.[131]

> Though seaweed has been a staple of East Asian diets for hundreds of years—South Koreans, for example, consumed 20.4 pounds of seaweed per capita in 2020—it remains a boutique food product in Western countries.
>
> ~ Smithsonian Magazine June 23, 2022

**Dulse and Yellowman** (John Murphy)
*Did you treat your May Ann to dulse and yellowman at the Ould Lammas Fair at Ballycastle -O?*

*Dulse is a purple, edible seaweed, I remember buying it at a penny a bag as a child when sweets were hard to get. It can also be stewed for a couple hours and eaten as a vegetable or with oatcakes. It is not known much outside of the north of Ireland – and it is great loss!*

*Yellowman is a different matter altogether. This toothsome, honeycomb, stick toffee is traditionally sold at the Ould Lammas Fair at the end of August.*

### **Hebridean Broth**[132] or Dulse Brooth

25 g dulse, dried
1 medium potato
25 g butter
1 tsp lemon juice
Salt and pepper
1¼ pint milk
Crusty bread

Place dulse in a bowl of water and leave for 5-10 minutes.
Drain and put into a sauce pan with fresh water and boil for 10 minutes. Peel and boil the potato and mash. When the dulse has cooked, drain it.

Mix in the mashed potato, butter and ½ teaspoon of the lemon juice. Season with salt and pepper.

Gradually stir in the milk and return to heat. Gently simmer for 20 minutes, stirring often. Check seasoning and if desired add rest of the lemon juice.

Serve with crusty bread.

### **Dulse Slaw** [133]

25 g dulse
50 g raisins
175 g white cabbage, shredded
1 medium carrot, grated
2 shallots, finely chopped

*Dressing*
4 tbsp mayonnaise
2 tbsp apple juice
Salt and pepper

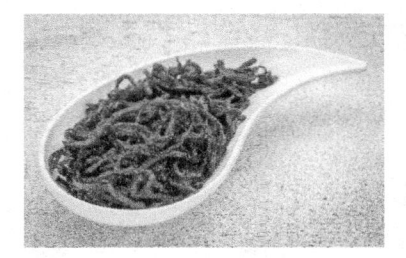

Soak dulse for 5-10 minutes in a bowl of water.
Put shredded cabbage, grated carrot, and finely chopped shallots into a large mixing bowl. Drain raisins and add to large bowl. Drain dulse, chop, and add to bowl.

In a small bowl mix together the dressing ingredients and then pour over and coat the salad thoroughly. Season, mix again, and serve.

**Bull Kelp Pickles** (Crystal Shepard)

Collect one or two bull kelp stalks, making sure they are firm. Remove the bulb at the base (air bladder) and leaves. Wash hollow portion of stem and bulb thoroughly clean of sand. Slice bulb and stem into half-inch rings. Rinse kelp rings again and toss lightly in salt. Slice one large onion and crush one clove of garlic. Rince kelp rings one more time and stuff into sterilized glass jars with onion and garlic. Put 1 teaspoon of lemon juice per jar. Make pickling brine by combining in a sauce pan and bringing to a boil: 2 cups of vinegar, 1 cup water, ⅔ cup sugar, and 4 tablespoons of pickling spice. Boil for 1 minute and pour into jars, covering kelp rings. Refrigerate for at least 48 hours before eating.

*Caution*: Seaweed can absorb heavy metals and chemical toxins, be sure you collect from unpolluted coastal areas.

## What Did Britons Eat in Ancient Times?

Ancient Britons were eating dairy, peas, cabbage, and oats, according to gunk trapped in their teeth. Scientists analyzed dental plaque found on the teeth of skeletons from the Iron Age to post-medieval times.

They found evidence of milk proteins, cereals, and plants, as well as an enzyme that aids digestion. Proteins found in ancient dental plaque have already revealed that humans were drinking milk as far back as 6,500 BC.[134]

Foods that grow wild in Briton include asparagus, blackberries, and wild herbs.

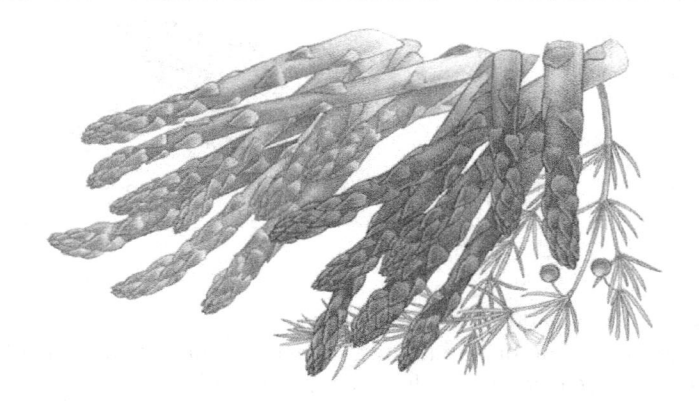

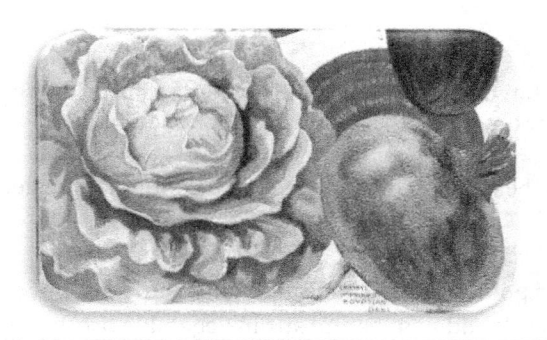

## Vegetables

### Shaved Apple, Fennel, and Celery Salad (Chef Christine Wokowsky)

2 celery stalks, peeled and sliced thin
1 fennel bulb, outer layer peeled and sliced thin (reserve a few fronds for garnish)
1 crisp apple, thinly sliced
1 tbsp olive oil
½ tbsp freshly squeezed lemon juice
Chopped assorted fresh herbs such as parsley, minutest, etc., along with fronds
Sea salt, to taste

*Dressing*
⅛ cup raw apple cider vinegar
¼ cup olive oil

Combine everything in a bowl, toss with olive oil and lemon juice. Season to taste. If you would like some sweetness, add a bit of honey.

### Asparagus Leek Soup (Chef Christine Wokowsky)

Serves 8 cups

1 bunch asparagus
2 knobs (tbsp) Kerrygold butter
2 cloves garlic, chopped
2 leeks, chopped
2 large red potatoes, peeled and diced
½ cup Cognac
Salt and pepper to taste
4 cups vegetable broth
Olive oil

Lemon juice

Combine everything in a bowl, toss with olive oil and lemon juice. Season to taste. If you would like some sweetness, add a bit of honey.

Melt butter over medium heat, add garlic and leeks, stir until they sizzle; cover to sweat the leeks – about 10 minutes.

Add asparagus stems and potato, stir to coat, sauté until soft. Pour in Cognac and stir until completely reduced. Add salt and pepper and stir in vegetable broth. Bring to a boil, reduce and simmer. Simmer until all vegetables are very tender, about 25 minutes.

While soup is simmering, steam the asparagus tips separately about 5-8 minutes; should be crisp and bright green. Soak tips in ice water to maintain color. Once cool, thinly slice tips lengthwise to be used as garnish.

Once vegetables are tender, purée in blender or with a hand blender. Stir in lemon juice. Serve immediately, garnished with a dollop of butter and asparagus tips.


**Asparagus, Roasted Red Peppers, and Garlic** (Tammera Karr)

1 bunch fresh asparagus
1 red pepper
1 cup fresh broccoli tops
2 cloves garlic
¼ tsp red pepper flakes
1 tbsp extra virgin olive oil
1 fresh lemon
1 oz feta cheese

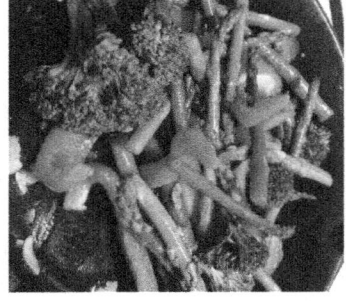

Wash and trim asparagus, using the top 4-5 inches that are tender. Wash and clean seeds out of red pepper. Trim broccoli to the tender stems and tops.

In a cast iron skillet warm oil over medium heat; add sliced garlic and pepper flakes. Let garlic toast and add vegetables. Toss vegetables with oil and garlic, cover with a lid, and allow to steam on medium low heat till vegetables are bright in color and tender but still crisp.
Crumble a little feta cheese on top before serving.


**Sautéed Brussels Sprouts with Chestnuts** (Chef Christine Wokowsky)

1 tbsp extra virgin olive oil
2 cups Brussels sprouts, ends cut off and quartered

1 onion, cut in half and sliced
½ cup red bell pepper strips
¼ cup shelled chestnuts*
½ cup vegetable stock or chicken stock
1 tbsp apple cider vinegar

Sauté onion in olive oil until translucent, add red pepper strips, and sauté another few minutes. Add Brussels sprouts, chestnuts, and stock. Cook on low to medium heat until done, about 10-15 minutes. Add apple cider vinegar when done.

*Feel free to substitute other nuts in place of the chestnuts.

## Brussels Sprout-Potato Hash (Chef Benjamin Qualls)

2 tbsp good olive oil
2 medium carrots, peeled and diced
½ lb small red potatoes, diced
8 slices uncured bacon, chopped
1 lb fresh Brussels sprouts, cleaned and quartered
1 bunch green onions, chopped
2-3 large cloves garlic, finely chopped
1 tsp whole thyme leaves
1 tsp whole rosemary leaves
1 tsp each sea salt and black pepper, or to taste
Chopped fresh parsley

In a large skillet, preferably cast iron, toss carrots and potatoes with two tablespoons olive oil. Sauté over medium heat for 5-7 minutes. Remove and set aside for later step.

Return skillet to medium heat; add chopped bacon and cook until crisp. Remove to drain on paper towel(s). Add Brussels sprouts to skillet; use a bit more olive oil, if needed, cook, and stir until slightly browned.

Add potatoes and carrots to skillet; stir in remaining ingredients. Cook and stir until all vegetables are browned.

Remove from heat and add cooked bacon, pour into serving dish; sprinkle with chopped parsley.

## Broccoli and Red Onions (Tammera Karr)

Lightly steam broccoli with red onions, mild chili peppers (seeded) and Roma tomatoes. Top with a dash of Parmesan cheese and a handful of pine nuts.

Cook time 10 minutes or until tender—don't overcook. Use amounts suitable for your family; it doesn't matter if you need one floweret or ten.

> *"Mediterranean food isn't supposed to be eaten in the car. It is meant to be savored. Its far-reaching flavors have the effect of slowing you down. Enjoying food in the presence of other people, at a table, with or without wine but with the pleasure of company, has got to be good for your health."*
>
> Martha Rose Shulman
> *Mediterranean Harvest*

### Sautéed Broccoli and Fresh Basil (Tammera Karr)

4 cup broccoli flowerets
½ cup fresh basil
2 cloves garlic, chopped
2 tbsp organic butter

In a cast iron skillet, gently melt the butter (low heat so as to not burn). Add fresh basil and garlic; let basil wilt. Add broccoli and cook on medium heat, tossing until broccoli is tender but not overdone.

Transfer vegetables to a platter, squeeze fresh lemon juice over vegetables, and sprinkle fresh coarse sea salt on top. Serve warm or cold.

### Best Ever Broccoli Soup (Brendan Karr)

Serves 3-4

4 cups chopped fresh organic broccoli (should be in 3 inch size to fit in the food processor)
3 cups of fresh water
3 tsp Celtic Sea salt
Fresh ground black pepper
Extra virgin olive oil

Place water, salt, and broccoli in a 4 quart sauce or stock pan. Bring to a moderate boil, stirring broccoli until tender and bright green.

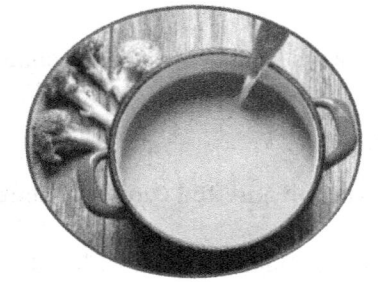

Place broccoli with broth from the pan in the food processor; you may have to do it in batches to not overload your processor. Process on purée until smooth; ensure you add enough liquid from the pot to make a medium-thick soup. Place in bowls, top with ground pepper, and a few drops of oil.
Serve hot.


**Hungarian Fried Cabbage and Noodles** (Chef Ben Qualls)
*Another of my grandmother's favorites. Also known as Krautfleckerl, this simple buttery caramelized cabbage recipe packs a lot of flavors. Goes well with a variety of meats.*

1 12 oz package egg noodles
1 large head green cabbage, cored and sliced thinly
6 tbsp butter
1 tsp pink Himalayan salt, divided
1 tsp paprika
Fresh ground black pepper to taste

Melt the butter over medium heat in a large skillet. Add the shredded cabbage, sprinkle about ½ teaspoon salt over it, and give it a stir. Cover and cook until the cabbage starts to wilt, stirring often.

In the meantime, cook the egg noodles in a pot of water according to the package instructions, then drain well.

Remove the lid and turn the heat up to medium high. Add the remaining ½ teaspoon of salt, and paprika; cook until the cabbage turns an amber color and starts to caramelize a bit. Stir in the pepper when the cabbage is just about finished cooking.

Finally, fold the sautéed cabbage mixture into the cooked noodles. Season with additional salt and pepper to taste and serve!


**Sopa De Ajo, Sopa De Borracho** - Garlic Soup (Kelsi Sitz)
Serves 6-8

1½ cups chicken or beef broth
3 large cloves garlic, minced
1 tsp salt
½ tsp black pepper
2 tbsp butter
2 tbsp olive oil
3-4 cloves, whole
3 tbsp chopped parsley

3 whole eggs, lightly beaten
3 large slices of dried sourdough bread, cut into cubes.

In a 3 quart pan, place all of the ingredients except the eggs. Cover and bring to a slow boil for about 15 minutes. Turn off the heat. Immediately add the egg while continuously mixing with a fork until there are strands of egg.

## Porru Sada: Leek Soup (Kelsi Sitz)

*Basque Heritage Cookbook by Kelsi Sitz was a Senior Project at Burns High School, Oregon, in 2008. Kelsi interviewed elder members of her family and community, collecting recipes and stories about the Basques who made Harney County their home. Many recipes she captured would be lost today without her effort to preserve her cultural heritage.*
Serves 4

6 medium potatoes, quartered
8 medium leeks, chopped
4 tbsp olive oil or bacon fat
1 clove garlic, chopped
Salt and pepper to taste
Water

In a large pot, bring 3-4 quarts of water to a boil. Add leeks, potatoes, and 2 tablespoon oil or fat. In a separate pan, sauté garlic in 2 tablespoons oil. Add to large pot when vegetables are done. Add salt and pepper to taste, and simmer for 15 minutes. Let cool and enjoy.

## Pakora plate - Potato, onion, banana, jalapeno fritters (Medha Mujumdar Murtyy)

*Every state in India has its own individual cuisine, a different language, and its own customs and traditions. Few things unite Indians as much as their love for Pakoda and hot ginger tea on a rainy day. This gluten-free snack can be found served hot with fried green chilies or garlic chutney on the streets almost anywhere in India. Several regional variations are most commonly made with onions or potatoes, including Pakodas made with ripe banana, spinach, and jalapeño.*

*Vegetables*
1 medium onion, sliced
1 medium potato, sliced
1 banana (medium ripe), sliced
1 jalapeño pepper, sliced

*Batter*
½ cup garbanzo flour (besan)
½ cup water
2 tsp hot oil
¼ tsp cardamom seeds (crushed fine)

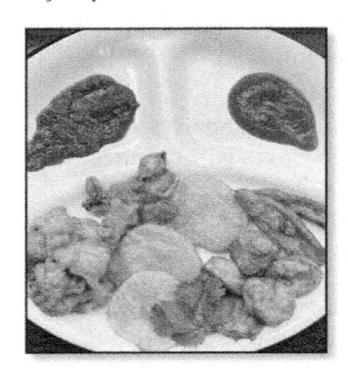

¼ tsp cumin seeds (crushed fine)
½ tsp turmeric
2 pinches of asafoetida
½ tsp salt
½ tsp red chile powder
1 pinch of baking soda
Oil for deep frying

1. Mix all spices in dry besan (garbanzo flour). Add 2 teaspoons of hot oil. Mix again. Add water and mix thoroughly while breaking lumps. Set aside for 5 to 7 minutes so that any remaining small lumps dissolve. Just before frying the fritters, add baking soda and mix lightly.

2. Heat oil in a frying pan for deep frying. Ensure the oil is hot (smoking point); otherwise, the fritters may soak up too much oil. Once the oil is heated to the right temperature, turn the heat to medium-high.

3. Add the potatoes to the batter and ensure that the potato slices are coated evenly with the batter. Deep fry on medium-high heat until golden brown. Remove onto a kitchen towel to drain off excess oil, if necessary.

Repeat this procedure with banana slices, jalapeño slices, and sliced onions.
You can also similarly make chicken pakoras, fish pakoras, spinach pakoras, etc.

Replace the vegetables with the meat of your choice.
Serve hot with mint chutney and/or ketchup.


### **Toasted Squash Seeds** (Tammera Karr)

Reserve seeds from the pumpkin, Hubbard, or sweet meat squash. Rinse seeds in cold water and rub off fibrous outer tissue. Rinse again and let drain on a towel. Spread seeds evenly on a cookie or jelly roll pan and sprinkle with fine sea salt. Bake at 350°F for 15-20 minutes.


### **Pumpkin Kibbeh** (Nour Danno)

6 cups of pie pumpkin (not carving pumpkin)
1½ cups bulgur
2 tbsp all-purpose flour
1 lemon
1¼ tsp salt
2 tbsp chickpeas
1 tbsp olive oil
1 medium onion
2 cups spinach

1½ tsp sumac
½ tsp salt
¼ tsp black pepper
12 cups of olive oil

*First, make the dough*
Peel, seed, and chunk the pie pumpkin, then cook it over high heat until soft and tender. Drain, then transfer to a large bowl, and mash it. Zest the lemon into the bowl, then add the flour, bulgur, and salt. Keep mashing until it's all mixed well. Set aside.
Next, make the stuffing. Chop the onion. Rinse and dry the chickpeas.

Heat 1 tablespoon olive oil over medium heat, then add the onion and cook until tender. Add spinach and wilt it. Add the chickpeas, sumac, salt, and black pepper. Once it's all cooked (everything is soft, but not soggy), turn off the stove and set aside.

*Finally, cook the kibbeh*
Put the oil in a large pot on the stove, but do not heat it yet.
With wet hands, take about 2 tablespoons of dough and shape into a ball. Hold it in the palm of one hand then press the thumb of your other hand into the center, making a bowl. Place 1 teaspoon of stuffing in the bowl and close the dough over it, shaping it into an oval. Smooth it with wet fingers and place on a baking sheet. Repeat with the remaining dough and stuffing.

After you have shaped half the kibbeh, begin heating the oil in a large pot over medium heat, and finish shaping the other half. Then, fry the kibbeh until dark brown and crispy.

Serve with a bowl of vegan yogurt on the side as a dip.


## West African Plantain and Okra Stew (Chef Christine Wokowsky)

1 tbsp extra virgin olive oil
1 onion, cut in half and sliced
4 garlic cloves, sliced
½ tbsp mustard seeds
1 tsp ground coriander
1 tsp ground cumin
1 tsp fennel seeds
1 small sweet potato, peeled and cubed; Yam, sweet potato, etc; any will do
2 cups vegetable stock
1 small BPA free can chopped tomatoes
1 cup sliced okra (fresh or frozen)
1 small green plantain, peeled and chopped
¼ cup cilantro

In medium pot heat oil over medium heat. Add onions and garlic, cooking until translucent. Add mustard seeds. Cook until they start to pop. After they've popped, add next three spices. Add remaining ingredients, cook until done, about 30 minutes. Garnish with cilantro.

Serve with 1-2 tablespoons of fermented veggies.


### Kale Sauté with Garlic and Lemon (Chef Benjamin Qualls)

1½ lbs (about 2 large bunches) kale*
2 tbsp olive oil
2 large cloves garlic, minced (use more if you wish)
Sea salt and black pepper to taste
Juice from 2 fresh lemons

Tear kale leaves into bite sized pieces; place in a large colander; rinse well under cold water. Fill a large pot with water. Add about ½ teaspoon salt and bring to a boil; add kale and cook for 4-6 minutes until crisp-tender. Drain well.

Heat olive oil in a large cast iron skillet over medium heat; add garlic and cook for about 1 minute. Add kale; season well with sea salt and black pepper. Cook, stirring often, until wilted and tender, 4-6 minutes.

Sprinkle with fresh lemon juice; toss to combine. Serve immediately.
*Collard or mustard greens work well also, blanch greens instead of boiling.


### Kohlrabi (adapted from a 1900 recipe)

1 kohlrabi root
1 tsp Celtic Sea salt
2 tbsp arrowroot powder
1 qt boiling water
2 tbsp organic or Amish butter or coconut oil

Wash, peel, and cut kohlrabi root in slices, and cook in rapidly boiling salted water until tender. Chop fine and cook the green tops in boiling water until tender; drain. Toss arrowroot powder through greens as evenly as possible. Reserve 1 cup of broth off greens.

(Greens will cook much faster than the root so do not add them into the same pan with roots for cooking).

Heat butter or coconut oil, add greens with arrowroot and reserved cup of kohlrabi broth. Add sliced tender kohlrabi, cook together, then serve.

*Note: Turnips and rutabagas can be prepared in the same fashion.*

## **Buttered Cabbage** (Tammera Karr)

Serves 6-8

1 lb fresh savoy cabbage
2-4 tbsp Kerrygold butter
Salt and pepper

Remove all the tough outer leaves of the cabbage. Cut the head into fourths; remove stalks from the center, then cut each across the grain into fine shreds.

Put 2-3 tablespoons water into your cast iron pan together with butter and a pinch of Celtic Sea salt. Bring to a boil, add cabbage and toss over medium heat, then cover and cook for a few minutes (don't overcook; this only takes 1-2 minutes). Toss again, add a pinch more salt and fresh ground pepper and top with a knob of butter (1 tablespoon) and enjoy.

For those with more time: Sauté ½ cup thinly sliced yellow onion in warm butter just before adding the cabbage. Eat alone or with steamed red potatoes and Irish bangers (sausages).

## **Red Cabbage and Apples** (Tammera Karr)

1 head red cabbage
1 cup red sweet peppers, minced
3 cups apples diced
¼ cup coconut sugar
2 tbsp real maple syrup
1 lemon (juice)
¼ tsp ground clove
½ tsp ground cinnamon
½ cup organic or Kerrygold butter
⅛ tsp Celtic Sea salt
1 pinch fresh ground black pepper

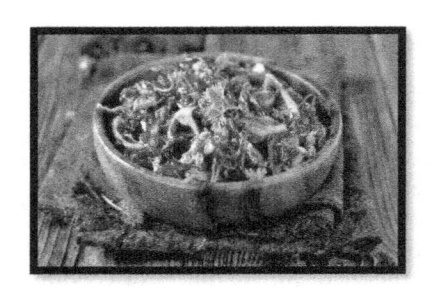

Shred cabbage, add minced sweet red peppers, season with salt and pepper, place in a greased casserole, and add dots or small chunks of butter. Add sugar, maple syrup, lemon juice, cinnamon, and clove to apples, and place on top of the cabbage.

*Topping*
1 cup gluten-free oat bran
½ cup finely chopped pecans
½ cup organic or Kerrygold butter

Blend ingredients together forming a crumb type topping; cover cabbage and apples. Bake in 350°F oven for 25 minutes.

## Cauliflower Kuku (Nicole Hodson)

*There are so many ways to enjoy Kuku – an endless variety of vegetables and meats can be used in this Persian style frittata. The sweetness of the cauliflower pairs beautifully with the richness of the eggs, making this my favorite KuKu. I can't overemphasize the importance of roasting the cauliflower and onion until they caramelize – this process renders tremendous flavor to the dish.*

1 medium to large head of cauliflower, cut into small bite-sized pieces
1 yellow onion, medium sliced
1½ tsp salt divided
½ tsp freshly ground pepper
¼ cup avocado oil
10 eggs
2 tbsp heavy cream

Heat the oven to 350°F.

Cover a baking sheet with tin foil. Place the cauliflower, onion, 1 teaspoon salt and pepper on the baking sheet. Drizzle with avocado oil and mix well.

Bake for 40 minutes, turning at least twice until caramelized. Remove from oven when very tender and let cool in a colander so excess moisture can drain off.

Reduce the oven temperature to 350°F. Oil a 9x13 inch high-sided baking pan, then fit with a piece of parchment paper.

Beat the eggs and heavy cream. Add in the cauliflower and onions and mix until well incorporated. Pour into the parchment lined cooking dish.

Bake for 45-50 minutes, until the top is set and a light golden color. Cool for 15-20 minutes before cutting.

This dish can be enjoyed warm or cold. I love it with a schmear of plain whole fat yogurt on top. It also makes a delicious breakfast on-the-go. *Nushe-joon!*

## Roasted Cauliflower with Pomegranate Glaze (Tammera Karr)

1 head cauliflower
Combine 1 cup pomegranate juice with the following:
⅛ tsp turmeric
⅛ cup raw honey

2 cloves garlic, chopped
Fresh basil leaves to taste

Wrap in foil and bake on the grill or in the oven 325°F until tender.

## Fennel and Delicata Squash Soup (Chef Christine Wokowsky)

4 cups vegetable broth
1 delicata squash, peeled, seeds removed and chopped
¾ cup collard leaves, ribs removed + chopped
1 fennel bulb, chopped (can sub 5 celery stalks, peeled, and chopped)
1 onion, chopped
3 cloves garlic, minced
1 tbsp coconut oil or extra virgin olive oil
4 fresh sage leaves or ½ tsp dried sage
1 tsp turmeric
½ tsp paprika
1 tsp dried parsley or handful fresh parsley, chopped
1 pinch of ground celery seed
Generous pinch of dried thyme
Sea salt and pepper, to taste

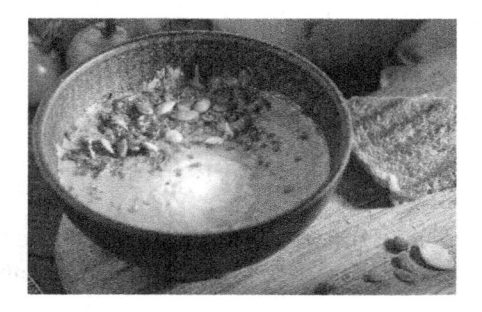

Heat a large sauce or soup pan over medium-low heat. Add onions and garlic, and sauté for 5-10 minutes. Add all the spices and herbs until well blended. Next, add vegetable stock and vegetables. Bring to boil. Lower to a simmer. Cook until done, about 30 minutes.

## French Onion Soup (Maria Brill) adapted by Tammera Karr

*Aunt Maria was a war bride from Alsace–Lorraine, France. She met my uncle Jack at the end of World War II when he was the driver for General "Ike" Eisenhower; it was love at first sight. This is one of the few recipes I have been able to translate from her French Alsace cookbook. Alsatian Minschterkaas (Munster) cheese comes from this region of France. Sweet with the flavor of long-simmered onions, this French onion soup also takes a savory note from reduced beef stock, bay leaves, black peppercorns, and thyme.*

1 tbsp clarified organic butter
1 lb onions, yellow winter, peeled and sliced thin
¾ lb white onions, peeled and sliced thin
¼ lb shallots, peeled and sliced thin
1 tsp unrefined Celtic Sea salt
2 bay leaves
3 sprigs thyme
1 tsp black peppercorns

1½ qt beef stock
1 cup dry white wine
4 slices day old sourdough bread
4 oz Munster cheese, shredded

Melt the butter in a heavy bottomed stock pot over medium high heat, then stir in onions and shallots. Reduce the heat to medium low and stir in salt. Cover and sweat the alliums, stirring frequently, until softened and translucent, about 10 minutes.

While the alliums sweat, tie bay leaves, thyme, and peppercorns together in a piece of cheesecloth or a small muslin bag, and add it to the pot. Stir in beef stock and wine, then simmer, uncovered, for 20-30 minutes or until the stock is reduced by one-third.

Preheat oven to 350°F.

Ladle into oven-proof soup bowls, top with a piece of day-old sourdough bread and 1 ounce of shredded cheese. Cover and bake for 20 minutes, then serve.

## Roasted Squashes Moroccan Style  (Chef Christine Wokowsky)

3 cups assorted 1 inch cubed squash (delicata, butternut, and kabucha)
2 tbsp extra virgin olive oil
1 medium chopped tomato
½ cup cooked chickpeas
2 tbsp green olives, chopped a bit
5 apricots, dried, cut in half
3 figs, dried, cut into quarters
5 apple rings, dried, cut into bite sized pieces
2 tbsp sliced or slivered almonds
2 tbsp pistachios
2 tbsp walnut pieces
½ tsp paprika
1 tsp cinnamon
¼ tsp cardamon
Pinch of cloves
Hefty pinch of nutmeg
Freshly ground black pepper and sea salt
Chopped mint and or cilantro

It is absolutely true that you do not need to peel the squash. In Japan they never peel kabucha. As the squash cooks, the skin gets soft as well. The exception would be Turban and Hubbard squash, which even after baking has a very tough skin. Spaghetti squash has an odd taste so it is not recommended to eat the skin.

Toss the cubed squash in 1 tablespoon olive oil, salt, and pepper. Roast in a 400°F oven until done, about 30 minutes. Next, transfer to a medium pot, adding all the rest of the ingredients. Cook together for about 15 minutes. Garnish with cilantro.

Add in 1-2 tablespoons fermented veggies.

## Tam's Tomato Soup (Tammera Karr)

3 pints tomato sauce
1 qt vegetable broth
1 small yellow onion or 2 shallots, minced
4 cloves garlic, minced
2 tbsp Italian herbs, minced
1 tbsp fresh parsley, minced
1 tsp Celtic Sea salt
Fresh ground pepper
3 tbsp extra virgin olive oil

Combine all ingredients in a 4 quart stainless steel stock pan, warm slowly on medium-low to a gentle boil, reduce heat, and simmer for 30 minutes.

Make grilled cheese sandwiches for on the side, or add a pinch of fresh Parmesan cheese and pinch fresh parsley on top.

## Zucchini Soup

Serves 6 (without cream)

1 tbsp olive oil
2 medium leeks, white and green parts, sliced
2 cloves garlic, crushed
1 medium celery stalk, diced
4 medium zucchinis, sliced
1 cup red potatoes, peeled and cut into 2 inch pieces
1½ tsp sea salt, divided
¼ tsp black pepper, fresh ground
½ cup dry white wine
3½ cups chicken broth or mushroom broth
2 tbsp fresh minutest leaves
2 tbsp fresh basil
¼ cup organic cream or coconut milk (optional)

Put the oil into a large sauce pan over medium heat. Add leeks, celery, and garlic. Stir over medium heat until vegetables soften, about 8-10 minutes.

Add zucchini and potato with 1 teaspoon salt and the pepper; stir ingredients together until well coated. Once coated, add the wine. Simmer until wine is just about evaporated. Add broth and increase heat to boil.

Reduce heat and simmer until all the vegetables are tender, about 20-30 minutes.
Add fresh herbs and blend in a Vitamix® or with an immersion hand blender until pureed. Add remaining salt at table to taste. If using cream or nut milk, add at the very end of blending, warm 5-10 minutes longer.


**Blitva -** Chard & Potatoes (The Peasant's Daughter*)
*A hearty and traditional peasant dish from the Dalmatian peoples of the Croatian coast. Blitva is a combination of potatoes, chard, garlic, and olive oil that is a perfect autumn and winter accompaniment to any meal but also a great unique side dish for your holiday Thanksgiving and Christmas dinners.*

1 bunch chard, any variety
4 lbs potatoes
1½ tbsp garlic, minced
¼ cup olive oil
½ cup butter
Sea salt & pepper to taste

Peel and wash the potatoes.
Set them to boil in a large pot of salted water and allow to boil.
As the potatoes boil, separate the chard stem and leaf. Chop the stems and leaves roughly.
After the potatoes have boiled for 20 minutes, add the chard stems to the water.
Allow the potatoes and stems to boil for another 10 minutes.
Add the chard greens and allow to boil until wilted; about 60 seconds.
Pour the potatoes and chard into a colander and allow to drain very well.

Heat the butter and olive oil on the stovetop over medium heat as the potatoes and chard drain. Use either the same pot you used to boil the vegetables or a different heavy bottomed one, which will double as a serving dish.

Add the garlic to the oil and butter mixture, allow to become fragrant (60 seconds).

Immediately add the potatoes and chard into the oil and butter. Add a big pinch of salt and lots of freshly cracked black pepper. Stir and roughly mash the potatoes. You can mash them into a finer puree if you like, but I prefer keeping the potatoes more rustic. It suits the dish better.
Allow to come to room temperature, check if salt and pepper is to taste, and serve.
* https://thepeasantsdaughter.net/

### Rainbow Chard and Pecans (Tammera Karr)

Chop 1-2 bunches of rainbow Swiss chard and add to warm skillet with 1 tablespoon olive oil. Add chopped pecans, toss with chopped nuts until wilted, add ¼ cup balsamic vinegar, toss and remove from heat. Cook time is less than 10 minutes.

### Spicy Green Soup (Chef Christine Wokowsky)

*One of the most flexible recipes I know of. Can be frozen and used at any time. Filled with liver cleansing and heavy metal chelating botanicals.*

4 cups water
3 medium garlic cloves
¾ cup firmly packed basil
1½ cups firmly packed cilantro leaves and stems
¼ cup lightly packed mint leaves
2 ginger, peeled and sliced into 1 inch pieces
3 tbsp extra virgin olive oil
2 small serrano chilies, stemmed
½ cup sliced almonds
1 tsp sea salt
Zest of 1 lemon
1 tbsp honey

Place the water in a sauce pan and bring to a low simmer. Combine all of the remaining ingredients in a food processor. Blend until smooth, thinning with a couple of tablespoons of cold water and scraping down the sides along the way, until the mixture becomes as smooth as possible. Taste and adjust to your liking; the paste should be strong and spicy.

Just before serving, add the paste to the simmering water and stir well. Make sure to not let this boil, keeping it to a simmer. Taste and adjust the seasoning; a bit more salt or a squeeze of lemon juice. Don't skimp on the lemon! It punctuates the flavors perfectly. Ladle into bowls with your chosen accompaniment and enjoy on its own or topped with any of the suggested toppings.

*Amazing, Endless Add-Ins*
Poached eggs, hot white beans, gluten-free soba noodles, brown rice, or quinoa.

Chopped black olives, 2 tablespoons fermented veggies, lemon wedges, toasted almonds, shaved green onions, roasted, sliced mushrooms, or other oven roasted vegetables.

Think shredded chicken, turkey, or small meat or lamb balls. Think shrimp, mussels, cod, salmon, or a twist on traditional tomato based Cioppini, the famous seafood soup from San Francisco, reminiscent of the French bouillabaisse.

**How to Cook Vegetables** (Theory and Practice of Cookery 1900-1912, pg 241)
*A New York Public text grades 6-8. Replicated as found in original form.*

390. People are not agreed on what are the best ways of cooking vegetables. Too many cooks think only of getting them soft, without regard to retaining their juices and salts. Vegetables cooked in water lose a large proportion of their foodstuffs. In carrots this loss may amount to 20 per cent of their whole value when they are cut into large pieces, to 30 per cent when they are cut small. Cabbage loses about one-third of its food value. Until we have more accurate knowledge, we can only try to make each vegetable palatable, endeavoring at the same time to keep it as nutritious as possible.

**General Rules for Cooking Vegetables**
391.    1. Cook vegetables whole when practicable. When not practicable, cut them into as large pieces as are convenient. If the cooking is to be served with the vegetable, the pieces may be smaller than would otherwise be desirable.

2. Use only as much water as is necessary to cover the vegetables. For small or cut-up vegetables that can be stirred, use just enough to keep them from burning, adding more as this cooks away.

3. Use the cooking water, if palatable, in sauces, soup-stock, cream-of-vegetable soup, etc. It contains much nutritive matter dissolved from the vegetables.

4. For vegetables cooked whole or in large pieces, keep the water boiling, that they may cook in the shortest possible time. Peas, beans and any vegetables served in the cooking water are better simmered.

5. Green vegetables keep their color better if cooked uncovered. The reason for this is not known. Cook onions and cabbage uncovered; their odor is less noticeable when allowed to pass off continually than when escaping occasionally in bursts of steam.

6. The time required to cook any given vegetable depends upon its size, age, and freshness. Old beets may be so woody that they cannot be cooked tender. Dried or wilted vegetables cook more quickly if first soaked in cold water. Think of the part water plays in cooking starch, and explain why this is so. *(The final question was for 6th-8th grade girls to answer in the New York State Public schools. 1912)*

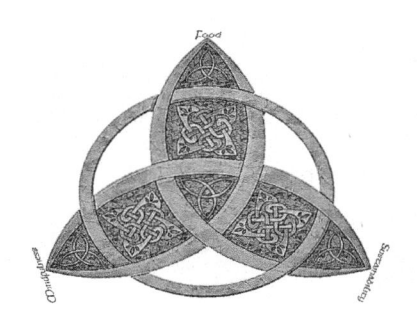

*While traditional Irish cooking stems in the main, from simple farmers, it also embraces the more sophisticated food served in the grand houses of the Anglo-Irish gentry.*

*From the dining-rooms of the great houses to the kitchen of the poorest cabins, and from pagan times right up to the present day, Ireland has had a strong tradition of generous hospitality. The best food was generally for guests, and the warmest hospitality was often to be found in the most humble of homes – the sort of wholesome, comforting dishes that nourished our ancestors for generations.*[135]

~ Darina Allen
*Irish Traditional Cooking*

---

[128] Seaweed: slimy, sexy and saleable; https://www.theguardian.com/uk/2007/jan/28/scotland.travelnews

[129] A Short History Of Dulse Seaweed by Mara Seaweed 2017: https://maraseaweed.com/blogs/news/a-short-history-of-dulse-seaweed

[130] A Sprinkle of Seaweed Could Deflate Gassy Cowshttps://www.nationalgeographiccom/people-and-culture/food/the-plate/2016/11/seaweed-may-be-the-solution-for-burping-cows/

[131] Irish Traditional Cooking by Darina Allen page 187

[132] Simply Seaweed by Leslie Ellis

[133] Healthy Recipes Seaweed by Cross Media Ltd

[134] The real cabbage soup diet by bbccom; https://ancientfoods.wordpress.com/page/1/

[135] Irish Traditional Cooking by Darina Allen page 9

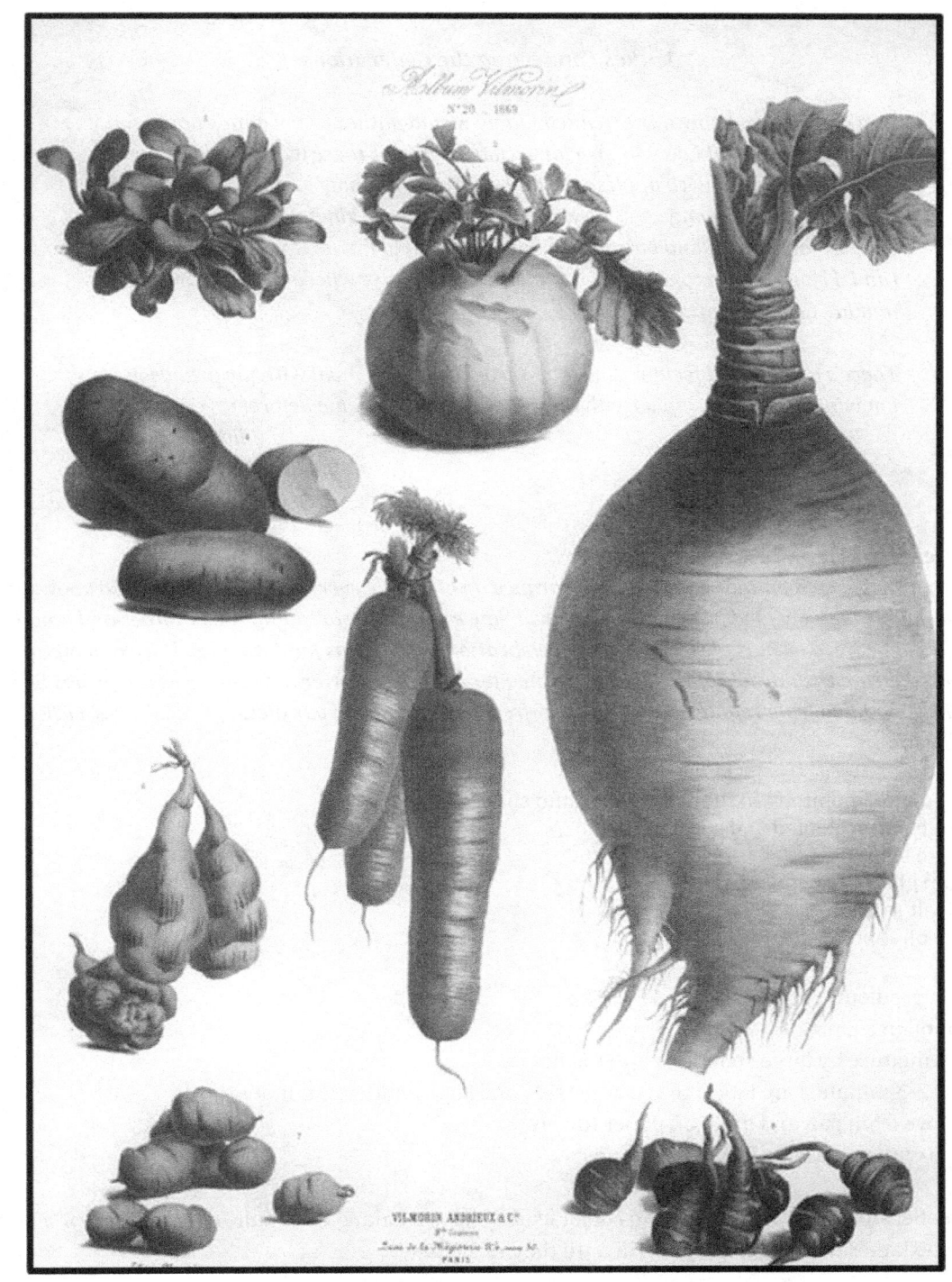

# Tubers & Roots

### Latkes Connecting the Generations

*As a child, I loved how our extended family would gather at my aunt's house for the holidays. Hanukkah was special because it meant there would be latkes and we could eat them with applesauce and sour cream. Some families are applesauce only or sour cream only, but we were definitely a both kind of family. Now my children are grown and one of them has a child of her own. It warms my heart (and, I confess, my stomach) to be invited to her house where she is the one making delicious latkes.*

*There's a delightful feeling that comes from sharing a meal with my grandson, knowing it's connecting us with the generations that came before.*

*~ Mira Dessy, NE*

### Latkes (Mira Dessy)

*Being Jewish, one food that makes an appearance on our table every winter is latkes, also known as potato pancakes. My food processor works overtime every year, shredding the potatoes and onion. Latkes are served as part of the Hanukkah celebration, which calls for eating foods fried in oil to commemorate the miracle of the oil that burned for eight days. Over the years, this recipe has been slightly modified from regular flour to gluten-free; depending on your dietary preferences, either will work.*

3 lbs of gold potatoes, scrubbed, peeled, and shredded
1 large onion, peeled and shredded
1 large egg
¼ cup gluten-free flour
Sea salt to taste
Olive oil (enough for frying)

Mix ingredients together.
Heat oil in a pan.
Drop mixture by large spoonfuls into the hot oil.
After 2-3 minutes, flip latkes to the other side and cook another 2 minutes.
Remove from pan and drain on paper towels.
Serve with applesauce and sour cream.

*Note:* Because these take a while to cook I usually have a baking tray in the oven set to 175°F and put the latkes in there to keep warm until they're all done.

**Is Food Art?**

Food, creativity, and art flow over many areas of human life. This story, shared by Confraria Gastronômica do Barão de Gourmandise, is a perfect example. *(Translated into English)*

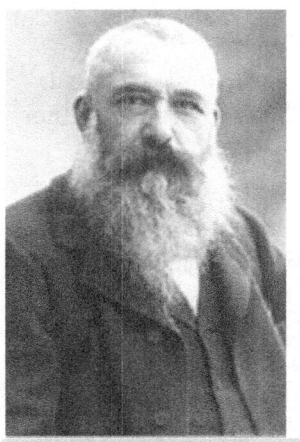

Claude Monet's Potato Pie

If you've ever visited Monet's house and studio in Giverny, France, you know one of the most exceptional rooms in their house is the large kitchen, clad in blue and white tiles and lined with copper pans.

The impressionist master was not only a painter but also a gourmand, savoring the full meals, of which he made abundant notes in his cooking diary. In The Monet Cookbook by Florence Genter (Prestel, 2016), you can discover some of the artist's favorite recipes, including this one for a rustic potato pie.

**Rustic Potato Pie** (Monet)

*For the dough*
500 g of wheat flour
250 g butter at room temperature
2 egg gems

*For the stuffing*
6 medium size firm potatoes
3 onions
1 small salsa dip
150 ml (a little over ½ cup) milk cream
1 whole egg
Salt and pepper to taste
Prep time 30 minutes

Start by preparing the dough: cut the butter into cubes and place in a bowl; add flour with 1 pinch of salt and mix with your fingertips until the mixture becomes thin bread crumbs. Combine the gems and make a ball out of the dough.

Place the batter on a baking sheet. Flour lightly. Press down dough with the palm of your hand, working from the center to the sides for a smooth dough. Repeat the process several times until dough is even. Turn it into a ball again, wrap it in plastic, and let it rest in the refrigerator for two hours. When you are ready to use the dough, preheat the oven to 180°C.

Peel the potatoes and cut them into thin strips. Soak potato skins in cold water. Peel the onion and cut into slices.

Remove the dough from the refrigerator and divide it into two uneven pieces. Place the larger piece on a floured surface and spread it out in a circle large enough to line the bottom and sides in a round, shallow ceramic form. The dough should overlap slightly on the sides. Open the second serving of dough into a circle slightly larger than the plate.

Loose the potatoes and dry them with a clean paper towel. Arrange them in the already-lined form with the single layer dough and sprinkle with the onion rings and chopped salsa. Season with salt and a good amount of pepper and then add the cream of milk (repeat until you finish the ingredients). Cover with the second circle of dough, joining the two sheets of dough together to seal the edges.

Make a scoop in the middle of the dough (to release steam during cooking) and carefully insert a funnel made from a small piece of aluminum foil. Beat the whole egg and brush the batter before going to the oven. Pie should take 2 hours to bake. If it goldens before that, cover it with a piece of lightly buttered paper.

Serve it up and enjoy it.

Also enjoy the blog on Monet's connection with gastronomy and you can check it out via the link:
http://confrariadobaraodegourmandise.blogspot.com/.../gen...

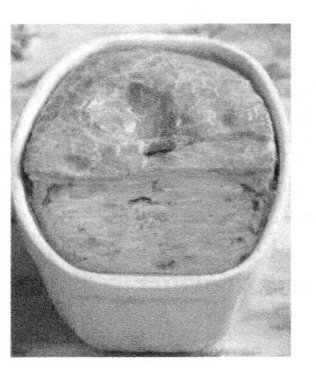

## German Potato Salad (Chef Benjamin Qualls)

8 potatoes, peeled and roughly chopped
½ cup chicken or vegetable stock, or more as needed
¼ cup white vinegar
¼ cup olive oil
1 large onion, chopped
¼ cup chopped fresh dill or 1 tbsp dried dill
6 slices cooked uncured bacon, chopped (optional)
Sea salt and black pepper to taste

Place potatoes in a large pot. Cover with water and bring to a boil. Reduce heat to medium-low and simmer until tender, 15-20 minutes; drain.

Combine chicken or vegetable stock, vinegar, and oil in a large pot; bring to a boil. Add onion to broth; cook to desired doneness, 2-6 minutes.

Remove pot from heat and add potatoes, dill and bacon (optional); stir *gently*, adding more stock if need to moisten salad. Season with sea salt and black pepper; serve warm.

### Purple Potato Salad (Chef Christine Wokowsky)

2-4 purple potatoes, depending on size, you'll want about 1 pound.
Handful frozen cooked peas, defrosted
¼-½ red bell pepper diced
½ cup dried arame
Small handful chopped cilantro

*Dressing*
1 tbsp apple cider vinegar
1 tbsp Dijon mustard
1 tbsp sesame seed oil
1 tbsp olive oil
2 tbsp pickled ginger, minced or
1 tbsp fresh ginger minced or grated
Sea salt and pepper to taste

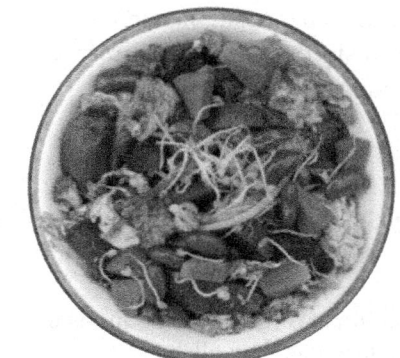

Soak arame in water in a bowl. Cook potatoes by steam or boil them, skin on. When done, remove and run cold water over them to stop the cooking process and cool them down so you can peel them.

Peel then dice and place inside a medium size bowl. Add peas, red bell peppers, drained arame and cilantro.

Make dressing by whisking everything together. Pour over the potatoes and veggies and toss. Serve at room temperature or slightly warm.

### Champ (old Irish adapted by Tammera Karr)

About 1½ lbs peeled old potatoes
Bunch spring onions (green onions)
½ pint whole milk
Celtic Sea salt and pepper
Kerrygold butter

Steam or boil the potatoes until tender. Drain boiled potatoes, cover with a dry tea towel, and return the pot to the heat to dry out the potatoes for a few minutes.

Meanwhile, simmer the chopped spring onions in the milk for 5 minutes. Mash the potatoes and beat until light and fluffy, season to taste and serve topped with knobs of butter. Young nettle tops or chives can be used instead of spring onions.

> Sweet potatoes originated in tropical America. There is similarity between terms for sweet potato in Polynesian languages and South America which supports the transfer that occurred from human movement more so than seed dispersal, resulting in prehistoric transfer(s) of sweet potatoes from South America (Peru-Ecuador region) into Polynesia by humans.[136]

## Spicy Sweet Potato Fries (Tammera Karr)
Serves size 4

3 medium organic sweet potatoes or yams
¼ cup organic olive oil
⅛ tsp organic cayenne pepper
¼ tsp organic garlic powder
Celtic Sea salt
Bake at 450°F for 20 minutes.

*Optional*
½ teaspoon organic Italian seasoning herbs.
Peel potatoes and cut each root into quarters, cut into French fries about ½ inch in size.
Place in a bowl, add olive oil and seasoning. Toss well for coverage on each fry.
Spread as a single layer on a baking sheet, drizzle leftover oil and seasoning from bowl over fries.

Place baking sheet in the preheated oven. Set the timer for 10 minutes.
Turn fries over after 10 minutes and cook for the remainder of the time.
Place fries on plates or serving dish. While still hot each person can add salt, pepper, or grated cheese to their serving.

Seasonings can be added or subtracted to suit taste.

## Sweet Potato Pudding

1½ cups sweet potatoes, boiled and mashed
2 eggs, beaten
½ cups coconut sugar
½ tsp vanilla
4 tbsp organic butter, melted
¼ tsp sea salt
1 cup organic whole milk or ½ & ½
½ tsp cinnamon

½ tsp ginger
⅛ tsp nutmeg
1 tbsp grated lemon rind

Blend eggs, sweet potato, sugar, vanilla, melted butter, salt, and milk. Stir in spices and grated lemon rind. Pour into a buttered casserole dish. Cover dish and bake at 325°F for 45 minutes. Remove cover and bake 15 minutes longer.


**Sweet Potato Noodles with Garlic & Kale** (Jeanine Donofrio)
Serves 4 as a side, 3 as a main

2 medium sweet potatoes, spiralized
1-2 tbsp extra virgin olive oil, enough to well coat the pan
3 garlic cloves, thinly sliced
¼ tsp red pepper flakes
2-3 tbsp water
4 cups baby kale (or thinly sliced lacinato kale)
Sea salt and freshly ground black pepper
Squeezes of fresh lemon juice, as desired

*Serve with*
⅓ cup fresh basil, sliced
Dollops of pesto (this recipe with basil in place of kale)
2 tbsp toasted pine nuts
Grated pecorino cheese, optional

1. Peel the sweet potatoes. Slice in half and cut the pointy tips off. Place into the spiralizer and spiralize into noodles. Alternatively, you can use a julienne peeler (although this is more difficult, so I recommend spiralizing).

2. Heat the oil in a large deep skillet over medium heat. Add the garlic and cook until the garlic slices are lightly golden brown, about 5 minutes, reducing the heat if necessary. If the olive oil is bubbling too much, turn the heat down; you do not want the garlic to burn. Add a few generous pinches of salt, red pepper flakes, and a few grinds of freshly cracked black pepper.

3. Add the sweet potato noodles and toss to coat. Let cook for 2 minutes, gently tossing and scraping down the sides of the pan.

4. Add 2-3 tablespoons of water and toss again to ensure that nothing is sticking to the bottom of the pan. Cover and let the sweet potato noodles continue for 5 more minutes or until they start to soften and are tender but still have a crisp "al dente" bite. Check and toss occasionally so that they cook evenly. Be careful not to overcook or they will start to break apart (this happens quickly).

5. During the last minute of cooking, stir in the kale so that it wilts into the noodles. Remove from heat and transfer to 3-4 bowls.

6. Serve with the fresh basil, a dollop of pesto, hemp seeds or pine nuts and pecorino cheese, if desired.

> Sweet potatoes may seem a quintessentially American food, but researchers have long debated the origin. David Dilcher and colleagues in India identified 57 million year old leaf fossils of the Morning Glory family, of which sweet potatoes belong.
>
> The research suggests the family originated in the late Paleocene epoch in the East Gondwana land mass that became part of Asia.

### Sweet Potato "Noodle" Pad Thai (Aysegul Sanford)
Serves 4

*Dressing*
3 tbsp unsweetened and smooth peanut butter
3 tsp tamari*
1 tsp sesame oil
1 tbsp maple syrup
1 tsp freshly grated ginger
2 cloves of garlic, minced
2 tbsp freshly squeezed lime juice
½ tsp salt
3-4 tbsp vegetable stock

*Pad Thai*
1 tbsp of olive oil
1 small onion chopped
1 red or yellow bell pepper seeded and sliced thinly
2 medium size sweet potatoes peeled and spiralized
¼ cup vegetable stock
½ cup edamame
3 tbsp chopped cilantro

*Garnish*
1 tbsp sesame seeds
1-2 stalks of green onions both white and green parts chopped
2 tbsp lightly salted peanuts coarsely chopped

1. To make the dressing: Whisk together all the ingredients of the dressing in a bowl, cover with plastic wrap, and refrigerate until you are ready to use it.

2. Heat olive oil in a large skillet on medium heat. Add in the onion and pepper. Cook, stirring frequently, until translucent, 5-7 minutes.

3. Add in the sweet potato noodles and vegetable stock and cook, stirring frequently, for 6-7 minutes.

4. Pour the dressing over the noodles and give it a large stir, making sure that the noodles are coated with the dressing. Cook 2-3 minutes until it is warm.

5. Off the heat, stir in the edamame and chopped cilantro.

6. To serve, divide the pad thai in 4 bowls and garnish each one with sesame seeds, green onions, and peanuts.

7. Serve immediately.
https://foolproofliving.com/sweet-potato-noodle-pad-thai/#wprm-recipe-container-13436

**Savory Creamy Root Soup**  (Tammera Karr)
*Perfect for folks who do not like beets or yams*
Yields 6 quarts

3 small beets, peeled and quartered
2 medium sweet potatoes or yams, peeled and chunked up
1 medium yellow onion, chunked up
3 medium carrots, chunked up
4 cloves garlic
½ cup dried or fresh mushrooms
2 large red potatoes, peeled and quartered
1 tbsp Italian seasoning
½ tsp celery seed
1 tsp caraway seed
1½ tsp Celtic Sea salt and pepper (add when you blend)
¼ cup extra virgin olive oil (add just before you blend)
2 qts chicken or vegetable broth
1 qt water

Combine vegetables, herbs, broth and water into an 8 quart stock pot. Bring to a boil, then turn down to simmer until vegetables are tender, about 45 minutes. Turn off heat, add oil, salt and pepper, stir.

Carefully ladle contents into a Vitamix® or other brand of blender (do not overfill your container!) and blend on medium speed for about 1 minute. Pour contents into a second stock pot and continue till all of the broth and vegetables are creamed. It is now ready to eat with some hearty bread and butter!

Place leftovers into leak-proof glass storage or reheatable dishes for lunch or dinner. Warm on low heat to prevent scorching.

**Potato Cheesecake** (*The New Cyclopaedia of Domestic Economy, and Practical Housekeeping, 1872, pg 435*)

Four ounces of butter, the same of pounds of sugar, six ounces of potatoes boiled and floured through a sieve, the rind on one lemon, and half of the juice, unless acid is desirable; mix these ingredients well together, with two eggs, and fill the tart-pan and bake it.

**Potato Cheese** (*The New Cyclopaedia of Domestic Economy, and Practical Housekeeping, 1872, pg 435*)

Potato cheese is celebrated in various parts of Europe. It is made thus: --- Boil good white potatoes, and when cool, peel them and rasp or mash them to a light pulp; to five pounds of this, which must be free of lumps, add a pint of sour milk and salt to taste; kneed the whole well, cover it, and leave it for three or four days, according to the season; then knead it afresh, and put the cheeses into small baskets, when then will par with their superfluous moister; dry them in the shade, and place them in layers in large pots or kegs, where they may remain a fortnight. The older they are, the finer they become. This cheese, it is said never engenders worms, and in well closed vessels, in a dry place, will keep for years. (*this recipe is from an Old English work*) – Original text included the mention of an Old English work.

**The Piperade** (Kelsi Sitz)

4 tomatoes
4 green peppers
4 onions
2 mild red peppers
2 garlic cloves
3 tbsp of olive oil, thyme, bay leaves, *Espelette pepper in powder, salt, pepper

Peel the tomatoes and the peppers. For this, scald the tomatoes, and place the peppers in the oven. Remove seeds from tomatoes and dice them. Remove seeds from the green and mild red peppers and cut them into strips. Cook the onions in olive oil for a few minutes, add the green peppers and the mild red peppers, mix and cook for 20 minutes. Then add the tomatoes, garlic, thyme and bay leaves. Mix, add salt, black pepper and the Espalette powder. Simmer for 20 minutes.

*The Espelette pepper (French: Piment d'Espelette French pronunciation: [pi.mã dɛs.pə.lɛt]; Basque: Ezpeletako biperra) is a variety of Capsicum annuum that is cultivated in the French commune of Espelette, Pyrénées-Atlantiques, traditionally the northern territory of the Basque people.


### Beetroot Raita (Medha Mujumdar Murtyy)

*Raita is a side dish made with raw or cooked vegetables mixed with yogurt and is the perfect way to soothe and balance an Indian meal rich in spices. The most common vegetables used in raita are tomatoes, onions, and cucumbers. This recipe using cooked beetroot gives the raita a beautiful pink color and a slightly sweeter taste.*

1 cooked and grated beetroot
½ small onion very finely chopped
1 cup Greek yogurt
¼ cup coarsely ground macadamia or cashew nuts
2 tsp finely chopped cilantro
1 green chile
Salt to taste
½ tsp sugar
1 tbsp ghee for tempering
1 tsp whole cumin seeds
1 sprig curry leaves (optional)

Mix grated, cooked beetroot with finely chopped onions, cilantro, coarsely ground cashew nuts, salt, sugar, and Greek yogurt. Heat 1 tablespoon of ghee until hot. Add cumin seeds, chopped chile and whole curry leaves and let the cumin seeds splutter. Pour this onto the mixture above. Mix thoroughly and raita is ready to serve.


### Lenten Borscht with Beans (Anastasiya Terentyeva)

Traditional Ukrainian dish
*It's my husband's favorite family recipe. We like it a lot as it's a great source of vitamins and fiber and it can be eaten for several days (less cooking and it tastes better the next day - all the vegetables are steeped in vegetable broth with spices; the original recipe is with meat like pork ribs and beef tail. It's not that hard. You may love it as it's an easy way of eating healthy vegetables like cabbage and beets in soup. Your digestive system will be happy with it. A very healthy easy way to enjoy food.*

100-150 g dry beans or 300-400g canned
2½–3 liters of water

4–6 potatoes
1 onion bulb
1 Bulgarian pepper
1 beet
1 carrot
2-3 tomatoes, peeled
300-400 g of cabbage
4 tbsp of vegetable oil
1 tbsp lemon juice
1 tsp of sugar
Salt to taste
Ground black pepper, to taste
2 dried bay leaves

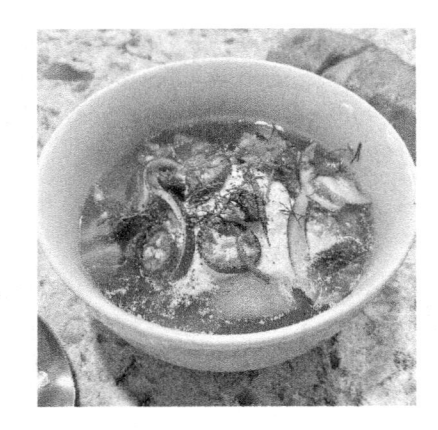

If using dry beans, sort them first and rinse in water. Then soak beans in cold water overnight. Drain the soaked beans in a colander, transfer to a sauce pan and cover with 2½–3 liters of water. Simmer for 30-40 minutes until almost soft.

Cut the potatoes into medium sized pieces and onion and pepper into small cubes. Grate the beets and carrots on a coarse grater or chop them into strips. Twist the peeled tomatoes through a meat grinder or chop finely. Finely chop the cabbage.

In hot oil, bring the onion to a golden color, add the carrots, and cook for a few minutes. Add the bell pepper and sauté for 3-4 minutes. Move the vegetables to a plate.

Pour oil into the pan and sauté the beets for 2-3 minutes. Add tomatoes, lemon juice and sugar, stir and simmer until vegetables are soft.

Put the potatoes into the pot with the boiled beans. If using canned beans, simply place the potatoes in boiling water. Boil potatoes until soft on the outside but still firm in the middle.

Add cabbage, bring to a boil, salt, and boil for 5 minutes. Put the sautéed vegetables into the pot and cook for another 5-7 minutes. (Add canned beans at this stage if using them). Add beets, bring to a boil again and boil for about 2 minutes.

Season the borscht with salt and pepper. Add bay leaves and let the soup simmer for 20-30 minutes.

I like to eat it with fresh onion, sour cream, and a little bit of fresh jalapeno pepper. But also, it can be served with fresh garlic.

> **UNESCO declares borsch cooking an endangered Ukrainian heritage**
>
> Often written borscht in English, the soup is widely eaten across Eastern Europe and is extremely common in Russia. But Ukraine considers it a national dish, or as UNESCO put it: "part of the fabric of Ukrainian society, cultural heritage, identity, and tradition."
>
> The soup's tangled origins possibly trace back to ancient Kievan Rus, which was summarily nationalized in the Soviet Union. The agency also noted how varied a dish borsch can be: featuring fish or mushrooms, though most commonly meat in addition to the typical base of beet, cabbage, tomato, and root vegetables, often served with sour cream, dill and bread or garlic rolls. [137]

### Parsnips with Ham and Basil (Tammera Karr)

*This recipe was developed for a cancer client going through chemo. Chemo changes the way foods taste; depending on the course; foods have a heavy metallic taste. This recipe provided a sweet and savory flavor that satisfied.*

1-2 medium organic parsnips
½ cup uncured ham or Canadian bacon chopped
½ cup chopped organic fresh basil
1-2 garlic cloves, minced
2 tbsp organic or Kerrygold butter
Pinch Celtic Sea salt

Peel and grate parsnips. Melt butter on medium-low heat in a cast iron skillet, and add chopped basil and garlic; when basil is wilted, add ham and parsnips. Toss all ingredients together, allow to brown golden on one side, then turn and brown the second side. Serve warm.

### Parsnip Cakes with Crispy Bacon (Tammera Karr)

Serves 4-6

1 lb parsnips
4 tbsp Kerrygold butter
Celtic Sea salt and freshly ground pepper
Seasoned spelt or gluten-free flour
1 beaten egg
Gluten free oat bran

Olive oil and butter for frying
Uncured beacon cut into ¼ inch cubes crisped in a little oil
Watercress for garnish

Peel parsnips with a vegetable peeler. Cut them into small chunks, and cook in a little boiling salted water until soft. Mash with butter, season with salt and pepper to taste. Wet your hands and shape the mixture into cakes. Dip each into flour, then egg, then oat-bran.

Heat a little olive oil with equal part butter in a skillet. Fry the cakes on a gentle heat until golden on both sides.

Serve hot with crispy bacon and fresh watercress.

**Potato Pancakes** (Tammera Karr)

2 cups raw red potatoes, grated
1 egg, beaten slightly
2 tbsp spelt flour or organic potato starch
1 tsp Celtic Sea salt
1 tsp black pepper, ground
1 small onion or shallot

Rinse and squeeze all water from grated potato. Combine with other ingredients and mix well. Drop by spoonful onto greased frying pan or griddle. Fry until golden brown on both sides. Serve with applesauce.

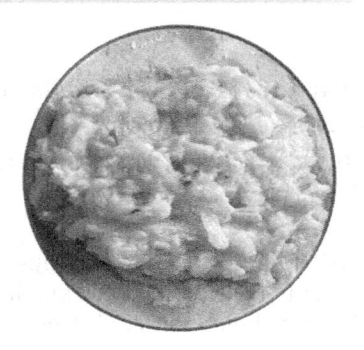

**Sautéed Radishes with Butter and Parsley** (Tammera Karr)

1 large bunch of radishes, sliced
1 good handful of radish seed pods from those that have bolted in your garden
2 tbsp organic butter
¼ cup fresh parsley, chopped
Salt

In a large skillet or sauté pan, melt the butter and add the radishes. Sauté over medium heat for about 5-7 minutes. You want the radishes to soften but still stay a little firm. Add the parsley and stir. Salt to taste. Serve immediately.

## Swede Turnip – Rutabagas

Serves 4-6

2 lbs rutabagas
Celtic Sea salt and lots of fresh ground black pepper
8 tbsp Kerrygold butter

Caramelized onions
1 lb yellow onions
3 tbsp extra virgin olive oil
Finely chopped parsley for garnish

Heat olive oil in heavy sauce pan, toss in the onions and cook over a low heat until they are soft and caramelized to a golden brown, about 35 minutes.

Peel the swede thickly to remove the total skin. Cut into 3x3 inch cubes and cover with water. Add a good pinch of salt, bring to a boil, and cook till soft. Strain off the excess water, mash the swede well and then beat in butter. Stir in the soft caramelized onions. Taste and season with lots of fresh ground pepper and salt to taste. Garnish with parsley and serve hot.


## Baked Turnips

3 cups organic turnips
1½ tsp Celtic Sea salt
1½ tsp coconut sugar
¼ cup organic butter
⅓ cup organic broth

Wash and peel turnips, place all ingredients in a glass or cast iron covered pan.
Cook at 325°F in the oven till turnips are tender (about 20 minutes).
Cooking time will vary based on the size of turnips.


## Yam and Ham Soup (Tammera Karr)

3 medium yams, chopped into chunks
3-4 cloves garlic, minced
½ cup chopped shallots
½ cup chopped celery with green leafy tops
1 cup uncured ham, chopped
1 stick organic butter
2 qts organic chicken broth
1 can organic coconut milk

Place all the ingredients into a Crockpot® or Instant Pot® cooker on ready to eat setting. Or cook in a conventional stock pot, bring to a slow boil, cover, and turn on low heat. Stir and serve with warm sourdough bread or gluten-free bread and organic butter. Warms up well and freezes also. Takes approximately 45 minutes.

### Diversity in Understanding Foods

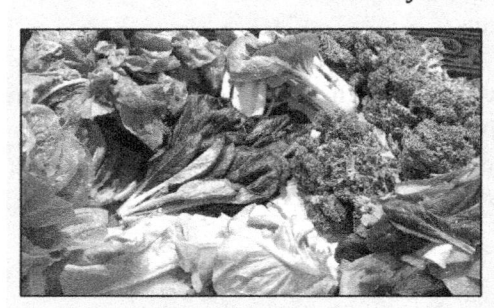

Not all vegetarians or vegans share the same beliefs on what foods are acceptable to eat. For those following Janism, all life is sacred and a scrupulous and thorough way of applying nonviolence to everyday activities, especially food, shapes their lives and is the hallmark of Jain identity. What does this mean for the modern chef or cook? Water must be filtered. Prohibited foods include honey, potatoes, onions, roots, bulbs, tubers, and food that have started to decay or are stored overnight. Consumption of most terrestrial vegetables is allowed (where the plants are annuals or leaves and fruit can be removed without harm). No meals after sunset.

---

136  S. D. S. Oliveira, I. B. Gois, A. F. Blank, M. F. Arrigoni-Blank, M. I. Zucchi, J. B. Pinheiro, C. E. Batista, A. Alves-Pereira, Genome-wide diversity in native populations of Croton grewioides Baill., a future crop with fungicidal and antioxidant activity, using SNP markers, Genetic Resources and Crop Evolution, 69, 5, (1965-1978), (2022). https://doi.org/10.1007/s10722-022-01357-y

137  UNESCO declares borsch cooking an endangered Ukrainian heritage
July 1, 20223:07 PM ET, NPR, retrieved Aug 2022: https://www.npr.org/2022/07/01/1109319174/unesco-declares-ukraine-borsch-ukrainian-heritage

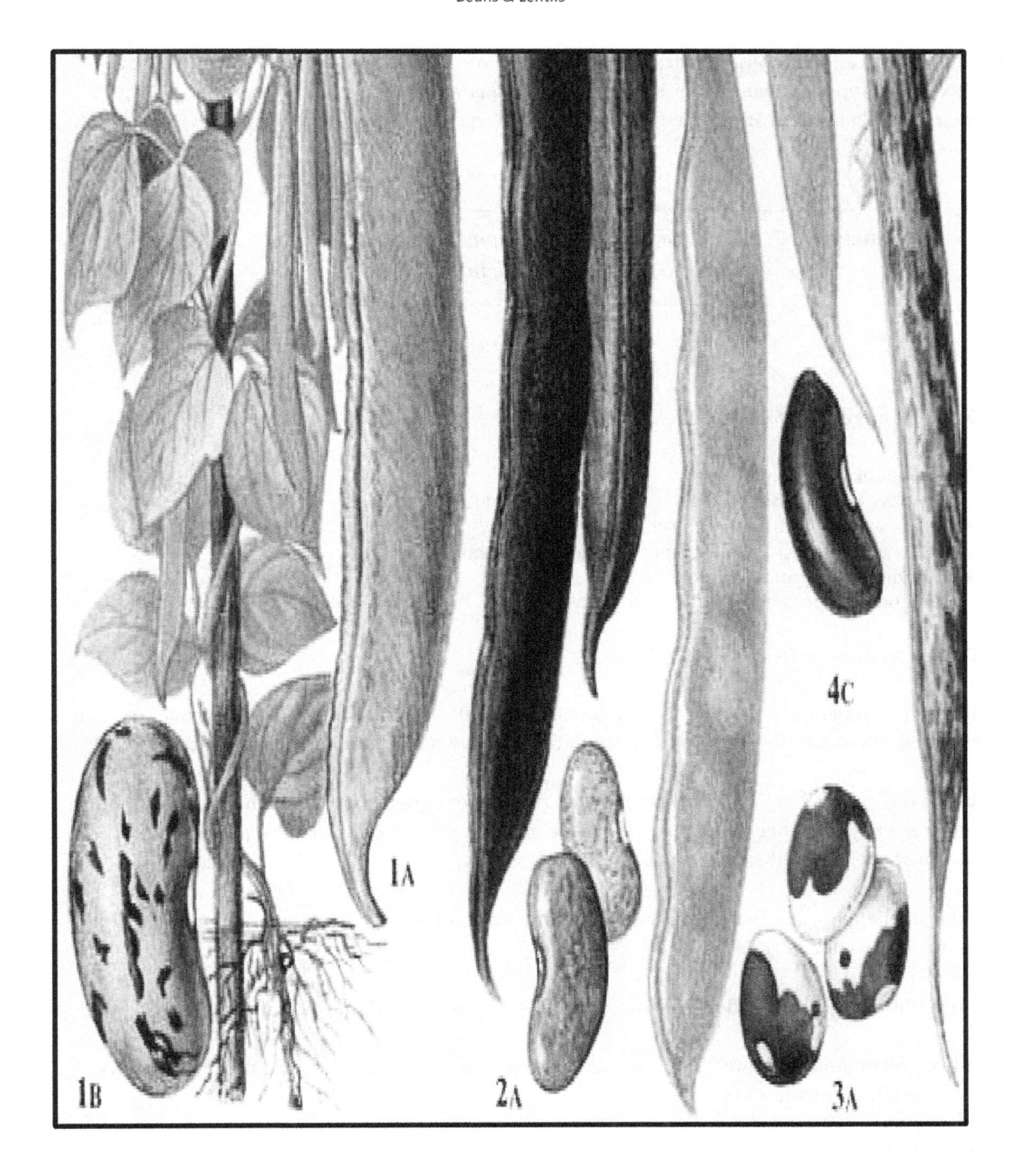

# Beans & Lentils

There are over one thousand varieties of beans (also known as pulses or legumes). There are three main types of beans; snap, shell and dry. Beans were discovered to have existed 20,000 years ago. The United States is currently the sixth largest producer of dry beans.

> **Principle 17**: *To reduce high lectin and phytic acid content, soak beans and quinoa before cooking under pressure.*

**Kuru Fasulye** (Nour Danno)

2 red peppers
4 tbsp olive oil (1 tbsp at the start, the remaining 3 later)
3 cups of water (1 early on, the remaining 2 later)
2 cans pre-cooked cannellini beans (white kidney beans)
4 tomatoes peeled and chopped
2 green bell peppers chopped

Preheat your oven to 400°F.

Chop the red peppers, place in a small roasting pan with 1 tablespoon of olive oil, cover the pan with foil, and roast the peppers for 40 minutes. Remove peppers from oven and let them cool.

While waiting for the peppers to cool, gather five dishes and peel and chop the tomatoes, chop the green peppers, dice the onions, mince the garlic (if you haven't bought it minced), and slice the mushrooms. Set them each aside in the five separate dishes.

Once the peppers are cool, blend them, any remaining oil, and 1 cup water until smooth (add more water if needed). Set aside.

On medium-high heat, add the remaining 3 tablespoons olive oil to a big pan.

Add diced onions and sauté for three minutes; add the minced garlic and sauté for one minute.
1 cup of sliced mushrooms
4 large garlic cloves minced
1 large white onion thinly chopped
5 tbsp tomato paste
½ tbsp zhug* (optional)
A pinch of salt
1½ tsp black pepper
1 tsp chile flakes

Add the chopped green pepper and sauté for three minutes; add the chili flakes and sauté for 30 seconds; add both the tomato puree and zhug (if you're using it) and sauté for two minutes; add the sliced mushrooms and sauté for one minute; add the peeled and chopped tomatoes and sauté for one minute; finally, add the salt, black pepper, and white beans. Stir and combine everything well.

Add the remaining 2 cups of water (or just enough warm water to cover everything) and bring that to a boil for a few minutes. Reduce the heat, cover, and simmer for at least 40 minutes.

* Zhug (also spelled "skhug" and "s'chüg") is a red pepper paste from the Middle East. Various American companies make and distribute and can be ordered online, and there are recipes for it online.

> "The art of cookery, when not allied with a degenerate taste or with gluttony, is one of the criteria of a people's civilization. We grow like what we eat; Bad food depresses, good food exalts us like an inspiration."
>
> ~ Fannie Merritt Farmer, 1911

### Feel Better Italian Soup (Nicole Hammond)

*My family were Italian immigrants who made a very successful living owning and operating a restaurant named The Casino in Albany NY for over forty years. I grew up in this restaurant, and much of my "free" time was spent cooking with relatives. Everything was made from scratch and only using the freshest ingredients possible.*

6 cloves of garlic
1 yellow onion
2 chopped zucchinis
¼ cup olive oil
1 tsp salt
1 tsp pepper
2 cups tomatoes chopped
1 cup chopped carrots
1 cup chopped celery
16 oz cannellini beans
2 cups arugula
1 qt low sodium chicken stock, bone broth, or vegetable stock
1 tsp sea salt
1 tsp red pepper flakes
Chopped basil, parsley, and oregano to taste

Sauté olive oil, garlic (crushing first and allowing allicin to be released), onions, zucchini, tomatoes, carrots, celery, salt, and red pepper.

Add chicken or vegetable stock, beans, arugula, and fresh chopped herbs and simmer for 30 minutes.

**Black Bean Chili** (Tammera Karr)
Serves 6-8; cook time 2-4 hours

1 lb lean ground pork, elk, or buffalo
2 tbsp organic extra virgin olive oil
⅓ cup organic ground chile powder
1 tbsp organic ground cumin
1 qt black beans (or four cups cooked from a pressure cooker)
1 qt beef mushroom broth (or 4 cups bone broth)
1 qt organic chopped tomatoes (or 4 cups stewed tomatoes)
½ pint chopped hot chiles (or ¼ cup chopped hot chiles of choice)
1 tbsp red chile flakes
2 tbsp organic Italian seasoning
¼ cup ground organic cocoa powder
2 tsp coarse grind Celtic Sea salt
1 medium organic sweet onion chopped
4 cloves Italian garlic chopped
1 organic orange sweet pepper chopped
*½ cup good Tequila

Add 2 tablespoons of extra virgin organic olive oil into a cast iron Dutch oven; a good stainless steel soup pot will work if you do not have an old Dutch oven. Add ground meat and brown.

Add all dry ingredients except coarse salt to the meat, and mix well to evenly distribute spices, cocoa, oil, and meat. Make sure there are no spices stuck to the bottom that may scorch.

Once meat, spices, and oil are combined, add chopped onion, garlic, and peppers. Mix well, add chiles with liquid, broth, and beans; next add pureed tomatoes.

Stir well.

Chile will be very liquidy at this point. Add tequila, and allow to cook over medium-low heat in an open Dutch oven for 2 hours, occasionally stirring to prevent sticking. As liquid concentrates with the beans, it will thicken. Turn heat to low, and cover with a Dutch oven lid to keep warm. Serve with gluten-free cornbread, blue corn chips, or tortillas.

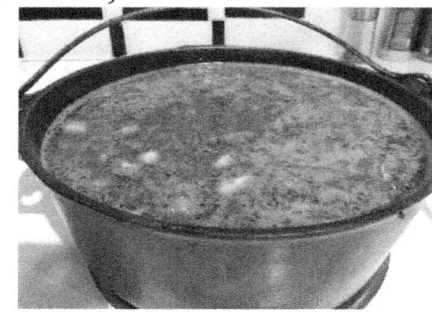

**Please use only locally sourced produce and clean meat for the best flavor.

*Tequila is optional, but it provides a traditional accenting flavor. The flavor remains, and the alcohol is evaporated during cooking.

### Alubias de Tolosa Stew - Basque Beans and Chorizo[138] (Tammera Karr)
*This is one of those old recipes and a favorite on cold days. Black pudding or blood sausage was available only on special occasions, and today few people eat, let alone make it. Over the years, I have modified my version for taste and practicality. The following is an original version.*

*For the beans*
500 g of dried Tolosa beans or black beans
1½ liters of fresh water
5 tbsp of extra virgin olive oil
1 large onion, finely chopped
Salt

*For the trimmings*
400 g fresh pork ribs, cut into 4 rib racks
200 g fresh pork belly
1 liter of chicken stock
200 ml white wine
Trimmings of the carrot and onion
200 g morcilla de Burgos (Spanish blood sausage) and/or 200 g soft cooking Basque chorizo
Extra virgin olive oil
2 garlic cloves, finely chopped
Whole guindillas peppers to garnish

In a wide sauce pan, place the pork ribs and pork belly with the white wine, chicken stock, and trimmings, and cook on low heat for 3 hours. In the last 15 minutes, add the soft chorizo and black pudding in whole pieces to finish cooking.

Place the soaked beans, onion, and oil in a large pan, and cover with water. Place on moderate heat, and bring to a boil. Lower the heat and simmer for around 2 hours and 30 minutes, preventing the liquid from boiling as it will make the beans break open. Shake the pot now and again to thicken the stew.

Remove all the trimmings. Keep the chorizo and black pudding hot. Heat a frying pan, and fry the pork belly and pork ribs on both sides for 3 minutes each until crispy. Finish in a preheated oven at 180°C/350°F for 5 minutes.

Heat the olive oil and fry the chopped garlic until slightly brown. Add to the tender beans, season the beans with salt.

Serve the beans in a large pot, with crispy pork belly and ribs, black pudding and chorizo, and some guindilla peppers to garnish.

## French Lentils Stew

Makes 6 cups

¼ cup extra virgin olive oil
1 onion, diced
2 cloves garlic, minced
2 carrots, diced
2 stalks celery, diced
1 bulb fennel, diced
1 tbsp chopped fresh parsley
1 can organic tomato sauce
1 bay leaf
3 sprigs fresh thyme
1½ cups French lentils
6 cups filtered water or rich broth
1 tsp Celtic Sea salt
Freshly ground black pepper to taste

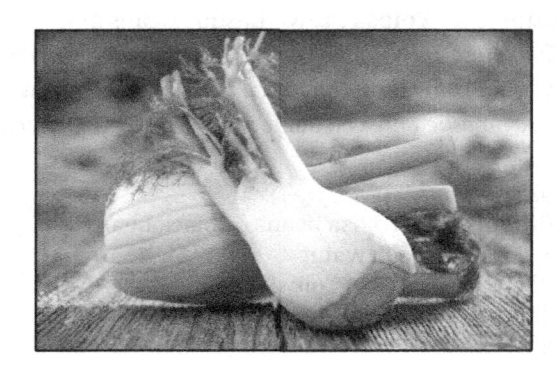

Use small green lentils as most other types can get mushy.

In a large, heavy pot, heat the oil over medium heat until shimmering. Sauté the onion, carrots, celery, and fennel until lightly browned, 7-10 minutes.

Stir in the tomato paste. Cook until it starts to brown, 2-3 minutes. Add the bay leaf, thyme, and lentils.

Stir in 6 cups of water or broth and bring to a boil over high heat. Reduce the heat to medium. Simmer until the lentils are al dente, 20-25 minutes.

Remove and discard the bay leaf and thyme sprigs. Season with salt and pepper.

## Teta's Lentil and Lemon Soup (Nour Danno)

*Teta is grandma in Arabic*

¼ cup of olive oil
2 medium onions
2 cloves of garlic
1 cup of black lentil
6 leaves of Swiss chard
2 medium potatoes chopped
2 cups of vegetable broth or water 1 lemon

In a medium pot, heat the olive oil. Thinly slice the onions and smash the garlic, then add them and cook until golden. Add the lentils and cook on low heat while you prepare the rest.

Wash and chop the Swiss chard, chop the potatoes, and add them both to the pot. Then add the vegetable broth or water and bring it all to a boil.

Check the potatoes and lentils occasionally. Once they are soft, the soup is finished cooking—turn it off and let it cool a bit, then squeeze one lemon in and stir.

**Split Pea Soup with Dulse** (Mira Dessy)
*This is a recipe that for me conjures up childhood in Connecticut. There's something deeply nourishing on so many levels when it comes to enjoying a thick, hearty bowl after being outside on a snow-laden winter day. As a child those snowy days were filled with playtime and I can only image how we looked coming inside all red-cheeked to sit in stocking feet at the kitchen table with a bowl of soup. As an adult it was a welcome way to warm up your insides after snow-blowing the driveway or building snowmen with the kids.*
Serves 6

Served either by itself or as a starter this soup is rich, flavorful, and tastes like comfort in a bowl.

2 carrots, diced
2 ribs celery, diced
1 onion, diced
1 lb dried split peas, picked over and washed
2 tbsp olive oil
1 bay leaf
1 tbsp fresh thyme
6 cups water
1 tsp sea salt
¼ tsp fresh ground pepper
2 tbsp dulse flakes

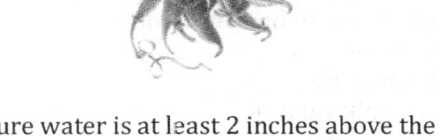

Place all ingredients except dulse into a pot, making sure water is at least 2 inches above the ingredients. Stir well to combine. Bring to a boil.

Reduce heat and simmer for 3 hours until slightly thickened.
Turn off heat and blend ingredients with an immersion blender.

Ladle into bowls, topping each bowl with 1 teaspoon of dulse flakes.

*By adding dulse, an edible seaweed from the North Atlantic or north Pacific regions, this recipe gets a wonderful boost of iodine and a slightly salty umami flavor. Dulse also offers several other nutrients that our bodies need such as vitamin C, alpha-carotene, beta-carotene, lutein, and zeaxanthin, and it contains all the essential amino acids our bodies need.*

## Italian White Bean Soup

Serves 4-5

1 tbsp organic extra virgin olive oil
1 clove garlic, minced
¼ cup onion, diced
1 30 oz can white kidney beans or Great Northern beans (do not drain)
1½ cups water
1½ tsp dried sage
¼ cup celery ⅛ tsp celery seed
¼ cup carrots, diced
½ cup fresh spinach, chopped or frozen
⅛ tsp ground black pepper
Celtic Sea salt

Sauté vegetables in oil with herbs. Add beans, water, and pepper to vegetables. Bring to a boil and cook for 20 minutes. Reduce heat, add spinach and simmer for 5 minutes. The total cooking time is about 25 minutes. Salt to taste after cooking.


**Tam's Refried Beans** (Tammera Karr) are fast to make with canned beans. Place one stick of organic salted butter or "clean" lard in a cast iron skillet, add one quart of canned pinto or black beans, warm and mash with a potato masher, and add Celtic Sea salt to taste. Beans are great in stews and soups and with rice and quinoa dishes.


## Nona's Pasta e Fagioli Soup (Miriam G. Zacharias)

1 cup ditalini or elbow macaroni
2 tsp olive oil
1 onion, minced
1 celery stalk, minced
1 carrot, minced
2 cloves garlic, minced
1 28 oz can of crushed tomatoes, including liquid
2 15 oz cans cannellini beans, drained
4 cups vegetable or meat stock
1 tbsp fresh thyme, minced or 1 tsp dried
1 bay leaf
Dash fresh ground pepper
Parmesan cheese, grated

In a large stock pot, heat the oil. Add the onion, celery, carrot, garlic, and sauté for 5 minutes. Add tomatoes, beans, stock, thyme, and bay leaf. Bring to a boil and simmer, covered, for 30 minutes.

Transfer ½ cup of the beans to a small processor or blender and puree. Return beans to pot and season with salt and pepper to taste. Bring liquid to a boil and add ditalini. Simmer until pasta is tender; add stock if the soup is too thick.

Garnish with basil and Parmesan cheese, and serve.


## **Yellow Split Pea Dhal** (Chef Christine Wokowsky)

4 oz yellow split pea
2 cups water
1 cup coconut water
1 stick cinnamon
2 slices ginger
1 tsp turmeric
1 small onion, finely chopped
2 cloves garlic, finely chopped
1 inch ginger, grated
1 tsp coriander
1 tsp cumin
1 tsp garam masala
½ tsp cayenne
1 tsp cumin seed
1 lemon, juiced
2 tomatoes, chopped
1 bunch cilantro, chopped

Rinse split peas. Bring to boil water, coconut water, cinnamon, turmeric, and ginger. Reduce heat and simmering for 30 minutes. Add split peas.

Heat oil in a frying pan and add cumin seed. Fry for 30 seconds and add onion, chile, and ginger. Fry until the onion is soft. Add garlic, coriander, garam masala, salt, and fry for a further two minutes.

Add tomato plus 100 milliliters of water and allow to cook for 20-30 minutes.
Add spice mix to split peas and stir. Squeeze in lemon juice and serve topped with coriander leaf.

Add in 1-2 tablespoons of fermented veggies.
Omnivores: Add protein of your choice.

### White Beans with Olive Oil & Parsley

1 30 oz can white beans, lightly drained
2½ tbsp extra virgin olive oil
⅛ tbsp ground black pepper
1½ tbsp fresh lemon juice
3 tbsp fresh parsley, chopped
¼ cup red onion, minced
2-3 cloves garlic, crushed
Celtic Sea salt

Place beans, oil, salt, and pepper in a sauce pan. Bring to a gentle boil. Reduce the heat to low. Add lemon juice, onion, parsley, and garlic. Stir and serve hot. Salt to taste.

### Broccoli and Chickpea Curry (Chef Christine Wokowsky)

2 tbsp extra virgin olive oil, ghee or coconut oil
1 small onion, diced
2 cloves garlic, minced
1 inch piece of ginger, grated
½ tsp curry powder
1 head broccoli, cut into florets
1 tomato, chopped
1 cup BPA free canned chickpeas
1 cup canned coconut milk
1 lime, juiced
1 bunch of cilantro, chopped
Salt

In a wok or large pan, sauté the onion, garlic, and ginger. Add the curry powder and salt to taste. Stir well.

Add the broccoli, tomato, chickpeas, and coconut milk. Let simmer for 5-10 minutes. Just before serving, add the lime juice and cilantro.
Add in 1-2 tablespoon of fermented veggies.

### German Lentil & Sausage Soup (Chef Benjamin Qualls)

1 tbsp olive oil
1 12 oz package organic nitrate free smoked sausage, sliced
3-4 medium carrots, chopped
5-6 ribs celery, chopped
1 large onion, chopped

2-3 cloves garlic, chopped
8 cups chicken or vegetable stock
1 tsp Worcestershire sauce
1 bay leaf
¼ tsp nutmeg
¼ tsp caraway seed
2 cups dried lentils, rinsed and drained
Sea salt and black pepper to taste

In a 6–8 quart stock pot, heat olive oil over medium heat. Add smoked sausage, cook, and stir until slightly browned.

Stir in carrots, celery, onion, and garlic. Cook and stir for about 5 minutes.
Add chicken stock, Worcestershire sauce, bay leaf, nutmeg, and caraway seed. Stir in lentils.

Bring mixture to a boil; reduce heat. Cover and simmer for 1 hour, stirring occasionally. Season with sea salt and black pepper.

## Lentil and Chorizo Casserole (Tammera Karr)

½ lb lentils, washed
1 bay leaf
1 tsp Celtic Sea salt
½ tsp dried thyme
¼ tsp ground black pepper
12 cups water
1 lb fried chorizo (cut into little slices and browned)
½ cup each chopped yellow onion, carrot, and celery
1 clove of Italian garlic, crushed
2 tbsp arrowroot or potato starch
1 cup chicken broth
½ cup of good red wine
1 tbsp extra virgin olive oil
2 tbsp butter, melted
1 cup fresh breadcrumbs

Place lentils, bay leaf, salt, thyme, pepper, and water in a cast iron Dutch oven and simmer until lentils are tender, about 30 minutes. (Drain off extra liquid, if any, at this point.)

Add browned sausage and vegetables and olive oil.

In a shaker, combine arrowroot with ¼ cup broth and mix well. Combine remaining broth with wine and thickening mix in a Dutch oven with lentils and sausage; stir well.

Combine bread crumbs in butter, cover the top of lentils and sausage, and bake at 350°F until the top is golden brown and the casserole is very hot.

*I found that, more than anything, my ancestors' work was guided by respect for the food they enjoyed.
Nothing was ever wasted; every bit was put to use.
This sparked creativity as well as resilience and independence.
Above all else, they were healthy and self-reliant.*[139]

~ Sean Sherman – The Sioux Chief
2022 Recipient of the James Beard Award

Antler spoons
*Cow Creek Band of Umpqua Tribe of Indians*, Canyonville Museum, Oregon

## Garam Masala

1 tbsp ground cumin
1½ tsp ground coriander
1½ tsp ground cardamom
1½ tsp ground black pepper
1 tsp ground cinnamon
½ tsp ground cloves
½ tsp ground nutmeg

Mix cumin, coriander, cardamom, pepper, cinnamon, cloves, and nutmeg in a bowl. Place mix in an airtight container, and store in a cool, dry place.

## Mutter Paneer (Medha Mujumdar Murtyy)

*This is an entrée that you will find on the menu card of almost every Indian restaurant in the world! This classic combination of peas and Indian cottage cheese has slight variations based on the region where it is eaten. The recipe is my healthier version that makes it possible to cook up this wonderful curry within minutes!*

¼ cup olive oil
1 cup tomato purée
2 cups cashew nut milk
500 g peas
250 g Paneer* block
2 tsp ginger garlic paste

3 tsp coriander
3 tsp cumin powder
3 tsp garam masala **
2 tsp Kashmiri Lal chile powder
½ tsp spicy chile powder
1 tsp chat masala***
1 tbsp crushed dried fenugreek leaves
¼ cup cilantro, chopped
2 tsp sugar
Salt to taste

* Paneer is a fresh cheese that is very common in Indian cuisine. Easy Paneer Recipe link: https://healthynibblesandbits.com/how-to-make-paneer/
** Garam masala is a spice blend – see recipe
 ***Chat masala - see recipe following

Heat oil in the pan. Add ginger garlic paste and sauté for a minute or until cooked. Add tomato purée and all the dry spices (coriander, cumin powder, Kashmiri chile powder, spicy chile powder, dried fenugreek leaves, and garam masala) except chat masala.

Sauté for 2-3 minutes, and add the peas, cashew nut milk, salt, and sugar. Cover and cook on low, medium heat until the peas are cooked and tender. Now add paneer cubed into 1 inch pieces or to your liking. Simmer for another 3 minutes, garnish with chopped coriander, and serve hot with chapatis or rice.

## Chat Masala

2½ tbsp cumin seeds
1 tbsp coriander seeds
1½ tsp fennel seeds
1½ tsp ajwain seeds, *also known as caraway seeds*
1 tbsp dried minutest
1 tbsp kala namak powder *
1 tsp sea salt
3 tbsp green mango powder
4½ tbsp tamarind powder
1 tsp whole black peppercorns
5 tsp Kashmiri red chile powder **
1 tsp ginger powder

* Kala namak is a kiln-fired rock salt with a sulfurous, pungent smell used in the Indian subcontinent. It is also known as "Himalayan black salt."
***Kashmiri red chile powder is mild and fruity. If you cannot find it and wish to substitute cayenne pepper, be sure to cut the amount used in the recipe by half.*

In a dry sauté pan over medium heat, working with one spice at a time, toast cumin, coriander, fennel, and ajwain until just warm and fragrant. Take care not to burn the seeds. Set each spice aside as it is done.

Combine all toasted spices with dried minutest, kala namak, salt, green mango powder, tamarind powder, black peppercorns, chile powder, and ginger powder. Grind to a fine powder. If using a spice grinder with a limited capacity, grind each ingredient in batches, then thoroughly combine in a small mixing bowl.

Store masala in an airtight container in a cool, dry place for up to 3 months. The masala's flavor is best the day after making once the spices have had a chance to mingle.

> **Principle 18:** *The care and kindness we show others should follow us into the kitchen. Small, meaningful adjustments made in relationships apply to recipes, too.*

### Rajma Masala (Medha Mujumdar Murtyy)

*When I was a child growing up in western India, I had not heard of Rajma. Over the years, that has changed much, and Rajma masala is now loved all over India. It is a competitor to its slightly more common cousin - chana masala. Made from red kidney beans in a tomato gravy, this staple of Northern Indian cuisine, often served with rice as "Rajma Chawal," has recently been voted by the Food Authority of India as the national dish of India!*

2¼ cups cooked red kidney beans
½ cup tomato purée
4 tbsp oil
½ onion, chopped medium
1½ tsp ginger garlic paste
1 pinch of asafoetida**
1 tsp cumin seeds
¾ tsp turmeric powder
2 tsp powdered coriander (seeds) and cumin powder
(Grind 1 measure of coriander seeds plus a ½ measure of cumin seeds to a fine powder.)
1½ cups water
1 tsp salt
¾ tsp Kashmiri chile powder

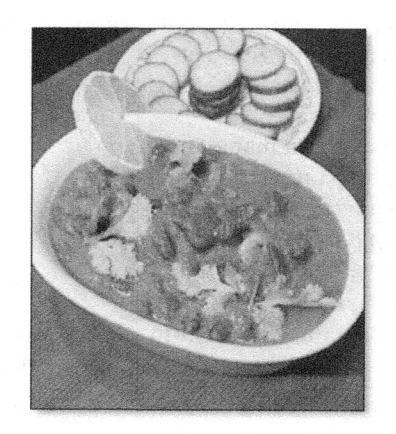

1½ tsp garam masala
1 tsp sugar

*** Asafoetida is the dried sap obtained from the roots of Ferula plants that are part of the celery family.*

Heat oil in a pot/pan. The asafoetida is to be added to the hot oil before adding cumin seeds and ginger garlic paste. Fry for about a minute or until the raw smell of garlic disappears. Add chopped onion and fry until translucent. Add tomato purée and fry for about 3-5 minutes. Add coriander-cumin powder, turmeric powder, and red kidney beans. Stir for a minute and add 1½ cups water.

Let the curry boil and at this point, remove ¾ cup of the curry plus liquid and grind it into a coarse paste. Return the paste to the pot; this will thicken the gravy. Add Kashmiri chile powder (more for color than spicy taste), garam masala, salt, and sugar, and let the curry boil again. Serve hot with rice or roti.

> *"Cookery is an art, a noble science; cooks are gentlemen."*
>
> ~ Robert Burton (1577-1640)

## Brown Kale with Chestnuts (European and American Cuisine 1906, pg 479)
*The following recipe is verbatim from the original text.*

Procure 3 nice heads of brown kale, remove the withered leaves and strip the kale from the stems, wash it thoroughly several times in cold water; place it in a sauce pan, cover with boiling water, set over the fire, and cook 10 minutes; drain in a colander and chop coarsely on a board; return the kale to the sauce pan, add 2 tablespoonfuls poultry fat or pure leaf lard; season with 1 even teaspoonful salt, 1 even teaspoonful pepper, and 1 fine-chopped onion, cover with boiling water, and boil till done, which will take 1½ hour. At the same time place 1 pound large chestnuts over the fire, cook 20 minutes; drain and remove the skin; return the chestnuts in a sauce pan to the fire, cover with white bouillon or broth, add 1 teaspoonful sugar, and boil till tender; then drain, add 1 ounce butter, and toss for a few minutes over the fire. Arrange the kale on a hot dish, around it lay the chestnuts, and around the chestnuts a boarder of small fried German potatoes.

**Ogokbap - Korean Five Grain Rice** (Yuan Wang, *Ancient Wisdom Modern Kitchen*, pg 130)
*This dish is traditionally eaten on a holiday in Korea, that celebrates the first full moon following New Year. Traditionally served with fruits and nuts and considered a national health food. The dish symbolizes a rich harvest in the year to come as well as five good things in life – longevity, wealth, good health, children, and a peaceful death.*

¼ cup dried black soybeans
¼ cup dried red beans
3½ cups water, plus extra for soaking
¼ tsp salt
¼ cup pearl barley or Job's tears
1 cup short grained white rice, uncooked
¼ cup millet
¼ cup pine nuts

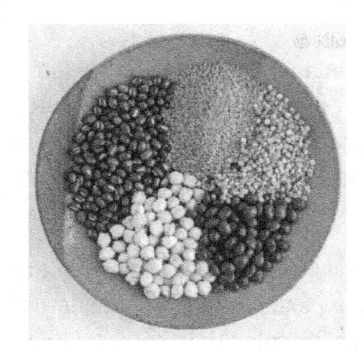

1. Soak all dry beans and grains for at least 6 hours. Except for regular short grain rice and sweet rice. Change water 2-3 times during soaking.
2. When beans and grains are fully soaked, drain and discard water. In your rice cooker/instant pot, add rice, all the soaked beans/grains. Then add water. (Use 1:1 dry grain to water ratio). Add salt.
3. Select mixed grain or brown rice setting. Manual time set at 45 minutes (based on your cooker or if doing on a conventional stove top).
4. while waiting for grains to cook, toast pine nuts in a dry skillet over medium high heat. About 3-5 minutes.

Sprinkle the pine nuts over grains as a garnish before serving.

*Tips & Notes*
Fully soak all beans and change water to make sure all beans are completely re-hydrated and any toxins (lectin) rinsed off.

*Adzuki red beans can cause some irritation for sensitive stomachs. Soak your beans overnight and pre-cook Adzuki beans if you want to make sure it doesn't cause any digestion issues for people with weak stomachs. But I have no issue so it should be fine for most.

---

138 Adapted and retrieved from https://www.bascofinefoods.com/spanish-recipes/alubias-de-tolosa-stew/

139 The Sioux Chef's Native Kitchen page 4

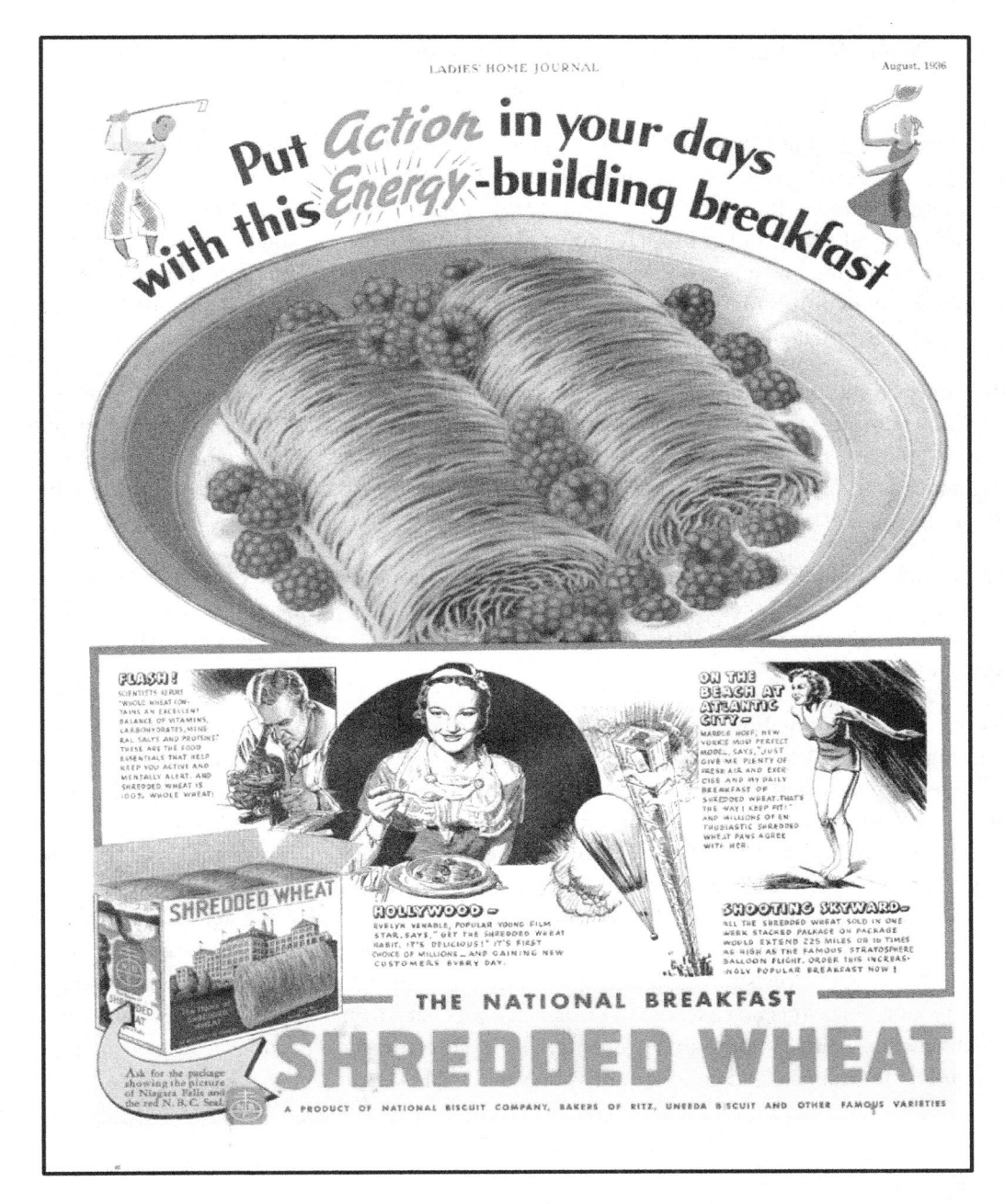

Popular magazine ads have been a source of recipes for over a century. Often, they were featured with a story, movie, or famous star of the day. In 1892, Denver Attorney Henry Perky discovered the health benefits of whole wheat and, together with William Henry Ford, developed a machine that could press whole wheat into tiny shred-like strips. Ladies' Home Journal, 1936.

# Grains

## What does it mean to be a modern-day eater when people aren't really growing their own food?

The conversation about grain and its role in human health can be confusing and contrary. Adding to the confusion is the reference to starches as carbohydrates separate from fruits and vegetables. There are three types of carbohydrates: sugars, starches, and fiber. All plants contain forms of sugar, and grains have some of the highest levels of soluble starches. Starches and fiber are formed when sugars are combined into more complex structures. Starches are complex carbohydrates found in plants. Plants with larger amounts of starch include legumes, cereals, grains, and some vegetables, including corn and potatoes.

All grains are starchy, including rice, oats, quinoa, bulgur, wheat, rye, barley, amaranth, millet, sorghum, triticale, wild rice, and cornmeal. These grains are refined by removing the bran and germ to increase shelf life, and they are often used to make baked goods, including bread, crackers, pasta, and tortillas. The grains and products made with them are considered starches or starchy foods.

A 2020 study in the *Journal of Food Science* looked at a sample of grocery store flours labeled as whole wheat and found that they contained up to 40% less of a specific whole wheat protein than the 100% whole grain standard. So how can the consumer be sure they are getting the flour they are paying for?

In times past, individuals grew their grain, threshed, and transported it to a local mill for grinding. As a result of the industrial revolution, food processing left the local community. It has taken almost a century for artisan grain mills to return to the landscape. *Scotland The Bread* launched its first three flours in the autumn of 2017, milled from varieties of wheat that were common in Scotland in the 19th century. How do you find the seed to revive and research long-forgotten wheat varieties? Modern food explores like Andy Forbes of Brockwell Bake Association in London search seed banks worldwide for viable seeds from history. Ancestral grains and seeds are essential sources of DNA information from which farmers can develop disease and drought-resistant crops. This may mean carefully germinating a small number of seeds to gain more. It is no easy feat to bring lost foods back from the past. It is, however, the safest way to regain lost foods and protect food supplies from insects and diseases no longer responding to chemical and genetic approaches of the 21st century.

### The Research

In 2014, the *James Hutton Institute at Invergowrie* tested 13 samples of wheat from the gene banks worldwide. The initial results revealed two things: 1) all the accessions named *Rouge d'Ecosse* were genetically identical despite decades in seed stores as far apart as Poland and the United States, and 2) all the "old" varieties had generally higher levels of nutritionally-important minerals and trace elements than the types of wheat grown commercially.

## Making Early Medieval Flat Bread

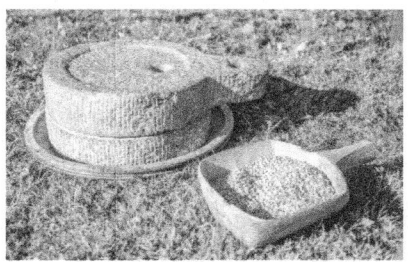

*A small rotary used to grind the flour. Vikings of Middle England*

Cereal husks have survived in the archaeological record, supporting that some bread was made from wheat, barley, rye, and spelt, and some from pulses (peas and beans) mixed with oat flour. Bread has been found in the Viking world, in burials at Birka, Sweden. There's a small biscuit-like bread full of protein found in a cremation burial in Jämtland, Sweden, that may have been mixed with blood (the protein) to make something akin to black pudding.

Leavened bread would require a large clay bread oven to get an even heat for the loaves to rise. Ovens are passively described in an 8th century biography of the abbot of Wearmouth and Jarrow called the *Life of Ceolfrith*. A simpler flatbread, or cake – *kaka* in Old Norse, and what Old English speakers would call *cycel* (pronozd '*kytchel*'), is where we get the words 'cake' and 'kitchen.' Cooked on hot stones, the hot ash of a fire, or on a frying pan or skillet.[140, 141]

## Heritage Grains and Native Preservation.

*Seeds are a vibrant and vital foundation for food sovereignty and are the basis for a sustainable, healthy agriculture. We understand that seeds are our precious collective inheritance, and it is our responsibility to care for the seeds as part of our responsibility to feed and nourish ourselves and future generations.*

*~Native Seed Keepers Network (ISKN)*[142]

Corn, initially used in reference to wheat, today is used almost exclusively by Euro-Americans as the name for maize in North America. Corn is, by volume, high in sugar, which is why it is a significant source of refined sugar in North America.

Is corn a carbohydrate?

Yes. All starches are carbohydrates along with fruits, vegetables, and pulses. Fruits, vegetables, pulses, and whole grains all contain starches. One medium-sized ear of corn contains 19 grams of carbohydrates; of that, 6.4 grams are sugar and 2 grams of fiber.[143]

## Some Surprising History

In 2020, a group of archaeologists in Mexico discovered a 1,300-year-old sculpture of the ancient Mayan Maize God *Hun Hunahpu*. This finding is helping researchers understand the mythical passage of the Maize God's birth, death, and resurrection. Maize, or corn, was more than food for the Mayan's; it was foundational in their beliefs. According to the *Popol Vuh*, the

Mayan's *K'iche'* language creation story, gods created humans out of yellow and white corn. Corn holds an important place in history for archaeology. Records indicate maize was domesticated about 9,000 years ago in Mexico and has also played an essential role in both Mesoamerican culture and the history of archaeology. As it turns out, 9,000 year old maize was one of the first archaeological finds to be carbon-dated. [144]

> *Nixtamalization, when done properly, spins corn into gold: taking something that's of little nutritional value and alchemizing it into a source of nourishment that has carried generations.* [145]

~ Andrea Aliseda

**Nixtamalization**

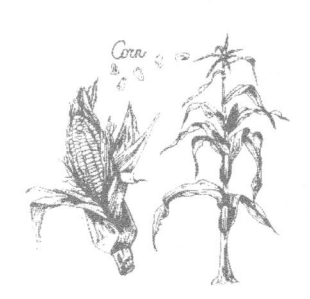

A 3,500 year old technology developed by Mesoamericans is still in use today, transforming maize from grain to sustenance. It's the backbone of approximately 605 Mexican dishes and is known in Mexico as nixtamal.

Andrea Alliseda explains: "The word nixtamal; pronounced by giving the letter *x* a soft *sh* sound, puts together two Nahuatl terms: *nixtli* meaning *ashes*, and *tamalli* meaning *cooked maíz masa*. When nixtamal first originated in 1,000 BC it was used to make tamales, wrapped and steamed *maíz* cakes, and *maíz* drinks, like the thick and warming *atole* and cool fermented *tejuino*. Tortillas came after."

The nixtamalization process significantly affects the nutritional profile of tortillas and related foods. The maize kernels are cooked with ash or calcium hydroxide (known as cal) and steeped in the cooking water. The alkaline quality of the mixture softens the kernels enough to make it possible to peel off their inedible external shell, known as the pericarp, making the corn more digestible. This followed by two washes to ensure the removal of organic components and excess alkali. Nixtamal is the product obtained after this process, and it is then ground to produce a soft dough named masa.[146]

Food inspectors in the U.S. required manufacturers to discard nixtamalized corn before the 21st century. Tortilla manufacturers could not demonstrate the safety of the nixtamalization process to regulators. Inspectors were concerned about the safety of the nixtamalization process, which lacks time and temperature controls familiar to them and instead the process relies solely on *pH* for pathogen control.[147]

### How to Make Nixtamal[148]

The standard ratio for nixtamal starts with the weight of the corn. Then, 1% of the corn's weight in *cal*, which is *calcium hydroxide*. Calcium hydroxide is sold as pickling or slaked lime in some places and in Latin markets.

*Note*: You can use wood ashes, but you will need considerably more to get proper nixtamalization, and it's very messy.

1) Bring water to a boil. Put the corn in the pot, cover with the boiled water by an inch, stir in the cal, and bring this mixture to a boil.

2) The corn will change color; usually, the color will switch toward yellow. Fascinatingly, red corn turns black. Cook the corn for at least 20 minutes. You are really simmering the corn vigorously.

3) Stir the pot every five minutes to keep the *cal* well distributed.

4) After 20 minutes, whole kernel nixtamal has formed and is suitable for several uses. For masa dough, you need to cook your corn for closer to 40 minutes. A bite test** will be necessary to determine if the nixtamal is done.

**After about 20 minutes of solid simmering, remove a kernel and bite it in half; it should be *al dente*. The center should look white and starchy, and the outer layer should start to get a gelatinous look. For flint corn the process take approximately 40 minutes.

> *"The first time I tried a corn tortilla made from real corn was when I lived in Mexico City. I nearly cried because it tasted so good, and because I've been deprived of the real thing for so long."*
>
> ~ Lesley Téllez
> *Nixtamal: A guide to masa preparation in the United States*

### A little more history

When reviewing English and American antique cookbooks dating from the 1860s through the 1940s, Tammera did not find a reference to nixtamal. The use of potash and *cal* are included in recipes for making hominy however. In addition, many foods such as hominy, were being commercially canned for home use by the end of the 19th century.

*Historical recipes are represented as found in the original texts.*

**Hominy** (*Home Comfort Cook Book,* 1864 pg 41)

Wash hominy thoroughly in one or two waters, put in the pan, and cover twice its depth with cold water: bring slowly to boiling point and let simmer – if large, 6 hours; if small or broken, 2 hours; as water evaporates, add hot water; serve with cream, fry in butter, or serve plain with boiled dinner. Hominy Flakes and Hominy Grits may be cooked like corn-meal mush but require cooking for about two hours.

**Hominy Balls** (*Home Comfort Cook Book,* 1864 pg 41)

Form cooked and cooled hominy into small balls about the size of a walnut with dampened hands: roll in fine, soft bread crumbs, dip into a mixture of beaten egg and 3 tbsp milk; roll again in crumbs, and fry in hot lard until browned; serve in place of potatoes. Any of the forms of hominy may be used. Farina may be used in the same way.

**Hominy Pudding** (*Household Cyclopedia,* 1873 pg 76)

This may be either baked or boiled. Mix the hominy (Indian corn bruised) which has been previously boiled, either in milk or water, with eggs, a little sugar, and nutmeg, a little chopped suet, and with or without currents and raisins, as preferred. Tie up in a basin, and boil two hours, or put into a pie dish, and bake in a moderate oven.

**Hominy** (*The New Cyclopedia of Domestic Economy and Practical Housekeeper. Adapted to all classes of society,* 1873 pg 453)

Wash the hominy clean, and boil it with sufficient water to cover it. It should boil from four to five hours over a very slow fire. Eat it with butter and molasses or with sugar and milk. It is considered extremely wholesome food, especially for children and delicate persons.

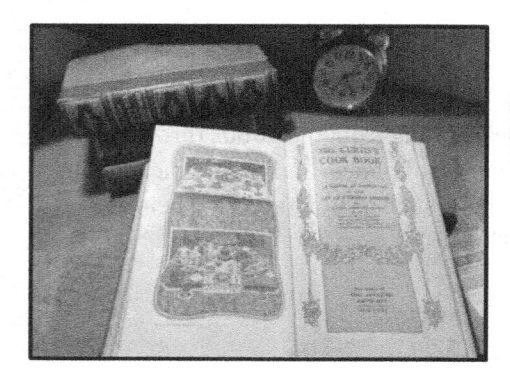

**Hominy or Grits Muffins** (*Mrs. Rorer's Cook Book,* 1886 pg 326)

Make and bake the same as plain muffins; add one cup of cold boiled grits to the batter.

**Hominy Griddle** (*Mrs. Curtis's Cook Book*, 1908 pg 58)

½ cupful boiled hominy
2 eggs
2 cupfuls sour milk
1¼ tsp soda
2 cupfuls flour
½ tsp salt

Warm the hominy and mix with it the well-beaten eggs. Sift in the flour and the salt, alternating with ½ cupful milk till the mixture is ready to beat; at last stir in the soda dissolved in a tbsp of warm water. Bake on a hot griddle. Eat with maple sirup (*spelling from the original source*).

**Raised Hominy Muffins** (*Mrs. Curtis's Cook Book*, 1908 pg 58)

1 cupful cold hominy
4 tbsp butter
1 cupful scalded milk
3 tbsp sugar
½ tsp salt
½ yeast cake dissolved in
¼ cupful lukewarm water

Warm the hominy in a double boiler and break it into grains in a mixing bowl, add milk, sugar, and salt. When it is luke warm, stir in the yeast and enough flour to make a thick batter. Let it stand overnight. In the morning fill gem pans ⅔ full, set to raise in a warm place, and bake in a moderate oven.

### *Preserving culinary culture and seeds*

The Navajo Robin's Egg Corn is grown by Diné Partner Farmer Michael Benally, who lives and grows food for his family on the San Carlos Apache Reservation. This traditional corn is used for tamales and soups and is high in fiber and iron.[149]

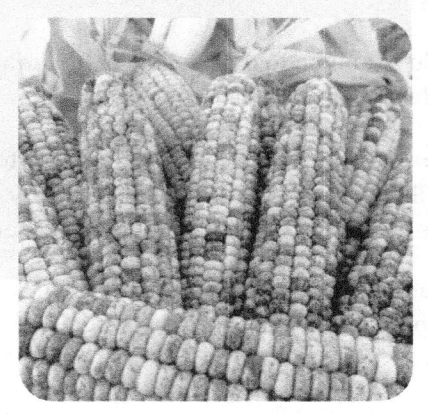

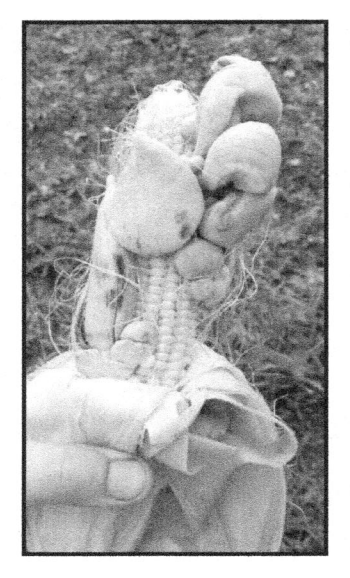

A delicacy in American Native cultures is *huitlacoche,* also known as corn smut. According to Mely Martinez, corn smut has been consumed in Mexico since before the arrival of the Spaniards. It is eaten, usually as a filling, in quesadillas and other tortilla-based foods, and in soups. Huitlacoche is more frequently consumed in central Mexico, where the climate is more humid. This fungus grows on corn when the humidity and temperature are right for it to infect corn and cause the kernels to expand. Huitlacoche does not need to be cooked to be consumed, so it is generally only sautéed lightly before being added to whatever dishes it is used in.

The number one way huitlacoche is prepared in Mexico is in the famous Huitlacoche Quesadillas. This is the most common way that you will find huitlacoche being eaten. Nevertheless, huitlacoche can be used in many dishes, like soups, tamales, tacos, crepes, lasagnas, and raviolis.[150]

### Huitlacoche Tacos (Mely Martinez)
Serves 8

2 tbsp vegetable or olive oil
1 lb huitlacoche rinsed and cut into bite-size pieces
¼ medium size white onion
2 small garlic cloves
4 epazote leaves
Salt to taste
8 corn tortillas, homemade if possible

In a medium frying pan, heat the oil over medium heat. Separately, finely chop the onion and garlic.

Add the onion to the pan and lightly sauté for 2 minutes, or until the onion becomes transparent. Add the garlic and continue cooking for 1 minute.

Next, add the huitlacoche and epazote to the frying pan. As you continue to cook, the huitlacoche will release a bit of liquid, so stir lightly. Continue sautéing for about 5 more minutes, after which the ingredients will be done. Do not overcook them; otherwise, they will become dry.

Place 2 tablespoons of the sautéed ingredients in each tortilla, and serve the tacos alongside a good raw serrano salsa.

> *"Maíz is a cultural creation."* It didn't spring up by accident—the cultivation of *maíz* was intentional.
>
> ~ Guillermo Bonfil-Batalla
> Anthropologist

**Polenta** (Chef Benjamin Qualls)

3 cups water
1 cup cornmeal
1 cup water
1 cup shredded cheese*
Sea salt and black pepper to taste

In a heavy sauce pan, bring 3 cups of water to a boil.
In a mixing bowl, stir together 1 cup cornmeal and 1 cup water.
Add cornmeal mixture slowly to boiling water, stirring constantly.
Reduce heat to low, stir in 1 cup shredded organic, raw cheese, and season with sea salt and black pepper.

Let simmer for 20-30 minutes; stir frequently.
*any shredded cheese you wish

**Green Corn Griddle Cakes** (*The American Woman's Cook-Book* by Ella M. Blackstone, 1920 pg 154)

Six ears of green corn, grated; stir in two eggs, one pint of milk, one pint of flour, two tablespoons of melted butter, a little salt, and one teaspoon of baking powder. Beat well and bake on a hot griddle.

**Hoe-Cake No.1** (*Century Cook Book* by Mary Ronald, 1897 pg 246)

Make the same mixture as for pone. Spread it on the greased hoe, or a griddle, making a round cake one and one fourth inch thick. Bake it on the top of the range, turning and baking it brown on both sides. Serve very hot. They are split and spread with butter when eaten.

> **Distinctively Southern Dishes**
>
> *The dishes in which the South excel, and which may be called distinctive to that section, are those made of cornmeal, of gumbo, or okra and those seasoned with sassafras powder or twigs. The cornmeal used in the South is white and course-grained (it is called there water ground), and gives quite a different result from that which is finer in grain and yellow in color, which is usually sold at the North. The hoe used for baking corn-cakes is an article made for the purpose, and not the garden implement usually associated with the name.*
>
> *~ Century Cook Book*, by Mary Ronald's, 1897, pg 246

## Pone (*Century Cook Book* by Mary Ronald, 1897 pg 246)

Sift a quart of white cornmeal, add a teaspoonful of salt; pour on enough cold water to make a mixture which will squeeze easily through the fingers. Work it to a soft dough. Mold it into oblong cakes an inch thick at the ends, and a little thicker in the center. Slap them down on the pan, and press them a little. These cakes, they say, must show the marks of the fingers. The pan must be hot, and sprinkled with the bran sifted from the meal. Bake in a hot oven for about twenty minutes.

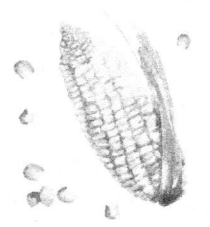

## Fried Cornmeal Mush

3 cups water
1 tsp salt
1 cup organic yellow cornmeal
1 cup "cold" water

Bring the 3 cups of water and salt to a boil in a large heavy-bottomed sauce pan. Stir in the cornmeal and 1 cup of cold water. Cook over high heat and stir constantly to eliminate lumps. When the mixture begins to thicken, decrease heat, and cook 5 minutes longer. Pour hot mush into a buttered loaf pan, and let cool. Cover and refrigerate for several hours. Invert pan and slide loaf out. Slice. Sprinkle pieces with flour. Fry on each side until crispy and golden brown.

Serve with organic butter and heated real maple syrup.

## Corn Griddle Cakes

½ cup organic yellow cornmeal
1½ cups boiling water
2 cups gluten-free flour mix or spelt flour
2 tsp baking powder
½ tsp salt
1 cup organic whole or nut milk
1 egg beaten
2 tbsp butter, melted

Place cornmeal in a small bowl and moisten with a little cold water to prevent lumps. Add moistened meal to the boiling water and boil for 5 minutes. Sift dry ingredients. Stir cornmeal mixture into dry ingredients. Add milk, egg, and butter. Beat.

Ladle onto hot griddle greased with fat. Fry on both sides until golden brown. Serve with hot real maple syrup or fruit compote.

## Mom's Cornbread (Norma Morgan) adapted by Tammera Karr

*My mom was strongly opinionated about cornbread. "None of that cakie stuff is real cornbread," she would say. And we were only allowed to use Albers® yellow corn meal. She insisted the only way to get a real crust was to cook the cornbread in a heavily greased cast iron skillet. Early on she used bacon grease, then later, it was Crisco®. Mom loved crumbling leftover cornbread in a glass and filling it with cold buttermilk.*

1 cup coarse organic corn meal
1 cup organic spelt flour
¼ cup organic sugar
1 tbsp baking powder
1 tsp Celtic Sea salt
1 cup organic buttermilk
⅓ cup extra virgin olive oil
1 egg lightly beaten

Heat oven to 400°F.

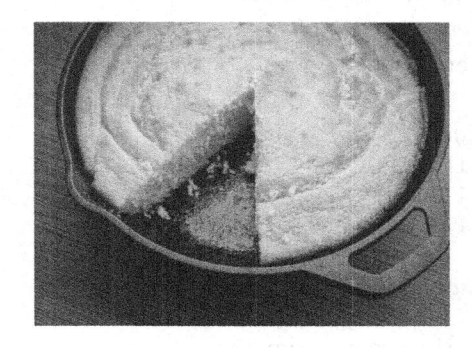

Combine and mix dry ingredients in a bowl, and form a well in the center. Combine egg, oil, and buttermilk in a smaller bowl and mix well; add to dry ingredients. Using a wooden spoon, gently mix liquid into cornmeal mix, do not overwork the leavening. Let set while buttering an 8-10 inch cast iron skillet, pour cornbread mix into skillet, and place in the oven for 20-25 minutes and golden brown top. Test for doneness with a thin knife blade in the center.

> "DNA probes and other technologies have been detailing the roughly 9,000-year process by which Native Americans transformed teosinte, the smallish semitropical grass with no ears or cobs, into maize, a productive, elaborate plant that can thrive in a cool temperate climate.
>
> In a 2003 analysis of cobs from Tularosa and locations in Mexico, researchers found that the earliest samples, some 6,300 years old, were apparently bred by people focused on boosting the crop yield by increasing the size of cobs and kernels. Later, in Mogollon times, growers were selecting for starch and grain qualities useful in making tortillas and tamales.
>
> The transformation of a weedy grass into one of the world's most important foodstuffs is far more complex than anything we can do today in a lab, even with all our genetic prowess. How the continent's first farmers accomplished that feat is a mystery." [151]

Smithsonian Magazine

### Semolina Dumplings (Chef Ben Qualls)

*This semolina dumpling recipe is very easy to make. It does not require many ingredients, preparation time, or advanced cooking skills. Making those fluffy dumplings is always a challenge. You have to figure out the right egg-semolina ratio and find the fine balance in order to make soft yet stable dumplings.*

Serves 4

*Equipment*
 1 Bowl
 1 Spoon
 1 Medium pot

*Ingredients*
 2 whole eggs
 3½ oz coarse semolina
 1 tbsp salt

In a bowl mix eggs with of semolina. Do not whisk the eggs, just stir gently.

Do not add any salt to the mixture. Put it in the refrigerator for about 5 minutes, the semolina will absorb some moisture, the batter will get thicker.

In a larger pot heat 1 liter of water, add 1 tablespoon of salt, and bring it to a boil.

Form small, ellipse-shaped dumplings using two tablespoons. Drop the dumplings in the boiling water and simmer for about 10 minutes. They will double in size. Remove, place them onto a plate, and serve in the hot soup.

> From ancient 7,400 year old rice in China to wild rice domestication in the Amazon 4,000 years ago, humankind on every continent has utilized this grain. [152, 153]

**Sweet Coconut Brown Rice** (Medha Mujumdar Murtyy)
*Narali Poornima (Coconut Day) is observed in the western state of Maharashtra in India during the full moon in late July or early August based on the Indian Hindu calendar. On this day, fishermen offer a coconut to the sea with prayers for their safety as they mark the end of the monsoon and the beginning of the fishing season. The day also coincides with another festival called Raksha Bandhan, celebrating the love between brother and sister and assurance of the brother's protection to the sister throughout life. Sweet coconut rice is a special delicacy that marks both these celebrations. Traditionally made with white basmati rice and sugar, the recipe is a healthier version made with brown rice and jaggery\* and tastes richer than the original version.*

2½ tbsp of unsalted butter
1 cup cooked brown basmati rice
¾ cup grated coconut (fresh)
½ cup jaggery
2-inch piece cinnamon stick
2 black cardamoms
5 green cardamoms
5-6 cloves
1 tsp freshly ground cardamom powder
6 walnut ¼ pieces

Cook brown basmati rice as per instructions [soaking basmati brown rice for 30 minutes]. Heat butter and add cinnamon sticks, black and green cardamoms, and cloves.

Sauté slightly until the spices release aroma.
Next, add the cooked rice, freshly grated coconut, and jaggery and mix it well.

Cook it on low, medium flame until the jaggery melts.

Continue stirring in between to ensure the rice does not stick to the bottom of the pan.
Add cardamom powder and chopped walnuts. You can also add saffron strands or a pinch of nutmeg powder as per your preference. Serve hot or cold as desired.

**Spiced Brown Rice Bowl** (Chef Christine Wokowsky)

1 tbsp extra virgin olive oil
1 cup cooked brown rice
½ onion, diced
1 clove garlic, minced
½ inch ginger, peeled and grated
1-2 leaves collard greens, ribs removed and chopped
1 small carrot, peeled and shredded
½ cup beans of your choice (pinto, black, lentils, etc.)
¼ tsp of any of the spices mentioned above

In a sauté pan over medium-low heat, add the olive oil. Next, add onions and sauté until translucent. Add garlic and ginger, and spices. Next, add the remaining ingredients, stirring to mix well.

**Meghli** (Nour Danno)
*A very healthy dessert*

2 cups of rice flour
6 cups water (2 cups to start, then the remaining later)
½ cup coconut sugar
1 tsp cinnamon
2 tbsp caraway
2 tbsp shredded coconut
2 tbsp pistachios
2 tbsp raisins
2 tbsp pine nuts

After the flour is done soaking, boil the remaining 4 cups of water in a large pot. While the water boils, prepare the sugar, cinnamon, and caraway and put them within reach of the stove.

Once the water boils, mix the soaked rice flour into the pot with a whisk. Keep the heat at medium and add the sugar and spices slowly; whisking constantly. Stir occasionally until it all thickens (about 50 minutes).

Pour into bowls, garnishing with the nuts, raisins, and shredded coconut.
Let them firm up and chill in the refrigerator for three hours, then serve.

**Quinoa and Watercress Salad** (Tammera Karr)

2 cups quinoa, cooked
2 Roma tomatoes, chopped
2 cloves fresh garlic, chopped
1 fennel bulb, chopped
1 watercress, good sized bunch chopped
2 sweet red, orange, or yellow peppers, chopped
1 Walla Walla onion, medium sized chopped
2 green chilies, medium sized chopped
½ cup pine nuts or pecans

*Mix to taste*
Olive oil, rice vinegar, Celtic Sea salt, black pepper, crushed garlic, turmeric, basil, and a dash of cayenne.

Mix everything together and eat fresh, warm, or cold. Keeps well refrigerated.

> *Quinoa* is a tall South American herb native to the high altitude of the Andes and characterized by small green clustered flowers and small fruits with a single seed. The name also is used for the edible, high-protein seeds, and dried fruits, which have served as a staple food for many people in South America since pre-Colombian times. Quinoa is a pseudocereal rather than a true cereal because, like amaranth and millet, it is not a member of the grass family.[154]

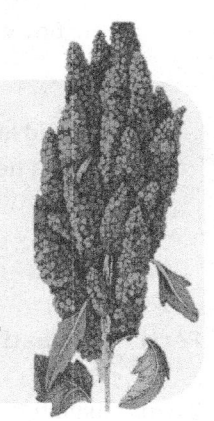

**Quinoa Salad** (Nicole Hammond)

1 cup cooked quinoa (cook for about 15-20 minutes)
1 cup shiitake mushrooms
2 cups chopped tomatoes
½ cup finely chopped red onion
½ cup finely chopped or matchstick carrots
2 cups arugula
½ cup shaved Parmesan or goat cheese

*For dressing*
¼ cup olive oil
¼ cup lemon juice
2 tsp sea salt
1 tsp black pepper

6 basil leaves chopped
2 cloves finely garlic

Toss everything together and serve with a balsamic glaze over the top.

> ### *The Aymara Spoke with the Stars* – Andean Legend
>
> The Andean legend tells us about a young boy that took care of the crops by Lake Titicaca. He watched over them because his people thought they were being stolen.
>
> One night, the boy discovered a group of country girls in the crops, so he made them go away. They turned into birds and flew away to the stars. Bewildered, the boy went looking for one of the stars on the back of a condor and he found her.
>
> She fed him with quinoa and when he returned to Earth, she gave him this seed so that he would feed his people.[155]

## **Persian Basmati Rice** (Nicole Hodson)

3 cups basmati rice
3 tbsp avocado oil
2 tsp Himalayan pink salt

Rinse the uncooked rice in warm water and swish in enough water to loosen the starch from the rice. Pour off water and repeat 4 more times.

Put rice in a pot and cover with at least 3 inches of water, add salt and bring to a boil. After a few minutes, check the rice by trying to break a grain in half with your fingernail. Once the rice breaks easily, remove it from the heat and drain the rice; do not rinse.

Meanwhile, dry the pot and return it to the stove on medium high heat. Add the avocado oil and wait until the heat causes ripples in the oil. Carefully add the rice to form a layer and cover the bottom of the pan. Add the remaining rice to form a pyramid in the center of the pot. Cook at this heat uncovered for 8-10 minutes; this will cause the rice to crisp up and create a golden crust, referred to as *Tah-dik* (means bottom of the pot).

Cover the lid of the pot with a kitchen towel – this is to prevent any moisture from escaping – and cover the pot. Turn the heat down and simmer for an additional 30 minutes. Serve with kabob, veggies, or anything you like and *enjoy!*


**Egyptian Tigernut Sweets** [156, 157]
*This recipe was on the tomb walls of Rekhmire, vizier of Pharaoh Tuthmosis III (Eighteenth Dynasty) from the 5th century BC. Ms. Manniche's translation comes from pictures on the tomb walls themselves.*

Grind a quantity of tigernuts in a mortar. Sift the flour carefully.
Add a bowl of honey to the ground tigernuts and mix it into a dough.

Transfer the dough to a shallow metal vessel. Place on top of the fire and add a little fat. Boil over a gentle fire until a firm paste is obtained. It must smell roasted, not burnt. Cool and shape into tall conical loaves.


**Kunun Aya Refresher** (Karen Langston)

1 cup raw tigernuts (I get mine from tigernutsusa.com)
Water for soaking
1 cup organic unsweetened coconut flakes or shredded coconut
1 inch fresh ginger
1-2 dates (I don't use any sweeteners as the tigernuts are sweet enough)
6 cups of filtered water
¼ tsp Celtic Sea salt

1) Place the tigernuts in a large glass bowl and add water; about 4-5 cups. Place on the counter and soak for 24 hours. Drain water and lightly rinse, then fill the bowl with another 4-5 cups of water and soak for an additional 24 hours totaling 48 hours.

2) Once soaked, pour the tigernuts and liquid through a colander and rinse well. Pick through and discard any tubers that are black or do not look good.

3) Add 6 cups filtered water, tigernuts, 1 cup organic shredded coconut, 1 inch piece of fresh ginger and dates if using, and ¼ teaspoon Celtic Sea salt in a high-powered blender.

4) Puree on high until smooth and creamy. Pour liquid through a fine mesh strainer, nut bag, or cheesecloth into a bowl; squeeze and strain the liquid into the bowl.

5) Pour milk into a glass jar and store in the refrigerator for up to 3 days. Shake before using because the beneficial resistant starch will collect on the bottom, which also contains all the flavor.

### Sherry's Tigernut Pancakes (Sherry Holub)

Makes 4 medium size pancakes.

2 eggs
¾ cup tigernut flour
¼ cup almond flour
¼-½ cup water (you can also sub in coconut milk, almond milk, hemp milk, whatever milk you prefer); adjust the amount for waffles or pancakes
1 tsp baking powder
1 tsp vanilla
¼ tsp salt

They come out fluffy and tasty.

### Greek Greens and Rice Salad (Chef Christine Wokowsky)

2 cups assorted leafy greens
¼ cup purple cabbage, cut thin
4-6 Kalamata olives
4-6 green olives
2 artichoke hearts in a glass jar
¼ cup garbanzo beans
¼ cup cooked quinoa or brown rice
1 tbsp each fresh oregano and basil leaves

A simple dressing of olive oil, red wine vinegar, a bit of Dijon, dried oregano and basil, sea salt, and freshly ground black pepper. You can also add sundried tomatoes.

> *"Cookery is naturally the most ancient of the arts, as of all arts it is the most important."*
>
> ~ George Ellwanger (1848-1906)
> *Pleasures of the Table* (1902)

### Brotchan Foltchep (Savory Irish Oat and Leeks)

2 lbs leeks
2 oz gluten-free oatmeal
2 pints of chicken stock
A knob of Kerrygold butter
2 tbsp fresh parsley, minced
Celtic Sea salt and pepper

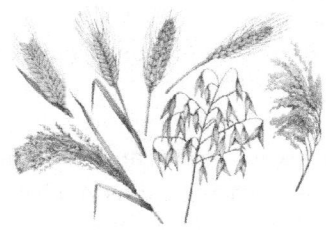

Bring stock to the boiling point, sprinkle in oatmeal, add butter and cook gently for half an hour. Add the washed and thinly sliced leeks, including some green parts. Simmer until the leeks are cooked, about 30 minutes more. Season to taste and serve sprinkled with minced parsley.

### Oatmeal Muffins (*The Great 20th Century Cook Book: Three Meals a Day: Cooking Table, Toilet, Health* by Maud C Cooke, 1902 pg 185)

1¼ cupfuls of sour milk
2 beaten eggs
1 level tsp of soda
2 tbsp of melted butter
¼ tsp of salt
Oatmeal to make a stiff batter

Beat the batter briskly; pour in buttered muffin rings and bake in a quick oven. Delicious eaten hot.

### Ezekiel Bread (Ben Rayl, *Comfortable Food*)

"Take also unto thee wheat, barley, beans, and lentils and millet, and spelt and put them in one vessel, Ezekiel 4:9  Ezekiel bread is sprouted, which increases digestibility and increases the bioavailability of nutrients.

2 cups water - warm
2 tbsp honey
¼ cup olive oil
1 package dry yeast - or 25 g fresh
1 cup wheat flour - or 1½ cups wheat berries
1 cup spelt flour - or 1¼ cups spelt grains
¼ cup millet flour - or ⅓ cup millet grains
⅛ cup green lentils - dry
4 tbsp kidney beans, dry
2 tbsp black beans, dry

¼ cup oat bran
¼ tsp salt

Measure the water, honey, olive oil, and yeast into a large bowl. Let it sit until foamy, about 5 minutes.

Stir the whole grains and beans until well mixed, then grind in a flour mill or blender and blend together with any grains you had that were already ground.

Add this flour mixture to the yeast mixture and stir until well combined - the dough will be very sticky and wet.

Pour the dough into a prepared loaf pan and let rise in a warm place for about 45 minutes, or until it reaches the top of the pan.

Bake at 350°F or 175°C for about 45-50 minutes, or until golden brown.

*Notes:*
Remember that flour may vary if the ingredient is in grain or already ground. If you can find it in grains, you have to add a little more to have the right amount. The idea is to have a bread dough that is NOT hard, more of a paste consistency (could be slightly sticky, but not too much, definitely not liquid!). That is why you add the flour to the liquid and not the other way around.

To grind the flour, I used a blender, it worked perfectly fine with all the grains; just make sure to let it run long enough so everything is broken into flour consistency (around 5 minutes). An important thing is not to put too many grains in the blender (never over 2 cups) because the weight of the grains will prevent the ones on the bottom from being ground. At the same time, be careful to not put too little in either because the speed of the blades will make the grains fly and then prevent them from being ground. It is all a matter of balance, if necessary, turn the blender off and use a spoon to mix the grains so the ones in the bottom are sure to be ground.

*In my recipe, I used kidney and black beans, but you could very well use pinto, soy, or any other kind of beans as you wish, just do not exceed the 6 tablespoons in total.*
*https://comfortablefood.com/*

> **History of Sourdough Bread**
>
> Until the development of commercial yeasts, all leavened bread was made using naturally occurring yeasts. In other words, all bread was sourdough, with its slower rise.
>
> Bread is older than metal; even before the bronze age, our ancestors ate and baked flatbread. There is evidence of neolithic grinding stones used to process grains, probably to make flatbread. The Egyptians discovered and recorded the use of leavening; there is some discussion about how this process happened and the degree to which there was an overlap between brewing and bread-making. What is not in doubt is that the ancient Egyptians knew both the brewing of beer and the process of baking leavened bread with sourdough, as proved by wall paintings and analyses of desiccated bread loaves and beer remains (Rothe et al., 1973; Samuel, 1996).[158]

## Salt Rising (Risen) Bread

*Starter 1*
¼ cup (57 g) milk
2 tbsp (14 g) cornmeal
1 tsp sugar

*Starter 2*
1 cup (227 g) hot water (120°F to 130°F)
½ tsp salt
½ tsp baking soda
½ tsp sugar
1½ cups (177 g) unbleached all-purpose flour

*Dough*
4 tbsp (57 g) soft butter
½ tsp salt
2¼ to 2½ cups (269 g to 298 g) unbleached all-purpose flour

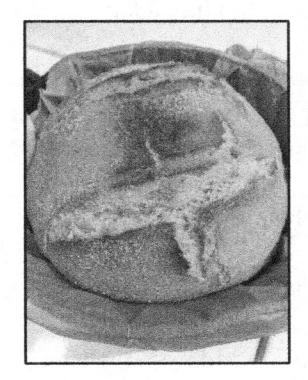

To make Starter 1: Heat the milk until it's nearly but not quite boiling; small bubbles will form around the edge of the pan, and you might see a bit of steam. This is called "scalding" the milk.

Cool the milk until it's lukewarm, then whisk together the milk, cornmeal, and sugar in a small heatproof container. The container should be large enough to let the starter expand a bit. Whisking vigorously will help prevent lumps.

Cover the container with plastic wrap, and place it somewhere warm, between 90°F and 100°F. We find our turned off electric oven, with the light turned on for about 2 hours ahead of time, holds a temperature of 95-97°F, perfect for this starter.

Let the starter rest in its warm place overnight or for 8-12 hours. It won't expand much but will develop a bubbly foam on its surface. It'll also smell a bit fermented. If it doesn't bubble at all and doesn't smell fermented, your starter has failed; try using different cornmeal or finding a warmer spot.

To make Starter 2: Combine the hot water (120-130°F) with the salt, baking soda, and sugar, stirring to combine. Add the flour, stirring until everything is thoroughly moistened.

Stir Starter 1 into Starter 2.

Cover the bowl with plastic wrap, and place it in the same warm spot Starter 1 was in. Let it rest until very bubbly and doubled in size, 2-4 hours. If it's not showing any bubbles after a couple of hours, move it somewhere warmer. If it still doesn't bubble after a couple of hours, give it up; you'll need to start over.

Transfer your bubbly starter to a larger bowl or the bowl of a stand mixer (or your bread machine bucket). Stir in soft butter, salt, and flour. Knead until smooth; the dough will be soft and fairly elastic/stretchy.

Shape the dough into a log, and place it in a lightly greased 8½ x 4½ inch loaf pan.

Cover the pan, and place it back in its warm spot. Let the loaf rise until it's crowned about ½-¾ inch over the rim of the pan, which could take up to 4 hours or so. This won't form the typical large, domed top; it will rise straight up, with just a slight dome.

Preheat the oven to 350°F.

Bake the bread for 35-40 minutes until it's nicely browned. Again, it won't rise much; that's OK.

Remove the bread from the oven; if you have a digital thermometer, it should read about 190°F to 200°F at its center. Wait 5 minutes, then turn it out of the pan onto a rack to cool.

Store cooled bread at room temperature for 5-7 days; freeze for longer storage.

> Bread has a long standing history, shaped by cultural movements in Ireland over the centuries. The first bread of the Gaelic Irish was actually a simple rustic oatcake. Oatcakes are still traditional in Northern Ireland. The Anglo-Normans brought wheaten bread when they settled in Leinster and Munster in the 1100s. Later, refined flours became the symbol of the wealthy, whilst rural communities still used whole meal brown flour for their homemade loaves.[159]

## Irish Soda Bread

3 cups Bob's Red Mill 1-1 Gluten Free Baking Flour, plus extra for work surface
¼ cup coconut sugar
1 tsp baking powder
1 tsp baking soda
½ tsp Celtic Sea salt
4 tbsp Kerrygold butter, melted
2 tbsp caraway seeds (optional)
1 cup currants
1 cup organic buttermilk
1 egg

Heat oven to 350°F. In the bowl of a standing mixer with the paddle attachment, combine flour, sugar, baking powder, baking soda, and salt. Add butter, caraway seeds, and currants. Combine just until incorporated.

In a small bowl, whisk together buttermilk and egg. Add to dough; mix just until incorporated.

Turn dough onto a lightly floured surface and fold it over onto itself two or three times, shaping it into a round 8 inch loaf. You can also use a tube pan to help shape the loaf. Transfer to a buttered cast iron skillet. If desired, score an "x" on the top of the dough.

Bake 45 minutes until well-browned and a toothpick inserted into the center emerges clean. Remove to a wire rack to cool completely before slicing.

> It is challenging to make yeast-leavened bread due to the climate in Ireland. Cooks, with the touch to make yeast bread, quickly became sought after by the Gentry, as did their bread. Soda bread is synonymous with Ireland.

## Traditional Irish Soda Bread [160]

3½ cup all-purpose flour, plus extra for dusting
1 tsp granulated sugar
1 tsp baking soda
1 tsp salt
1½–2 cups buttermilk or soured milk (coconut or rice milk)

*Hint — To make your own soured milk, gently heat milk until warm. Remove from the heat, add the juice of ½ lemon and leave at room temperature overnight.*

Preheat the oven to 450°F

Mix flour, sugar, baking soda, and salt into a large bowl.

Pour in most of the buttermilk, leaving about ¼ cup to use as needed. Using your fingers, bring the flour and liquid together, adding more buttermilk, if necessary. *Don't knead the mixture, or it will become heavy. The dough should be soft but not too wet or sticky.*

When the dough begins to stick together, remove it from the bowl and place the dough onto a floured work surface, and form into a ball. Pat the dough down into a circle, about 1½ inches thick, and cut a deep cross. Place on a baking sheet or in a greased cast iron skillet.

Bake for 15 minutes. Turn down the heat to 400°F for an additional 30 minutes. When done, the loaf will sound slightly hollow when tapped on the bottom and be golden in color. Allow to cool on a wire rack until you are ready to eat.


## Libby's Buttermilk Baking Mix (Libby Karr, 1930)

4½ cups white spelt flour or Bob's Red Mill Gluten Free All-Purpose Flour
¾ cups buttermilk blend powder
2½ tbsp baking powder
½ tsp baking soda
1½ tsp Celtic Sea salt
2 tbsp coconut sugar
1 tsp cream of tartar
1 cup organic butter, lard, coconut, or red palm oil

In a large bowl or food processor, blend the dry ingredients. Cut in coconut or palm oil with a pastry cutter or in your food processor until it looks like small crumbs.

Store in an air-tight container.

**Drop Biscuits or Dumplings** (Libby Karr, 1950)

1 cup Libby's Buttermilk Baking Mix
¼ cup cold water, plus 1 tablespoon water

Gently stir together; it should be like cookie dough. Use a soup spoon to make large drops of batter into rolling boil broth or onto a buttered cookie, jelly roll, or cast iron pan.

Bake at 425°F for 11-12 minutes. Depending on the elevation, you may need to finish browning the top with a broiler.

**Pancake Mix** (Libby Karr, 1955)

8 cups sifted spelt flour
4 tsp Celtic Sea salt
4 tsp baking powder
10 tsp organic lard or Kerrygold butter
¾ cup powdered milk

Mix well and store in a sealed glass jar.

To make pancakes: 1 cup of mix, 1 egg, and water.
Mix egg and ¾ cup water, and whip the egg into the water.
Combine egg and water with dry mix, and stir until combined.
Heat cast iron griddle; test by flicking a drop of water on the surface; it should sizzle. Add a thin layer of oil to the griddle surface with a pastry brush or paper towel, then pour the batter onto the surface. When bubbles appear on the surface of the pancake, flip and cook on the other side.

*A little history*

The waffle irons of today have their history in the 15th century Netherlands. Offshoots of the wafer waffle iron with long handles and propped over the fire were used in the American colonies. In 1854, cast iron waffle *furnaces* developed the divided grid pattern. By the early 20th century, the waffle iron was electric and used at the table for dinner or breakfast.[161]

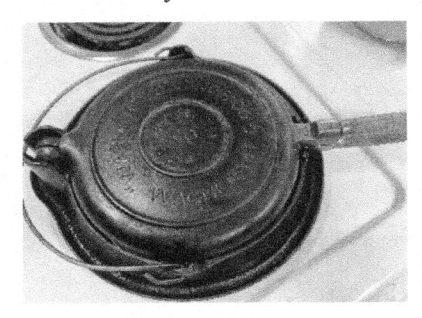

Wagner Cast Iron Waffle Iron
Patent July 26, 1892
Michael Karr collection

**Plain Waffles** (*Mrs. Rorer's Philadelphia Cook Book: A Manual of Home Economics*, 1886 pg 328)

1 qt of sifted flour
1 tsp of salt
3 eggs
2 oz butter
½ cup of yeast or ½ a compressed cake
1½ pints milk

Rub the butter into the flour, add the salt, then the milk --- which should be scalded and cooled, and the yeast; beat thoroughly and continuously for three minutes; cover and stand in a warm place for two hours, or until very light. Then beat the eggs separately, add to the batter first the yolks and then the whites; let stand fifteen minutes. Have the waffle iron gradually and thoroughly heated. Dip a small paint brush in melted suet and brush the iron until every part is well greased. Pour the batter into a pitcher, so that you may fill the iron quickly. Open the iron, pour the batter from the pitcher into the iron until you have covered the elevations, close the iron quickly and turn it over. Bake about two minutes, or until a nice golden brown; then remove them carefully, place on a hot dish, and serve quickly.

**Rice Waffles** (*Mrs. Rorer's Philadelphia Cook Book: A Manual of Home Economics*, 1886 pg 328)
Make the same as Plain Waffles, adding one cup of boiled rice with flour.

**Grits Waffles** (*Mrs. Rorer's Philadelphia Cook Book: A Manual of Home Economics*, 1886 pg 329)
Make the same as Plain Waffles, adding one cup of boiled grits with flour.


**Waffles** (*A Thousand Ways to Please a Husband with Bettina's Best Recipes*, 1917 pg 326)
Serves 6

1¾ cup flour
2 tbsp sugar
1 tsp salt
3 tsp baking powder
2 well-beaten eggs
¾ cup milk
1 tbsp melted butter

Mix and sift the flour, sugar, salt and baking-powder. Add the eggs and milk. Beat two minutes. Add the butter. Bake in well-greased waffle irons.

**Waffles** (*The American Woman's Cook-Book* by Ella M. Blackstone, 1920 pg 154)

Take one pint of sour milk, three tbsp of melted butter, three eggs, beaten separately, a tsp of soda, dissolved in a little warm water, add a little salt, and stir in enough flour to make a stiff batter. Bake upon waffle irons.


**Buckwheat Waffles** (Michael Karr)

*This recipe is an adaptation of my mother's waffle recipe and others from the 1940s. I prefer Bob's Red Mill Buckwheat flour; it is less refined and has a more robust flavor.*
Yields 4

1 cup buckwheat flour (fine grind)
½ tsp Celtic Sea salt
2 tsp baking powder
½ tsp baking soda
1 tbsp coconut sugar
3 large eggs (separated)
1¼ cup buttermilk or rehydrated buttermilk powder (using buttermilk powder may require adjusting the liquid quantity)

Sift flour, salt, baking powder, baking soda and sugar together.

Beat egg yolks and add milk. Stir egg yolks and flour together. Beat egg whites until they form stiff peaks. Fold egg whites into the mixture gently, do not overwork.

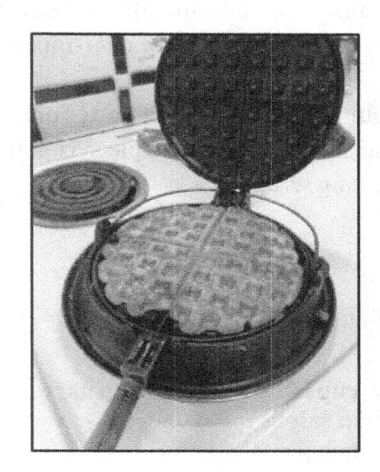

Cook in a waffle iron of your choice. Using butter to grease the waffle iron is preferred by this cook.


### Buckwheat – a pioneer food

Buckwheat, unlike grains from the grass family, contains all eight essential amino acids in excellent proportions; including lysine. Because of that, buckwheat is a surprisingly rich source of protein. One cup of buckwheat delivers 23 grams of high-quality protein and is gluten-free.

**Buckwheat Pancakes** (Norm Michaels)
Serves 4

1 cup organic buckwheat flour
2 tsp baking powder
1 tbsp organic coconut sugar (optional)
1 egg
1 ¼ cup water

NOTE: Buckwheat flour, when combined with liquid, easily thickens. Extra water, milk, or ½ & ½ may be added to thin the batter to personal taste.

Combine dry ingredients, and mix well. Add egg to buttermilk and whisk together gently, add to dry ingredients. Do not over-mix as it will kill the leavening properties of the baking powder.

Pour desired rounds of batter onto a heated cast iron griddle, cook each side till golden brown and serve with real maple syrup, fruit compote, molasses, or let cool and use as a tortilla for making wraps.


**Buckwheat Grits** (Liz Lipski)

2½ cups fine buckwheat grits
½ tsp salt
1 pinch paprika
1 egg
2 cups boiling water
2 tbsp organic butter, ghee

Mix salt, paprika, and grits with egg, and place in a dish in the oven to brown. Pour and stir in as much water as it will take, add fat, cover, and bake for 20 minutes or until tender.

*Note:* This can be used as a rice side dish with chicken, fish, or lamb.


**Buckwheat Naan Bread** (Tammera Karr)
Yields 4

¾ cup buckwheat flour or arrowroot starch
3 tbsp coconut flour
¼ tsp salt
1 egg
1 cup full fat coconut milk or ½ & ½

2 cloves garlic, finely chopped

Combine flour or arrowroot starch, coconut flour, and salt in a medium bowl, and mix to combine.

In a separate bowl, whisk an egg with coconut milk, add the wet mixture to the dry mixture and stir until well incorporated. Allow to sit on the countertop for 5-10 minutes for the batter to thicken.

Heat a 9 inch pan over medium-low heat and add a little bit of oil to it, then spoon about ⅓ cup of batter into the pan and cook on each side for 2-3 minutes.

Sprinkle with fresh or roasted garlic and drizzle with olive oil; serve warm.


## Buckwheat Rye Bread

2½ cups white spelt flour
1 cup buckwheat flour
1 cup dark rye flour
2 tsp Celtic Sea salt
1 tsp yeast
1 tbsp blackstrap molasses
1¼ cups water, approximate

Combine molasses and warm 100°F; set aside.

Combine all dry ingredients, form a well in the center and add water and molasses. Stir together, turn out onto a floured surface, and knead in all flour plus ¼ cup more. The dough should form a ball but will still be sticky.

Place dough in a large bowl, cover with a tea towel and set aside out of cool drafts. Let proof for 4-6 hours. This allows the grains to absorb more moisture and the yeast to grow.

Turn dough out on a floured surface and knead out air while working in ¼ cup more flour. Form into round peasant loaves, place in a cast iron Dutch oven, or divide and place into loaf pans. Place in a warm oven (100°F) and let double. Bake at 400°F, for 30-35 minutes.

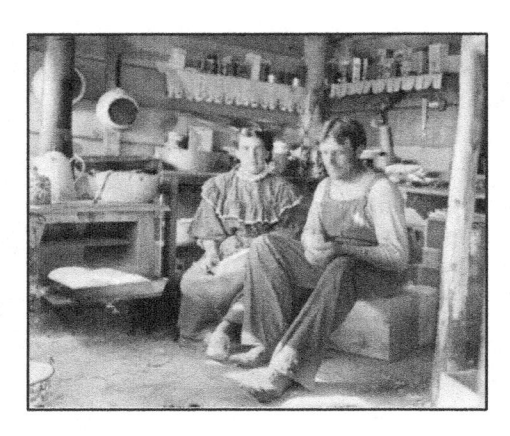

Mrs. Johnstone's cookbook came with some old-time advice, as well as recipes:

*To keep a husband, he must not be stewed, basted, roasted, scorched, soaked, chilled, parboiled, nor beaten; but endeavor to reach his heart three times daily, by following the directions given in the foregoing recipes, and the happiest results are promised. A Collection of Her Own Recipes Faithfully Tested in Montana*, Butte Miner, 1905 pg 73

## German Caraway Bread

2 cups scalded milk
2 tbsp organic sugar
2 tbsp organic butter
1 tsp salt
1 measure yeast
½ cup lukewarm water (100°F)
2 tbsp caraway seeds
6 cups rye flour
1½ cups spelt flour

Add sugar, butter, and salt to scalded milk. Add yeast, caraway seeds, and water when the mixture is warm. Stir. Add in rye flour and knead while incorporating spelt flour. Return to bowl, cover, and let rise until mixture has doubled in bulk.

Shape into loaves, put in buttered pans, add a couple of shallow slits with a sharp knife on top, cover, let rise, and bake in a hot oven. (375°F)

## Norwegian Rye Bread

1 cup graham flour
¼ cup brown sugar
3 cups rye flour
1 tbsp salt
1 measure of yeast
Hot water

Mix dry ingredients. Pour and beat in as much hot water as the flour will take, making a stiff batter. Cover, let stand until lukewarm. Add yeast, dissolved in 1 cup of warm water. Knead wheat flour in until it holds its shape. Let proof till double in bulk. Punch down and shape into loaves, let double in size once more, and bake at 375°F for 1¼ hours.

**Scotch Oat Cake**

1 cup boiling water
½ tsp salt
1 tbsp lard
Oatmeal
¼ tsp soda

Add salt, soda, and lard to boiling water, then stir in oatmeal until the dough is stiff enough to knead. Roll very thin, cut into squares, bake slightly on the griddle, then dry in the oven on low heat.

**Grain-Free Granola** (Tammera Karr)

1 cup dried cranberries
1 cup slivered almonds
1 cup shredded coconut, unsweetened
1 cup pumpkin seeds
½ cup 65% extra dark chocolate chips
1 cup pecans, coarsely chopped
3 tbsp butter
½ tsp Celtic Sea salt
¼ cup pure maple syrup
3 tbsp raw honey

Mix all the ingredients thoroughly, and spread on parchment paper inside the cookie sheet. Place in a 300°F oven, and stir every 10 minutes until the mixture is lightly browned. Cool and store in an air tight container.

**Amaranth Pilaf** (Tammera Karr)
*One of the perks of being a forest biologist is the opportunity almost every day to be out in the forest and meadows where I can forage for wild foods. Amaranth is a gluten-free seed that can be used for cookies and porridge. I use this cold for lunch or as a side with dinner.*

3 cups water
2 cups amaranth leaves, trimmed and washed
1 cup amaranth seed plus 2 tbsp more for reserve
1 sweet onion, chopped fine
2 cloves garlic, minced fine

2 tbsp good olive oil
2 tbsp butter, clarified
¼ cup pecans, chopped
¼ cup almonds, blanched and match stick slivered

In a skillet, sear amaranth leaves and heat olive oil. Add onion and garlic and sauté for about 5 minutes.

Add 1 cup of amaranth seed and toast in clarified butter in a small pot. Add garlic and onion and toast all for 3-5 minutes. Add 3 cups of water, stir, cover with a tight-fitting lid, and reduce heat to low for 25 minutes. Let stand with the lid on for an additional 15 minutes.

Place seared amaranth leaves on a platter with fresh thin slices of sweet onion around the edges. Arrange cooked amaranth in the center of the leaves and onion slices. Toast the remaining 2 tablespoons of amaranth seeds and sprinkle over the top.

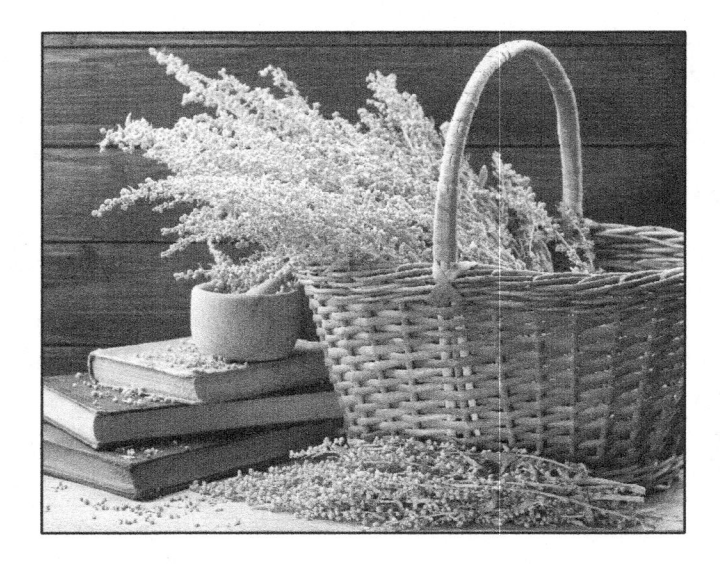

140 Daily Life in Anglo-Saxon England by Sally Crawford November 2008, https://oldenglishteaching.arts.gla.acuk/Units/2_Life_in.html

141 Retreved July 2022: https://vikingsof.me/blog/making-early-medieval-flat-bread/?fbclid=IwAR3oR-lum9vHNNG2aeluF36d0ozPJwmHWUzrkGF2ESnwqXpvyQaonCKsR-w

142 Native Seed Keepers Network: https://nativefoodalliance.org/our-programs-2/native-seedkeepers-network/

143 Retreved July 2022, https://www.nutritionvalue.org/Corn%2C_raw%2C_white%2C_sweet_nutritional_value.html

144 https://inah.gob.mx/boletines/11262-a-stucco-head-of-the-young-maize-god-associated-with-a-ritual-deposit-unearthed-in-palenque Retrieved 6-13-2020

145 Unlocking Nixtamal by Andrea Aliseda, Retreved July 2022: https://www.epicurious.com/ingredients/what-is-nixtamal-article

146 Cereal Grains for the Food and Beverage Industries, Publishing, 2013, Pages 67-115e, ISBN 9780857094131, https://doi.org/10.1533/9780857098924.67. (https://www.sciencedirect.com/science/article/pii/B9780857094131500024)

147 Chapter 4 - Quality Assurance for Corn and Wheat Flour Tortilla Manufacturing, 2015, Pages 97-123, ISBN 9781891127885, https://doi.org/10.1016/B978-1-891127-88-5.50004-9. (https://www.sciencedirect.com/science/article/pii/B9781891127885500049)

148 *How to Eat like a Human* by Bill Schindler pg 158-59

149 Native Seeds/SEARCH (NS/S) is a nonprofit seed conservation organization based in Tucson, Arizona. https://www.nativeseeds.org/pages/history-mission

About the Seeds: https://www.nativeseeds.org/pages/safe-seeds-organic-practices-gmos

150 Retreved July 2022: https://www.mexicoinmykitchen.com/huitlacoche-tacos/

151 What Ancient Maize Can Tell Us About Thousands of Years of Civilization in America Read more: https://www.smithsonianmag.com/smithsonian-institution/ancient-maize-thousands-years-civilization-america-180970543/#PO9kTBXW7tsTqeGS.99

152 7,400-year-old rice grains discovered in central China; https://ancientfoods.wordpress.com/2018/03/22/7400-year-old-rice-grains-discovered-in-central-china/

153 Amazon farmers discovered the secret of domesticating wild rice 4,000 years ago; https://ancientfoods.wordpress.com/2017/10/29/amazon-farmers-discovered-the-secret-of-domesticating-wild-rice-4000-years-ago/

154 Quinoa retrieved July 2022: https://www.newworldencyclopedia.org/entry/Quinoa

155 The Spanish Academy, Origin of Quinoa: Retrieved July 2022, https://www.spanish.academy/blog/10-authentic-peruvian-recipes-with-quinoa-you-wont-believe-7/

156 Tigernut Processing: Its Food uses and Health Benefits;
https://scialert.net/fulltext/?doi=ajft.2011.197.201

157 Ancientfoods - Exploring the origins and history of food&drink around the world.
https://ancientfoods.wordpress.com/2012/03/23/tigernuts/

158 https://www.sourdough.co.uk/the-history-of-sourdough-bread/

159 A Little History Of Irish Bread, Retreved July 2022: https://goodfoodireland.ie/uncategorized/bread-saint/

160 https://www.almanaccom/recipe/irish-soda-bread-4

161 Oxford Companion to American Food and Drink, 2007, pg 613

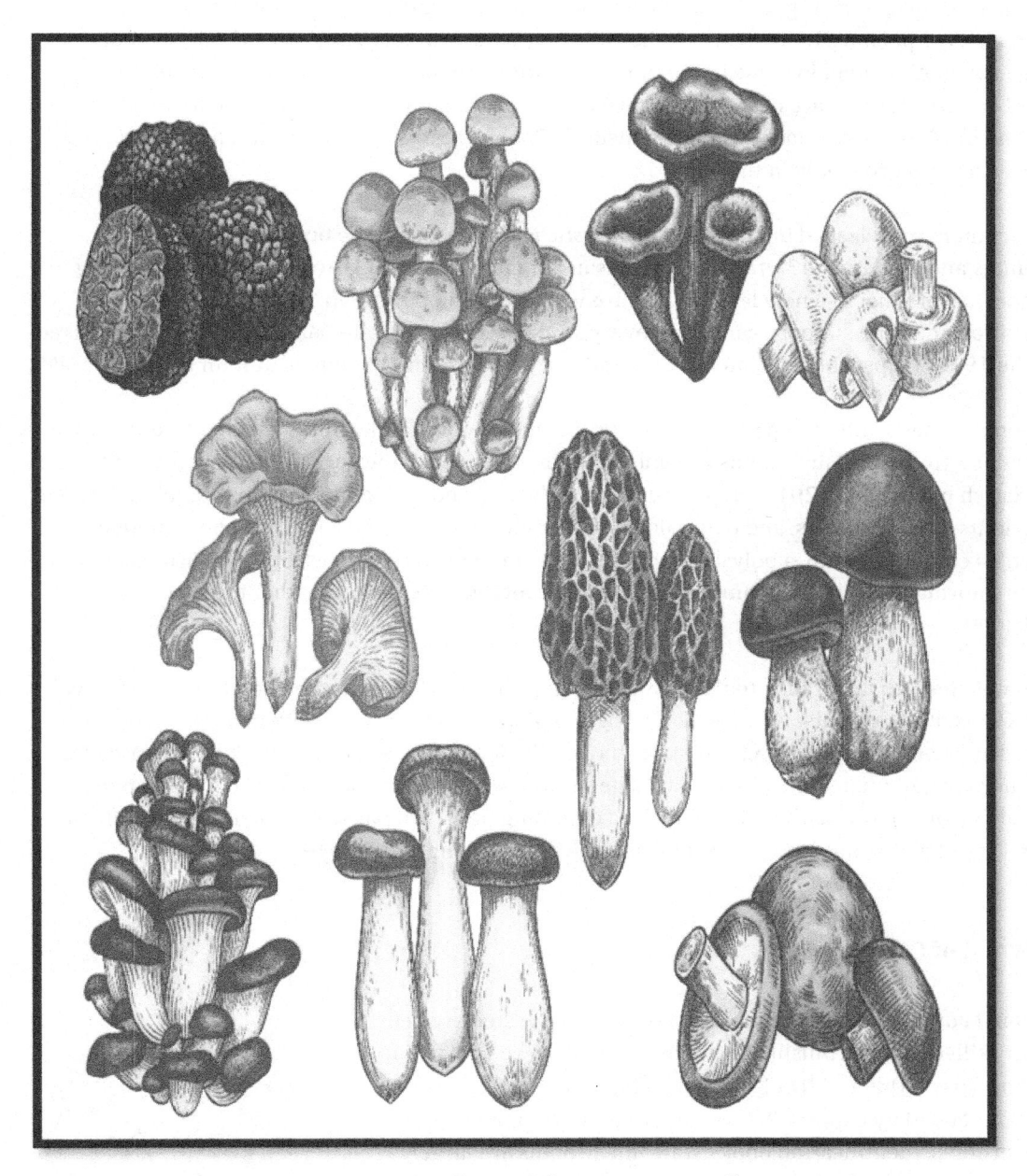

# *Umami ~ the 5th Taste of Fungi*

Fungi, in all of its forms, goes beyond much of our understanding of food. Fungi are powerful medicines or poisons. In many ways, they are the poster child for *Food as Medicine*. Humans have been consuming fungi for time immemorial. According to the *Oxford Companion to American Food and Drink*, there are over 38,000 varieties of fungi that have mycelia and a distinctive cap, of which 2,000 are considered safe to consume. To the great chagrin of cooks and researchers, most varieties grow only in the wild.

A documentary released in 2020 titled *Fantastic Fungi,* based on the books written by Paul Stamets and *Finding the Mother Tree* by Susan Simmard, catapulted awareness of the healing properties of fungi to a new level. Fungi are well established for their health benefits for cognition, immune support, cancer recovery, and rewiring the brain pathways. Research started in the 1960s on psychedelic mushrooms and was dusted off and resumed at John Hopkins.[162, 163]

When it comes to fungi, especially in the form of mushrooms and truffles – well, you either love them or hate them. Mushrooms are unique in the food world; they are neither meat nor plant. Research published in 2014 supported this conclusion, and stated mushrooms contain the same nutrients as meat, plants, and dairy along with "a unique nutrient profile."[164] These unique profiles comprise chitin, a polysaccharide, and the unique sterol, ergosterol. Mushrooms have been informally categorized among the "white vegetables" described as the "forgotten source of nutrients."

Umami, the fifth taste, adds to the flavor of both flesh and plant-based dishes. In the early days of the 19th century, chemist Kikunae Ikeda tried to pinpoint why *dashi* (broth made from seaweed and dried fish flakes) had such a distinct flavor. Ikeda found the seaweed in *dashi* contained the amino acid glutamate. In 1909, Ikeda suggested the savory sensation triggered by glutamate should be one of the basic tastes that give something flavor, on par with sweet, sour, bitter, and salt. He called it *umami*, riffing on a Japanese word meaning *delicious*.[165]

## A Word of Caution

When it comes to fungi, the majority are wild harvested. Even if you are a skilled forager, mushroom identification can be tricky. <u>If In Doubt, Toss it Out</u> and <u>NEVER Eat Wild Mushrooms Raw</u> are recommended by experts. These rules don't just apply to wild mushrooms. Identification books state mushrooms are largely undigestable until cooked. Morels are a good example; these mushrooms are poisonous when raw or undercooked. Any mushroom past its prime, in a state of decay, can cause food poisoning.

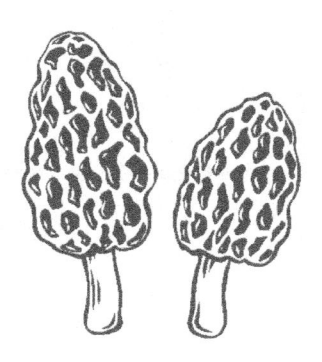

| Nutrient Contribution[2] per USDA Food Group Serving Size[a] | | | | | | |
|---|---|---|---|---|---|---|
| Food Kingdom | Underconsumed Nutrients[b] | | | | Other Values | |
| | Potassium, mg | Fiber, g | Vitamin D, IU | Calcium,[c] mg | Protein,[d] g | Calories |
| **Fungi/mycology** | | | | | | |
| White button mushrooms 1 cup sliced, stir fried (no added fat) | 428 | 1.9 | 9 | 4 | 3.9 | 28 |
| Portabella mushrooms UV exposed 1 cup, sliced, grilled | 529 | 2.7 | 634 | 4 | 3.9 | 35 |
| **Plants/botany** | | | | | | |
| Carrots 1 cup, sliced, cooked | 367 | 4.7 | 0 | 47 | 1.2 | 55 |
| Broccoli 1 cup, chopped, cooked | 457 | 5.1 | 0 | 62 | 3.7 | 55 |
| Potato 1 cup, boiled in skin | 591 | 2.8 | 0 | 8 | 2.9 | 136 |
| Banana 1 cup, sliced | 537 | 3.9 | 0 | 8 | 1.6 | 134 |
| Multi grain whole-grain bread one 1-oz slice | 65 | 2.1 | 0 | 29 | 3.8 | 75 |
| **Animals/zoology** | | | | | | |
| Ground beef 80% lean: 20% fat, 3 oz, broiled | 258 | 0 | 2 | 20 | 21.9 | 230 |
| Milk 1% fat, without added vitamins A and D, 1 cup | 366 | 0 | 2 | 305 | 8.2 | 102 |
| Milk 1% fat, with vitamins A and D added, 1 cup | 366 | 0 | 117 | 305 | 8.2 | 102 |
| Yogurt, whole milk, plain, 1 cup (8 fl oz) | 380 | 0 | 5 | 296 | 8.5 | 149 |

Abbreviations: DGA, Dietary Guidelines for Americans; USDA, US Department of Agriculture; UV, ultraviolet.
[a]USDA food group amounts/quantity equivalents in footnote to Appendix 7. Although protein is given in 1-oz equivalents, 3 oz is used in the table to indicate a more commonly consumed portion. http://www.health.gov/dietaryguidelines/dga2010/DietaryGuidelines2010.pdf.
[b]The 2010 DGA identified potassium, fiber, vitamin D, and calcium nutrients of concern for the general population and recommended dark green, red, and orange vegetables in the USDA Food Patterns. White potatoes are included in the table as a popularly consumed "starchy" vegetable. Bananas included as America's favorite fresh fruit. http://www.ers.usda.gov/data-products/chart-gallery/detail.aspx?chartId=30486#.U45kkPldVNY.
[c]Mushrooms are not a source of calcium, but mushrooms exposed to UV light to increase vitamin D content would help calcium utilization.
[d]Protein is not considered an underconsumed nutrient. However, protein in mushrooms have a moderate protein quality score 0.66 with 70% digestibility. Nutrient Profiling of Mushrooms. Mushrooms and Health Report 2012. Mushrooms and Health Web site, http://www.mushroomsandhealth.com/mushrooms-health-report/nutrient-profile/. Accessed April 12, 2014.

https://www.ncbi.nlm.nih.gov/pmc/articles/PMC4244211/bin/nt-49-301-g002.jpg

| Food | Naturally Occurring Free Glutamate IMP and GMP When Known),[a] mg/100 g | Sodium,[2] mg/100 g | Potassium,[2] mg/100 g |
|---|---|---|---|
| Fresh shiitake mushrooms | 71 (0 GMP) | 9 | 304 |
| Dried shiitake mushrooms | 150 GMP | 13 | 1534 |
| Potatoes flesh/skin, raw | 102 | 6 | 421 |
| Sweet potatoes, raw | 60 | 55 | 337 |
| Tomatoes, red/ripe | 246 | 5 | 237 |
| Chinese cabbage, raw | 100 | 65 | 252 |
| Carrots, raw | 33 | 69 | 320 |
| Parmesan cheese, dry grated | 1200 | 1529 | 125 |
| Soy sauce (shoyu) | 780 | 5493 | 435 |
| Beef ground, 80% lean, raw | 10 (80 IMP) | 66 | 270 |
| Pork tenderloin, raw | 2.5 (122 IMP) | 53 | 399 |
| Chicken ground, raw | 1.5 (76 IMP) | 60 | 522 |

Abbreviations: GMP, Guanylate; IMP, Inosinate.
[a]Umami Information Center, www.umamiinfo.com.

https://www.ncbi.nlm.nih.gov/pmc/articles/PMC4244211/bin/nt-49-301-g004.jpg

### Hungarian Mushroom Soup (Chef Ben Qualls)

*An incredibly rich and satisfying soup with a depth of flavor that is a meal in itself. Not my grandmother's this time. Discovered this recipe on my own. Have made it several times at the care facility where I work. Residents were initially hesitant, but once they tasted it, they really enjoyed it.*

2 tbsp butter
1 large yellow onion, finely chopped
1 clove garlic, minced
12 oz cremini or white button mushrooms, sliced or diced, your choice
2 tbsp genuine imported Hungarian paprika
1½ tbsp chopped fresh dill (fresh is highly recommended, or 1½ tsp dried dill)
1 tsp pink Himalayan salt
Freshly ground black pepper to taste
3 tbsp butter
2 tbsp all-purpose flour
1 cup whole milk
2 cups quality beef broth or vegetable broth
1 tbsp tamari or soy sauce or Worcestershire
½ cup sour cream
Chopped fresh dill or parsley for garnish
Extra sour cream for serving

In a heavy pot or Dutch oven, melt 2 tablespoons of butter. Add the onions and cook until translucent and just barely beginning to brown. Add the garlic and cook for another minute. Add the mushrooms and cook for 5-7 minutes until the mushrooms release their juices. Transfer the mushroom mixture to a bowl and set aside.

Melt 3 tablespoons of butter in the same pan and stir in the flour, constantly whisking for 6-7 minutes or until the mixture is a rich, caramelized brown. Add the milk, broth, and soy sauce, still whisking continually until the mixture is smooth. Add the paprika, dill, salt and pepper. Stir in the mushroom mixture. Bring to a boil, reduce heat to medium, cover and simmer for 15 minutes, stirring occasionally.

Stir in the sour cream and heat through. Serve immediately with a dollop of sour cream and a sprinkling of chopped dill. Serve with crusty bread.

Works well as a sauce, too. Just add an extra tablespoon of flour to the roux.

**Tomates Farcies** - Basque Tomatoes Stuffed with Foie Gras, Duck Confit, and Chanterelles

10 large vine ripe tomatoes
Kosher salt
¾ cup rendered duck fat or vegetable oil
2 lbs bone-in lamb shoulder
Freshly ground black pepper
14 oz duck foie gras, cut into ½ inch cubes
3 confit duck legs, bones removed, meat roughly chopped
8 oz chanterelle mushrooms, roughly chopped
2½ oz Parmigiano-Reggiano, finely grated
½ cup black truffle juice, optional
Piment d'Espelette
3 cloves garlic, smashed flat
3 sprigs thyme
1 bay leaf
1 cup chicken stock
3 tbsp plus 1 tsp balsamic vinegar
Juice of 1 lemon

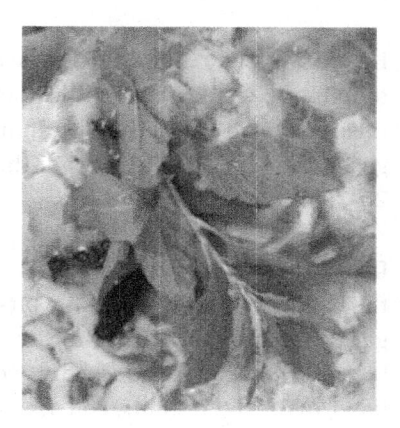

Using a paring knife, cut ½ inch off each tomato top and set aside. Using a melon baller or small spoon, scrape the insides from each tomato into a bowl, being careful not to tear through the skin. Sprinkle the insides of the tomatoes with salt, then invert onto a rack set over a baking sheet and let drain for 1 hour.

Meanwhile, heat the oven to 300°F. In a medium Dutch oven, warm ¼ cup duck fat over medium-high heat. Season the lamb shoulder with salt and pepper, then add to the pot and cook, turning, until golden brown on all sides, about 12 minutes.

Transfer the pot to the oven and cook, turning the meat once halfway through, until tender and falling off the bone, about 2 hours. Transfer the lamb to a rack and let cool. Shred the meat from the bone and transfer to a large bowl, discarding the bone.

Warm a large nonstick skillet over high heat. Add half the foie gras and cook, undisturbed, until dark brown on one side, about 30 seconds. Shake the pan to ensure that the foie gras doesn't stick to the bottom, then continue cooking until it is cooked to medium-rare, about 1½ minutes more. Using a slotted spoon, transfer the foie gras to the bowl with the lamb, drain off all the fat, and return the skillet to the heat. Repeat with the remaining foie gras, draining off all but ¼ cup fat from the skillet.

Add the duck to the skillet and cook, stirring occasionally, until warmed through, about 2 minutes. Using a slotted spoon, transfer the duck to the bowl with the lamb and foie gras, and return the skillet to the heat.

Add the chanterelles and cook, stirring, until they give off their liquid and are golden brown, about 4 minutes. Scrape the chanterelles and any fat left in the skillet into the bowl with the duck and foie gras, then stir in the Parmigiano and truffle juice, if using. Season the filling with salt and piment d'Espelette.

Heat the oven to 275°F. In a large baking dish wide enough to fit all the tomatoes snugly, arrange tomatoes cut side up. Equally divide the filling among the tomatoes, then cover each with its reserved top. Drizzle the remaining ½ cup duck fat over and around the tomatoes and scatter the garlic, thyme, and bay leaf over the top. Bake until the tomatoes are tender and the filling is hot, 20-25 minutes.

Using a large spoon or spatula, gently transfer tomatoes to a serving platter. Pour the stock into the baking dish, scrape up any bits that are stuck to the pan, then pour the pan liquid, herbs, and garlic into a small sauce pan. Stir the balsamic vinegar and lemon juice into the pan, bring to a boil, and cook until reduced to ⅓ cup, about 5 minutes. Pour the sauce through a fine sieve into a bowl, discard the solids, and season with salt and piment d'Espelette to taste. Serve the tomatoes warm, with a spoonful of sauce on each, and extra sauce on the side.

### Mushrooms Sautéed (Tammera Karr)

6 large crimini mushrooms
6 chanterelle or small portabella mushrooms
2 tbsp organic butter
1 tbsp extra virgin olive oil
2 garlic cloves, minced (let rest for 5 minutes before adding to oil)
3 shallots chopped

Warm butter and oil in cast iron skillet, add shallots and garlic, sauté till tender. Add sliced mushrooms and toss the mixture together; let mushrooms sweat till they reabsorb their liquid. Add salt and pepper to taste.

### Creamy Mushroom Soup (Tammera Karr)

1½ qt organic chicken broth
1 can organic coconut milk
7 tbsp organic or Kerrygold butter
4 cups sliced Portobello mushrooms
1 cup shallots thinly sliced
3 medium cloves garlic
1 tbsp arrowroot
1 cup dry sherry or white wine
2 bay leaves
½ tsp thyme leaves
Kosher salt and freshly ground black pepper

1 tbsp organic olive oil

In a 4 quart pan, add olive oil and heat on medium low. Add shallots, garlic, herbs, and mushrooms, toss and heat on medium till mushrooms release juices.

Remove from heat, and puree mushrooms and herbs into ½ of the chicken stock in a Vitamix or food processor. Return contents to pan and add ½ of the remaining broth and coconut milk. Bring soup up to a slow boil. In a separate bowl, add last of the broth, and whisk in arrowroot powder and wine.

Turn heat to low, add remaining broth and wine, and simmer for 15 minutes. Stir soup to ensure it does not stick on the bottom, and slightly thickens. Serve in bowls with a dollop of butter and salt and pepper.

**Roasted Chanterelle Mushrooms with Caramelized Fennel** (Tammera Karr)
*Chanterelle mushrooms grow wild in the woods of the Pacific Northwest, along with oyster, chicken and many others. When it comes to mushrooms, I'm too chicken to try wild harvesting, so I buy from mushroom growers at a local farmer's market.*
4 servings

8 large chanterelle mushrooms, approximately
¼ cup olive oil, plus more for tossing the mushrooms in
Celtic Sea salt and freshly ground black pepper
1 medium fennel bulbs, cored and cut crosswise into thin half-moons (freeze or save stalks for vegetable stock)
¼ cup chopped fresh basil
½ cup poultry broth or reduced sodium store bought chicken broth or vegetable stock

Preheat the oven to 450°F. Lightly oil a large jelly roll pan.
Place the mushrooms on the baking sheet after tossing to coat with oil in a bowl or plastic bag. Roast for 10 minutes. Turn them over and continue roasting until tender, 3-4 minutes. Season to taste with salt and pepper.

Heat ¼ cup of oil in a cast iron skillet over medium-high heat. Add the fennel and cook, stirring occasionally, until golden brown and tender, about 10 minutes. Stir in the stock and basil and bring to a boil. Season to taste with salt and pepper. Transfer the mushrooms to a cutting board and cut them into ½ inch thick pieces. Transfer to a serving platter. Pour the fennel sauce over the mushroom slices and serve hot.

## Chanterelle's and Green Beans

1 lb fresh green beans
6 oz chanterelle mushrooms
2 tbsp dry sherry
¼ cup walnuts or pecans
3 slices cooked bacon chopped up
Salt and pepper

Add chopped bacon to a cast iron skillet and brown on medium-low heat till crisp and oil from bacon has been released. Add chanterelles and toss with bacon, let mushrooms cook until they have released juices, add nuts and green beans, toss well together, add dry sherry and cover, turn heat to low and cook for 15 minutes.

## Mushroom Stir Fry (Chef Christine Wokowsky)

1 lb fresh mushrooms, assorted (shiitakes, crimini, portabella, button, etc)
1 onion, diced
1 cup purple cabbage, thinly sliced
Splash of coconut aminos or Bragg's liquid aminos
Hefty pinch of white pepper
½ tsp garlic powder
Dulse for sprinkling on top for garnish
½ cup cooked brown, black and purple rice or quinoa

In a wok with ¼ cup of either extra virgin olive oil or coconut oil or ½ olive and ½ coconut, sauté the mushrooms stirring the whole while so they don't create excess moisture. Add onions and cook until translucent.

Add the purple cabbage. Serve in bowls with rice or quinoa. Sprinkle Dulse on top.

## Matsutake Cracker Hors d'oeuvre (Crystal Shepard)

*Matsutakes are nutty and rich, smelling reminiscent of the Ponderosa pine bark and Doug fir needles littering the ground where they grow. Matsutakes are one of the few mushrooms that don't marry well with dairy products. Most mushrooms are well complimented by cheeses and cream sauces, but not these. However, a grating of a nice dry parmesan is the exception in these "crackers".*

10-20 firm matsutakes, stems removed (save for other recipes)
Olive or toasted sesame oil
Chunk parmesan cheese
Green onions, slivered

Salt and pepper

Lay caps out, gills up on a baking sheet. Drizzle each lightly with your oil of choice and sprinkle with salt. Bake for 10 minutes at 375°F. Check for the mushrooms to stop losing moisture (sweating) and for the moisture to evaporate from the pan. Add a light grating of parmesan cheese and a sprinkle of black pepper. Bake for 5 more minutes, then turn on the broiler. Pull matsutakes out when cheese begins to brown. Top with slivered green onions and serve.

### Mushroom Medley-Miso Soup (Yuan Wang)[166]
Serves 4-6

3 oz shiitake mushrooms, fresh
3 oz maitake mushrooms, fresh
3 oz oyster mushrooms, fresh
2 tbsp dark sesame oil
¼ medium onion, diced
7 oz firm tofu, cut into ½ inch cubes
1 green onion, chopped into ¼ inch pieces
3½ *dashi* soup stock
4 tbsp white miso paste

1. Slice mushrooms into ½ inch pieces.
2. In a pot heat sesame oil. Add onion, and sauté until translucent and golden.
3. Add the mushrooms, tofu, green onions, and sauté for 2 minutes.
4. Add soup stock and bring to a boil, then simmer for 2 minutes. Turn off heat.
5. Remove 4 tablespoons of stock and mix it with the miso paste in a bowl, make sure there are no lumps.
6. Gradually pour the miso mixture into the stock pot and stir before serving.

### Scrambled Eggs with Shaved Oregon White Truffle (Crystal Shepard)

4 eggs
1 Oregon White Truffle
Shallots, cut for garnish

Whisk the eggs and fry; sprinkle with shaved Oregon White Truffle and shallots.
Serve with toast. Alternatively, store your truffles in a glass container with eggs (in shell) for 24 hours; the eggs will absorb the aroma and flavor through the shell from the truffles.

**Rose Oyster Mushroom with Epazote & Chipotle Soup** (Denise Couturier Maitret)
*Inspired by the traditional indigenous recipes of Cuetzalan in the Puebla region of Mexico.*
Serves 8

8 cups salted natural chicken or hen broth (preferably from organic, free range chickens, Cornish or wild game hens), or simple vegetable stock made from organic vegetables if possible

1 lb rose oyster mushrooms, stalks and stems removed and reserved for future stock (any mushrooms or wild mushroom medley can be used, although cooking times may vary)

⅓ cup olive oil (you can also use avocado oil, ghee, raw butter or a mixture of these)
1 medium or 1½ small white or yellow onion, finely diced
2 stalks organic celery, finely diced
3-5 cloves of garlic (depending on size and preference), minced
8 small red potatoes, peeled and diced into 8 pieces each

4-6 stalks fresh epazote herb (you can use parsley, thyme, marjoram, or cilantro if epazote is unavailable, although the taste of epazote gives this soup its unique flavor)
1-2 dried, roasted and seeded whole chipotle peppers
1 dried, roasted, seeded, and chopped chile ancho pepper (dried poblano chile)
White pepper and/or nutmeg to taste (optional)


*To prepare mirepoix* (vegetable mixture)
Boil potatoes in 1 cup of broth for about 15 minutes or until soft; do not overcook.
Sauté onions and celery, waiting until translucent and soft before adding minced garlic. Do not let it brown. Add to boiled potatoes.

With the heat turned to medium, add chopped rose oyster mushrooms to mirepoix and stir until all ingredients are well incorporated and mushrooms begin to soften and shrink. Turn down heat and simmer for 20-30 minutes, stirring occasionally and tasting for softness. Mushrooms should not be chewy.

Add remaining 7 cups of heated stock. Stir and simmer for 10 minutes.
Taste and add salt accordingly.

Add chipotle and epazote. Cover and simmer 10 minutes.
Add dash of white pepper and nutmeg to taste if desired.

*Suggested toppings*: avocado, cream (raw, organic, or dairy-free), blue or purple maize chip strips, lime slices, cilantro, extra epazote

*Prepare toppings.*
To serve, ladle soup into large bowls, add a teaspoon of roasted and chopped chile ancho, a few avocado slices, a dollop of cream of choice, a side of sliced Mexican lime, and fresh epazote and cilantro as garnish.

> Oyster mushrooms are one of the most popular wild mushrooms. They often grow on the sides of tree trunks. Oyster mushrooms should be cultivated from hardwood; the ones growing on softwood are poisonous.
>
> Pink oyster mushrooms are one variety of oyster mushrooms. They can also come in white, brown, golden, and blue colors. All fade to creamy gray when cooked. Pink oysters have a surprisingly short shelf life, and can disintegrate within 12 hours. Should you buy some, cook them immediately.
>
> A 100-gram serving of oyster mushroom contains 3 g protein, 6 g carbohydrate, 2.3 g fiber.
>
> Oyster mushrooms may be beneficial for your heart due to beta-glucans, which are fibers that make up the cell walls of yeast and fungi.

**Triple Mushroom Mélange** (Yuan Wang, *Ancient Wisdom Modern Kitchen*, pg. 128)
*In Asia mushrooms are traditionally associated with longevity.*

½ cup fresh enoki mushrooms
2-3 large shiitake mushrooms
½ cup fresh king oyster mushrooms
2 tbsp olive oil
2 cloves garlic, peeled and minced
1 cup vegetable broth
1 tbsp kudzu, powder, or arrowroot powder for thickener
2 tbsp water
Salt

Slice trimmed and cleaned mushrooms into ½ inch pieces.
Heat olive oil in skillet, and add minced garlic, sauté until garlic becomes fragrant (about 30 seconds).

Add mushrooms and sauté for 2 minutes.

Add vegetable broth and cook loosely covered, for another 8 minutes.

In a small bowl mix kudzu or arrowroot with 2 tablespoons of water, removing any lumps, then add the mixture to the pan of mushrooms and broth. Stir well to prevent lumps forming, add salt and serve.

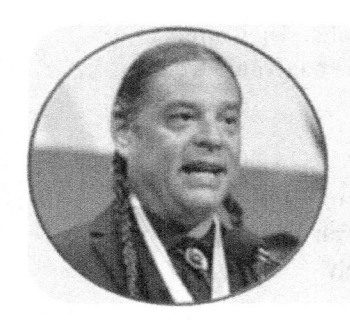

*"I tasted how food weaves people together, connects families through generations, is a life force of identity and social structure."*

~ Sean Sherman – The Sioux Chief
2022 Recipient of the James Beard Award

---

162 https://www.jhunewsletter.com/article/2020/09/hopkins-launches-clinical-trial-for-psilocybin-mushrooms Retrieved 6-11-2022

163 https://hub.jhu.edu/2016/12/01/hallucinogen-treats-cancer-depression-anxiety/ Retrieved 6-11-2022

164 Jo Feeney, M., Miller, A. M., & Roupas, P. (2014). Mushrooms-Biologically Distinct and Nutritionally Unique: Exploring a "Third Food Kingdom". Nutrition today, 49(6), 301–307. https://doi.org/10.1097/NT.0000000000000063

165 https://www.bbccom/future/article/20190503-the-mystery-taste-that-always-eluded-us Retrieved 6-11-2022

166 Ancient Wisdom, Modern Kitchen, Recipes from the East for Health, Healing, and Long Life, pg 74

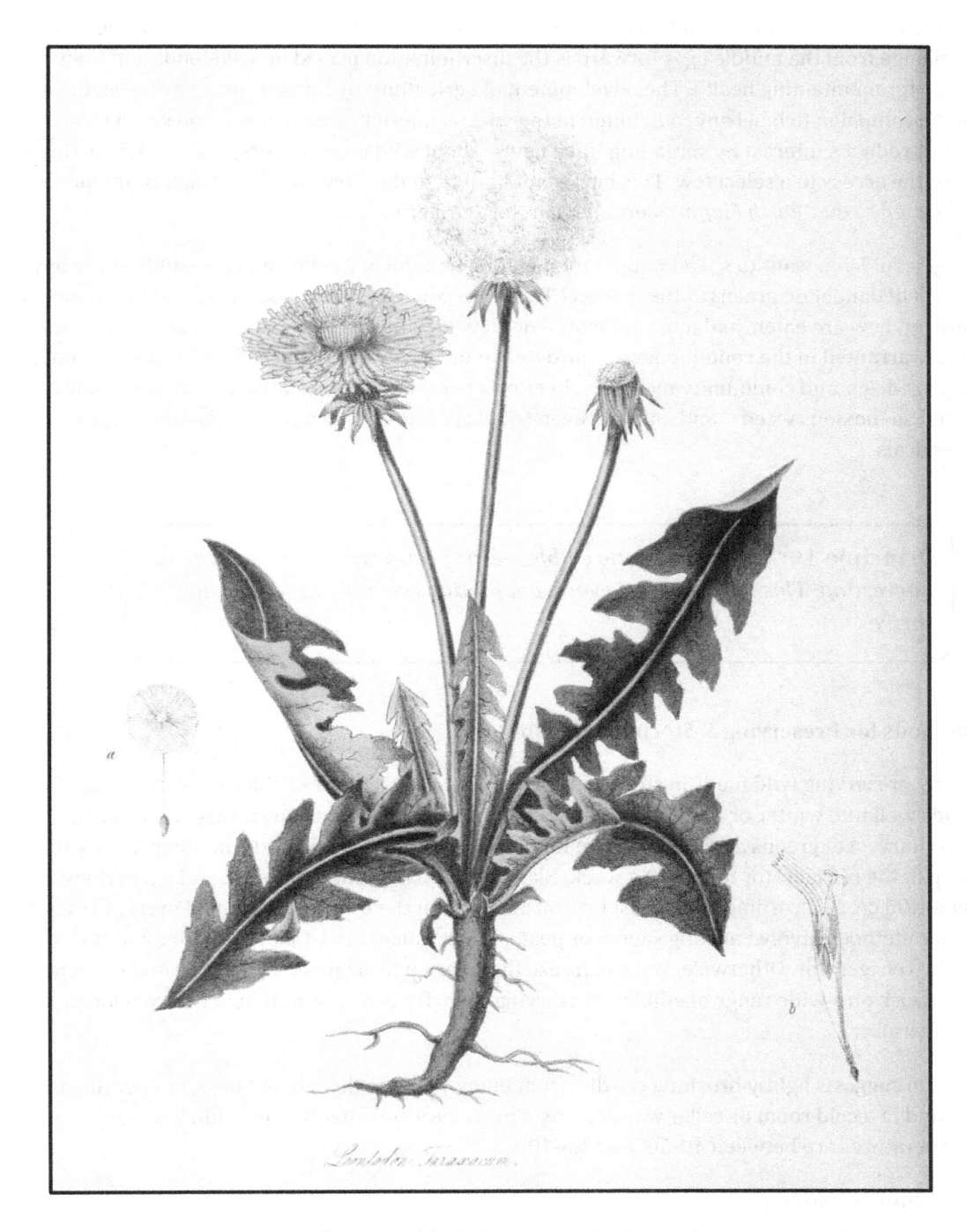

# The Wild Side of Food

Edible plants are not new; humans have been hunting and gathering from the beginning. The challenge from the middle ages forward is the discrimination placed on wild foods and their value for maintaining health. The development of agriculture by humans may have been the start of the campaign to label any food found in the wild as inferior or poisonous. You could increase your product's interest by spreading "fake news" about wild greens, roots, grains, and berries. Or limit the access to a select few. This bias is not limited to the "New World." Still, it is undoubtedly relegated to the "*Earth Muffin*" stereotype in North America.

Why would you want to spend hours foraging for a handful of food when you could simply buy a bunch of dandelion greens at the market? There are countless wild foods available to the modern forager. Few are eaten, and most are feared or viewed with suspicion. In truth, the skepticism is well warranted in the contemporary world due to the heavy use of herbicides by state, county, city agencies, and community members. In efforts to eradicate non-native plants, especially those listed as "noxious weeds" and animals, even tribal agencies have embraced the use of toxic chemicals.

> **Principle 19:** *Targeting exotic edible weed species is guaranteed ethical harvesting. This helps control exotic populations so native species can thrive.*

## Methods for Preserving & Storing Wild Edibles

Safely preserving wild foods in sterilized containers extends the shelf life so one can enjoy these foods well into winter or the starvation spring months. For short-term storage, wash and pat dry your harvest of greens and loosely wrap them in a towel in a sealed food container. They will keep in the refrigerator for about a week. Blanching and freezing are also useful when there is a bountiful crop, according to botanist Crystal Shepard on the Umpqua National Forest in Oregon. Other methods involve making sauces or pesto. Fresh sauces are usually kept for about five days in the refrigerator. Otherwise, you can freeze them for up to six months. Pickling and fermenting also work on a wide range of edibles, preserving them for 3-6 months if kept in a cool location or refrigerator.

Crystal suggests lightly brushing the dirt from bulbs, hanging them in net bags, or covering them in sand in a cold room or cellar wooden box. This is easy and effective, providing the temperatures are between 40-50°F or 4.5-10°C.

## The Human Journey

Due to time and a devaluing of native peoples' ancestral foods, a growing volume of foraging information has been lost. *A Note:* All peoples have moved and settled from the earliest humans migrating across Africa into the Siberian steps, across oceans following the air and sea currents.

With each step, we have brought tools, skills, and seeds. Humans have been changing the planet for a long time by accident and intent.

In the modern world, relatively few individuals have begun the journey back to foraging wild foods; however, there is a resurgence of interest. We can learn about ancestral foods with a measure of reassurance; if harvested, prepared, and cooked correctly, an exciting banquet of color, texture, and flavor from nature and the past can be enjoyed. Foraging wild foods connects us to nature, origin, cultures, and potential healing through foods, long forgotten. (Thayer, 2015)

In the spring of 2022, while visiting the John Day Fossil Beds-Painted Hills Unit in Central Oregon Tammera struck up a conversation with a fellow traveler. She asked if the lady was enjoying her visit and she enthusiastically replied, "It is all so big." Recognizing the traveler had an accent, Tammera inquired where home was. "Holland," the traveler said, "my whole country fits in a small area of this state!" Tammera agreed and, when asked, shared where she hailed from also. "Oh, this is like your garden," the traveler replied.

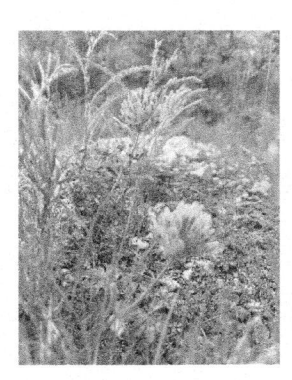

At first, I didn't think much of the comment Tammera later shared. The following day at Big Summit Prairie, Tammera recalled her visit days before with the Wallowa and Grant County Museums curators. Independently, they talked about how area Indian bands or family groups actively cultivated food resources in Oregon, Idaho, Washington and Montana plains, prairies, forests, and deserts.

"I slipped on my boots and headed out of our handy hideout travel trailer door to take pictures of wildflowers. I was soon struck by the abundance of edible plants in specific areas. Is this by natural design or a residual cultivation pattern from migrant peoples? The longer I surveyed the landscape, the more it looked and felt like a garden for the body and spirit."

> **Principle 20:** *Ethical harvesting reduces and assists the species you harvest so they can continue growing successfully, ensuring future harvests are abundant for foragers, including animals.*

### Broad-Leaf Maple Flower Fritters (Crystal Shepard)

*One of the perks of being a botanist is being out in the woods daily and knowing when the first spring treats are almost ready. If you like young asparagus, the texture and light greenness of maple flowers will delight you the same as it does me. I like to find trees on slopes with easy to access branches and pick when the flowers are just starting to open. Once they are too mature, they become fibrous. If you spread your flowers out for a bit before cooking, most of the little forest denizens will depart on their own. I like to serve these on a weekend morning with a little homemade maple syrup.*

2 cups of maple flowers
4 eggs cracked and stirred into a bowl with a splash of water and a little salt
Butter
Black pepper and maple syrup

Lightly sauté maple flowers in butter, keeping them moving so that flower petals do not brown. When stems become tender, spread flowers out evenly in pan and pour egg mixture over, covering with a lid for a few minutes. When egg is beginning to slightly dry and bubble on the edges, flip over and turn off heat. Frittata will continue cooking. After a couple of minutes, transfer to plate and top with fresh black pepper and a drizzle of maple syrup.

*Some of the following recipes are from American Indian Nations; out of respect, we have presented the recipes as we found them.*

### Bitterroot Pudding (Julia Rock-Above of the Crow Nation)

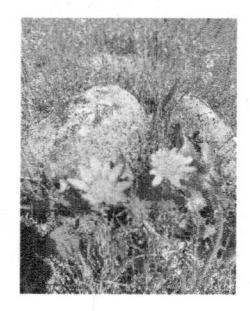

Use about ½ cup of bitterroot roots per serving. Par-boil the roots for a few minutes. Drain and add fresh water. Cook until tender. Sweeten with wild honey to suit taste. Add 1 teaspoon bone marrow per serving. Thicken with the scrapings from the inner side of a fresh skin.

Note: Before European cooking came west, the people of the Crow Nation used honey or a sweetening plant to sweeten the food. Bone marrow was a favorite enrichment of the food.

*Julia Rock-Above Ground received this recipe from her mother and grandmothers who received it from the ancestors back through time. Captain Meriwether Lewis gathered samples of the plant to take back to the states in 1806. Bitterroot was named Montana's state flower in 1985.*

### Elderberries and Rosehips Syrup

½ cup of elderberries
½ cup of rose hips
2 cups of water
1 tsp of cinnamon
Pinch of freshly grated nutmeg
Raw honey to taste

Simmer the elderberries and rosehips in 2 cups of water for 20 minutes. Strain well.

Whisk in the cinnamon and nutmeg.

Add honey to taste while the mixture is still warm. Mix well.
This syrup can be used for colds and sore throats, drizzled on ice cream, bananas, or pancakes.

## Elderberry Infused Honey

Raw honey
Dried elderberries
Dried elderberry flowers
1 glass storage jar

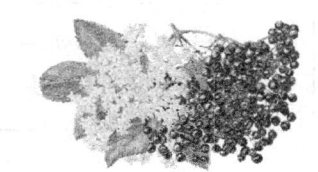

Take a glass jar and fill ¼ of the way with dried elderberries and flowers.

Pour honey over the berries and flowers, filling to the top. Affix lid.
Set the elderberry honey in a sunny area for two weeks. If the honey is thin, flip the jar every few days. If honey is thick, stir to ensure the best infusion.

After two weeks, strain honey and save the berry and flower mixture for tea.

## Oregon Grape or Elderberry Jelly

6 cups cleaned Oregon grape berries (or wild elderberries; with these, we are less picky about stems and leaves)

Place berries in a 4–8 quart stainless stock pot with 2 cups of water.
Bring contents to a boil, then turn down and simmer for 15 minutes. Use a potato masher or emersion blender to mash berries releasing the juice.

Place a Foley food mill over a second stock pot. In 1-2 cup increments, turn the berries and juice through the food mill to separate the seeds. Remove the seeds from the mill before straining another batch.

Once finished, measure your juice with pulp. It should yield about 3 cups. Add a little water to bring your volume to 3 cups if necessary.

In a large pot (jelly and jam like to splash so we use a 6 quart pan to reduce mess) on the stovetop, add 3 cups juice, 1 ounce of Certo® (about ½ of a liquid package) or Ball pectin and the juice of ½ lemon. Stir well to incorporate pectin. Increase heat, stirring consistently to prevent scorching.

Bring juice to a rapid boil once more, add 3 cups organic sugar, and return to a rolling boil - boil for exactly 1 minute. Any longer and you will have rock candy.
Remove from heat.

Place the jelly in clean hot ½ pint canning jars, wipe the top of the jars clean, cover with lids, and can in a water bath for 10 minutes. If any lids do not seal, refrigerate for up to three weeks.

> **Principle 21:** *Consider the nutrition or medicinal benefits for which you are harvesting a plant.*

### Wild Huckleberry Bars

1 cup chopped, pitted dates
½ cup almonds
½ cup pumpkin seeds
2 tbsp chia seeds
⅓ cup frozen fresh huckleberries
½ cup protein powder
½ cup almond butter

Place all ingredients in a food processor and process until well combined.
Press into an 8×8 inch pan and refrigerate 1 hour.
Cut into 6-8 bars and store in the refrigerator until ready to eat.

### Sarvisberry Pie

4 cups fresh sarvisberries
1 cup organic sugar
3 tbsp flour
Dash salt
½ tsp cinnamon
¼ tsp ginger
⅛ tsp clove
Juice of ½ lime
Juice of ½ lemon

Line a 9 inch pie plate with pastry. Combine fresh berries with sugar, flour, and salt. Add cinnamon, and spices to mix, add to pie shell, dot top with butter and cover with second pie

crust. Place vent slits in top after crimping edges. Bake in a 400°F oven 35-40 minutes (place a pizza pan or cookie sheet under pies to catch juices).
Serve warm with cream.

> Chokecherry (*Prunus virginiana*) grows wild in the Pacific Northwest and can be used for both food and medicine. The bark can be used as a powerful cough sedative - especially useful for those dry, spasmodic coughs. Chokecherries especially shine as food. If you've ever popped one into your mouth, you'll immediately understand astringency. Chokecherries have higher levels of antioxidants then blueberries or goji berries.[167]

## Chokecherry Syrup
6 pints

Cook cleaned ripe chokecherries in enough water to cover berries until cherries are soft. Strain juice through a cheesecloth or fine sieve. (Reserve the pulp for jam.)
7 cups juice
2 tbsp pectin (Sur-Jel or Certo®)
7 cups sugar

Mix pectin and juice in a large kettle and heat to a rolling boil. Boil one minute. Add sugar and mix thoroughly. Bring to a rolling boil and boil for one minute. Pour into sterilized jars and seal.

## Chokecherry Jelly Recipe
Makes about 6 pints

8½ lbs of berries
7 cups water
½ cup lemon juice
2½ cups sugar
9½ tsp of pectin
9½ cups water

Bring the berries and water to a boil and then lower to a simmer.

Continue to simmer for fifteen minutes while crushing the berries with a berry masher, potato masher or large spoon.

Use a Fully Food Mill for mashing, strain and squeeze out the juice from the berries.
Yield roughly 9½ cups of juice. Next, add the ½ cup of lemon juice to the berry juice.

And then add the remaining water to the juice.
In a separate bowl mix the pectin and sugar.
Next, bring the juice to a boil and add the sugar mixture.
Stir the mixture vigorously for a couple of minutes.
Turn off the heat and put into sterilized jars and water bath process for 10 minutes.

## Rose Hip Jelly

*Juice:*
1 pint cleaned rose hips
Peelings from 2 medium sized tart apples
Cover with water in a sauce pan and cook until tender, then crush and strain through a jelly bag.

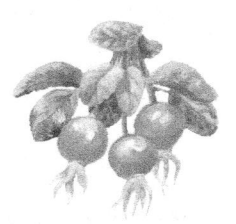

Mix 2 cups of juice with 2 cups sugar and bring to a boil. Add ½ cup lemon juice and boil for 15 minutes. Test for jelly every few minutes. Do not over-boil as the liquid toughens if boiled too long. Pour into jelly jars and seal with paraffin.

## Buffalo Berry Jelly

Pick berries after they have been frosted several times. Float leaves and other debris off berries. Place clean berries in an enamel or stainless steel kettle and barely cover with water. Bring slowly to a boil over medium heat and boil gently for about 15 minutes, stirring occasionally. Pour into a jelly bag and squeeze. Do not be concerned about murky appearance of the juice. Follow the directions of your favorite pectin, using 5 cups juice and 7 cups sugar to each box of pectin.

## Dandelion Wine

*There is a family secret involving my sister when she was at Crane high school in eastern Oregon and dandelion wine. Every time I hear or read dandelion wine; I remember my sister and a smile and even an out loud laugh happens.*

1 qt dandelion flowers (greens will make bitter)
1 gallon water

Soak blossoms for 24 hours, then strain. Add 3 oranges and 3 lemons quartered. Add 1 pound raisins, 3pounds granulated organic sugar (6¾ cups) and ½ cake of fresh yeast. Let ferment 7-8 days; while fermenting, stir 1-2 times daily with a wooden spoon. Strain liquid into ½ gallon growler jugs and let settle at least 6 weeks; siphon into bottles and cork.

### Dandelion Jelly (tastes like honey)

1 qt dandelion blossoms
2 qts water
1 package pectin
5½ cups organic sugar
2 tbsp fresh orange rind grated

Pour blossoms into a large sauce pan with water. Bring to a boil, add orange rind and continue boiling for approximately 4 minutes. Strain mixture through a cheesecloth, pressing out 3 cups of dandelion liquid. Return 3 cups of liquid to pan. Add pectin and let boil, stirring constantly. Gradually stir in sugar and boil 5-6 minutes more. Skim foam from jelly. Pour into sterilized jelly glasses, and place seals and rings on jars.

Process in boiling water bath for 5 minutes.

### Dressing for Dandelion Greens

1 egg, beaten
¾ cup coconut sugar
¼ cup spelt flour
1 tsp salt
¼ cup bacon fryings (oil and uncured minced brown bacon)
½ cup apple cider vinegar
2 cups water
¼ lb uncured natural beacon, crisply fried and broken into bits
2 hard-boiled eggs, sliced

Combine egg, sugar, flour, salt, bacon fryings, vinegar and water in a sauce pan. Bring to a boil. Cook 3-4 minutes. Cool. Pour over dandelion greens that have been washed, drained and patted dry. Garnish with sliced hard-boiled eggs and bacon bits.

### Fried Dandelion Blossoms
Harvest chemical free blossoms. Dip fresh blossoms in beaten, salted egg. Drop into a skillet with several tablespoons of organic ghee or clarified melted butter. Brown quickly on both sides. Eat immediately. (Blossoms will be tough if allowed to cool.)

### Dandelion Greens (Lorrie Amitrano)

Dandelions and garlic were plentiful in many dishes growing up. We would pick young dandelion greens before they begin to blossom, then they are be tender and a tad less bitter.

Wash and rinse well.
They can be tossed raw into a salad with olive oil and red wine vinegar. They can be tossed into a pan with olive oil, potatoes, onions, garlic and sausage or scrambled eggs, salt and pepper.

*Other options*
They can be steamed over rapidly boiling water only until bright and tender and tossed with olive oil, onion, garlic, salt and pepper for a side dish.

Steamed dandelions can be tossed with soft butter, onion, sea salt and fresh ground pepper.

Be creative; what sounds good? Adding onion brings a sweetness that works well with the bitter flavor.

### Dandelion Greens (1902)

Select dandelion greens early in the spring before they begin to blossom. Wash thoroughly, and remove roots. Cook in a large amount of rapidly boiling water only until tender. Drain. Season with Organic or Kerrygold butter, Celtic Sea salt and fresh ground pepper. Serve with a sweet balsamic, apple or rice vinegar, or serve raw as a salad with salt, pepper, and vinegar.

### Dandelion Risotto Soup (Roseanne Romaine)
*This is a delicious soup using Arborio rice, bitter greens and natural smokey ham cooked up in a base of chicken stock.*
Serves 8

1 cup diced natural smoked ham
2 small shallots diced
3 cloves garlic diced
1 large bunch of dandelion greens, chopped 1 inch strips
2 small carrots, diced
1 bay leave
2 tbsp extra virgin olive oil
1 cup white arborio rice
8 cups homemade chicken stock 1 whole lemon juiced
1 tsp sea salt
2 tsp black pepper

*Cooking instructions*
Bring 4 cups of salted water to boil, add dandelion greens and cook for 5 minutes. This will create a less bitter green once added to the soup. Discard water and drain greens, rinse well with cold water and set aside.

Preheat a heavy bottom soup pot. Add olive oil and bay leaf. Add shallots, carrots and garlic and cook until translucent. Add rice and cook while stirring constantly for two minutes or until the rice takes on a bit of color. *Do not brown the rice. Add the ham and stir, allow the ham to crisp a bit. When ham is cracking add lemon juice and deglaze the bottom of your pot.

Add 6 cups of warm chicken broth, stir well, add salt and pepper to taste. Stir well and allow the soup to come up to a boil, add the cooked dandelion greens, lower heat, place a cover over ¾ of the pot and allow to simmer for 30 minutes, you may want to add the last two cups of broth as the soup simmers, depending on how thin or thick you want your soup to be. After cooking for 30 minutes, check the texture of your rice, if it is still al-dente, allow to simmer for 10 more minutes, adjust the seasoning to your liking and add more broth if you want to. Serve along with a side a fresh green salad and perhaps some Parmesan crisps.

*Serving instructions*
This is a very hearty and satisfying dish; a 6-8 ounce serving is satiating.
*Note:* You can vary the veggies in this recipe. I am keeping it nightshade-free but I think some red peppers would be delicious as well as mushrooms.

### Dandelion Love

*The few memories I have about my Sicilian grandmother's cooking, besides it always smelling amazing, is that it was varied, and there was always something simmering or braising. The dish my mom made that always stood out in my memory is a dandelion soup she would make during family holidays. The bitter taste to my young palate was quite off-putting, so I did not voluntarily partake of this soup; as I grew older, this chain of thinking and my eating changed.*

*The actual recipe used by my grandmother is now lost. I am sure the loss of traditions and recipes like this is felt by many of us. However, I am happy to say that there is a shift toward exploring traditional foods and recipes, even if it's not the exact, original recipes. I hope this continues, and we can all start sharing the knowledge and love we have for the foods of our ancestors. I believe strongly that food is medicine; therefore, we can heal this aching world through food.*

*~ Roseanne Romaine*

## Timpsila, or "Indian Turnip"

Timpsila was probably the most important wild food gathered by the Lakota. In 1805, a Lewis and Clark expedition observed Plains Indians collecting, peeling, and frying prairie turnips. The Lakota women told their children, who helped gather wild foods, that prairie turnips point to each other. When the children noted which way the branches were pointing, they were sent in that direction to find the next plant. This saved the mothers from searching for plants, kept the children happily busy, and made a game of their work.

Prairie turnips were so important, they influenced the selection of hunting grounds. Women were the gatherers of prairie turnips and their work was considered of great importance to the tribe. In 1804, Lewis and Clark called it the "white apple" and their French boatmen called it *pomme blanche*. In 1837, while crossing the James River basin, Captain John Fremont refers to it as *pommes des terres*, or the ground apple.

The tuber can be eaten raw, cut into chunks, boiled in stews, or ground into a fine flour. The flour can then be used to thicken soups or made into a porridge flavored with wild berries. Mixed with berries, water and some tallow, the flour can be made into cakes, which when dried, make a durable and nutritious trail food.[168]

Additional Information can be found at **American Indian Health and Diet Project**:
https://aihd.ku.edu/foods/prairie_turnip.html

## Watercress Dressing

*Watercress is versatile, it can be used as a salad green with Romaine lettuce or fresh spinach, steamed and eaten as a vegetable, and in soups for a subtle, peppery flavor, in sandwiches and wraps.*

½ cup extra virgin organic olive oil
⅓ cup apple cider vinegar (this should be the raw form with "mother")
1 tsp Celtic Sea salt
Dash fresh ground black pepper
½ cup chile sauce
1 cup watercress fresh fine chopped

Blend oil, vinegar, chile sauce, salt, and pepper, until creamy. Add watercress. Ready to serve with a spring green salad.

## Old Fashioned Irish Watercress Soup

Serves: 4-6

6 tbsp Kerrygold butter
2 medium Yukon gold or red potatoes
1 cup chopped leeks (white only)
3 cups vegetable or chicken broth
1 cup ½ & ½ or cream
2 bunches watercress

Slice the leeks and sauté in butter in a heavy pot on medium heat. Peel and chop potatoes and add to leeks, and give a good stir. Pour in the broth, bring to a boil, cover and cook until the vegetables are soft (about 20 minutes). Remove the coarser stems from the watercress and chop the rest, leaving a few sprigs for garnish. Add to the pot and cook uncovered for 4-5 minutes. Do not overcook or watercress will lose color. Purée in a blender, return to pot, add cream, and reheat slowly. Adjust seasonings. Serve decorated with reserved sprigs of watercress. Add salt and pepper to taste.

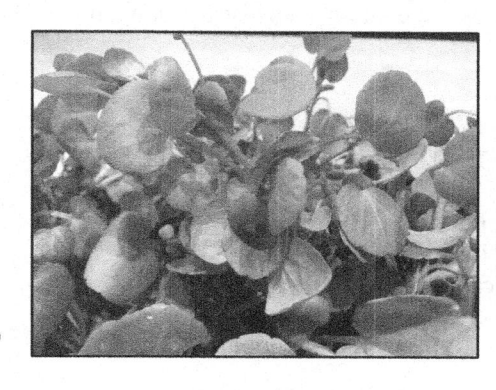

## Steamed Purslane (Mely Martinez)

*Purslane is considered a succulent. It's believed to arrive at the Mediterranean from Asia. It appears in the cuisines of Spain, Greece, and Italy. In Mexico, it is sold at the municipal markets, and people commonly forager them from their local surroundings. Other names for Purslane (Portulaca oleracea,) is little hogweed, pusley, fatweed, and pigweed. In Spanish, "Verdolagas" and they taste a little bit tart. You can eat them raw in salads before their small yellow flowers appear, after that, you can use them in stews or steamed.*[169]

Serves 2

2 cups purslane
1 clove garlic
1 tbsp olive oil
2 tbsp Cotija cheese or Parmesan
Salt and pepper to taste

Fill a small sauce pan or wide skillet with 1 cup of water, and add the garlic clove. Turn the heat to medium high.

Bring the water to a boil, add the purslane, and reduce the heat to low. Cover the sauce pan or skillet and keep cooking for 6 minutes. The cooking time will also depend on the tenderness of the purslane. If it has long, and woody stems it will take more time to cook compared to tender small leaves and steams.

Remove it from the heat and drain. Season with olive oil, salt, and pepper. To serve dust with the Cotija cheese or if you don't find it, Parmesan cheese is a good substitute. Just remember that these two kinds of cheese are salty, no need to add much salt to the purslane.

### Nettle Broth (old Irish recipe)

2 pints of nettle tops
2 lbs beef stew meat
Scallions
1 cup barley
Celtic Sea salt and pepper

Bring the meat and barley to a boil. Simmer on low heat for 2 hours. Add the chopped scallions and nettles, cook for another hour.
Season to taste.

### Stinging Nettle Sauté (Crystal Shepard)
Serves 2

1-2 tbsp lard (or butter or olive oil)
1 slice of bacon, minced
1 small onion, thinly sliced
2 cups tightly packed fresh nettle leaves
2 tbsp balsamic vinegar (or to taste)
Salt and pepper to taste

To prepare the fresh stinging nettle leaves simmer them for about two minutes in boiling water and then drain. Let them cool slightly, then chop them up.

In a medium sized skillet, heat the lard. When hot, add the bacon and onion slices. Cook until the bacon is cooked through and the onions are translucent.

Add the prepared nettles. Mix well. Drizzle with a couple tablespoons of aged balsamic vinegar. Season with salt and pepper to taste. Serve hot.

### Irish Moss Lemonade (1891)

¼ cup Irish Moss
2 cups water

1 lemon, juiced
Sugar, organic to taste

Wash, clean and soak Irish Moss in cold water to cover until soft. Clean and wash once more, add the 2 cups boiling water and cook 20 minutes, until dissolved, in a double boiler, then strain; add lemon juice and sugar to sweeten.

Good for delicate digestion.

> **Recipe for Happiness**
> *SRM Trail Boss Cookbook 1990*
>
> *2 heaping cups of patience*
> *2 handfuls of generosity*
> *1 heartful of love*
> *Dash of laughter*
> *1 head full of understanding*
>
> *Sprinkle generously with kindness. Add plenty of faith. Mix well.*
> *Spread over a period of a lifetime and serve everybody you meet.*

## Mugolio: Pine Cone Syrup (Chef Alan Bergo, Hungarian traditional recipe)

*Foraging is my therapy and connection to nature, as well as something that feeds me. In searching for ingredients, I found myself and what it means to be truly happy.*
Serves 8

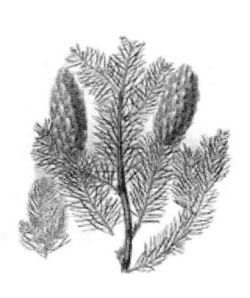

Dark, rich syrup infused with the essence of pine. Makes a little under 2 cups. This is a small amount; you can scale the recipe using the same proportions as needed. For large batches, just combine pine cones with approximately twice their weight in non-white sugar. Use as a condiment, breakfast syrup or dessert.

2 cups (8 oz) young red pine or other pine cones (soft enough to be cut with a knife)
2 cups (16 oz) organic brown sugar or other brown sugar, just not white which is dry and makes a clear syrup

*Maceration*
Combine the sugar and pine cones and pack into a quart jar, then allow to macerate (age) for 30 days. Put the jars in a sunny place where they will get warm during the day, which will help ward off mold.

During the first few weeks of maceration, open the jar occasionally to release carbon dioxide as the mixture will ferment vigorously. Shake it occasionally to help it on it's journey.

As the cones release their water, the volume of the contents in the jar will decrease. If you have more cones and sugar, you can add it to fill up the jar.

*Finishing and storing*
After the maceration is complete, scrape the sugar slush and pine cones into a pot, bring to a brisk simmer and heat through to melt the sugar, then strain and bottle.
All you need to do is bring the temperature up and melt the sugar, if you reduce the syrup too much it will crystalize after it cools. For the amounts listed, it should take about 5-10 minutes.

The syrup is stable at room temperature since the fermentation lowers the *pH* but will keep the best flavor in the refrigerator. It can also be water bath processed.

*The Forager Chef James Beard Award Winer:* https://foragerchef.com/mugolio-pine-cone-syrup/

## Wild Rice Salad

*Apple cider vinaigrette*
6 tbsp apple cider vinegar
¼ cup wild honey
¾ cup extra virgin olive oil, or clarified organic butter (melted)
Celtic Sea salt and fresh ground pepper

Combine all ingredients, whisk or blend and let rest for 1 hour or up to 10 days refrigerated.

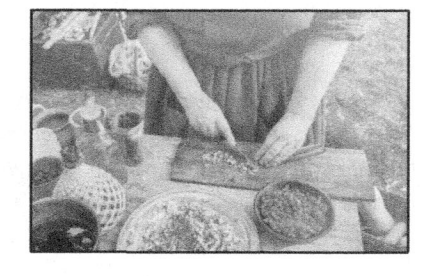

*Salad*
6 cups homemade vegetable stock or organic brand
1½ cups wild rice
1 carrot, peeled and cut into 2 inch matchsticks
3 tbsp dried cranberries
1 plum (Roma) tomato, finely diced
4-5 scallions (green onions), including green tops, finely chopped
½ cup pine nuts, toasted and cooled
½ cup raw pumpkin seeds, toasted and cooled
3 bunches washed watercress stemmed

Combine stock and wild rice. Bring to a boil, and then reduce the heat to simmer. Cover and cook until tender (45-55 minutes). Spread the rice on a baking sheet and let cool.

Scrape the rice into a large bowl and add the carrot, cranberries, tomato, scallions, pine nuts, and pumpkin seeds. Toss to mix.

Add ½ cup vinaigrette and toss and coat. Cover and refrigerate for at least 1 hour. Divide the watercress among salad plates and top with the wild rice.

*This adapted recipe comes from the traditional Ojibwa of the North American Great Lakes.*

## Chickweed Salad

2 cups chopped young chickweed greens
1 cup chopped young watercress leaves
¼ cup chopped wild onion bulbs and flowers
1 oz chopped buds, flowers and green pods of fanweed, shepherds purse and tumbling mustard

Mix all ingredients and toss: add favorite dressing.

## Wild Greens Pie

Use pigweed, lambs quarters, sorrel, purslane, chickweed, nettles, dandelion leaves, or cows cabbage.

Make pie crust and place in the bottom of pan.
Fill pie crust with 1 cup of cooked greens. In a sauce pan, beat 2 eggs, a teaspoon salt, dash of pepper, ¾ cup organic whole milk. Place over low heat, do not boil. Pour while hot over greens. Top with ½ cup sharp cheese grated. Bake at 350°F for 30 minutes. Serve hot.

## Cattails on the Cob

Use as young cattail flowers as possible, but they're still palatable after they turn brownish and start releasing pollen. Remove leaves. Drop in a pot of boiling water for 8-10 minutes. Drain well and serve with melted butter, salt, and pepper. The water you cooked them in will probably have turned yellow from the pollen from male flowers. Save it, it is full of pure pollen protein. Use it in soup, or add a little salt and broth and drink.

## Cattail Pollen Dumplings in Sweet Onion Soup

*Combine*
⅔ cup cattail pollen and flowers
¼ cup wheat germ

½ cup cracker meal
¼ cup powdered milk
½ cup flour
2 tsp baking powder
½ tsp salt

Add: 1 egg plus water to make ½ cup and 2 tablespoons melted butter. Drop from a wet spoon into simmering soup.

*Soup*: Sauté sweet onions until tender. Add broth, seasoning and simmer.

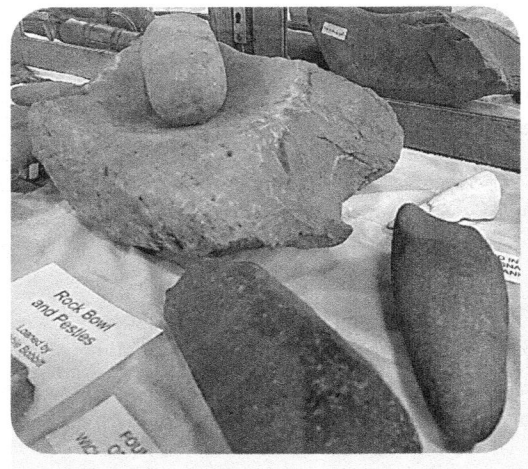

### Foods of Northwest Tribes

*Those living along the Northwest coast such as the Bella Bella, Bella Coola, Chinook, Coosans, Haida, Kwakiutls, Makah, Nootkans, Quileutes, Salish, Tillamook, Tlingit, and Upper Umpqua were supported by a vast amount of foods from the ocean and the lush land. Salmon was a major source of food, along with trout, halibut, and herring; followed by acorns, hundreds of different plants, whales, otters, seals, bears, beavers, lynx, deer, small game, ground squirrels, rabbits, and hares.*

*Devon A. Mihesuah,*
*Recovering Our Ancestors' Gardens: Indigenous Recipes and Guide to Diet and Fitness*
*(University of Nebraska Press, 2005)*

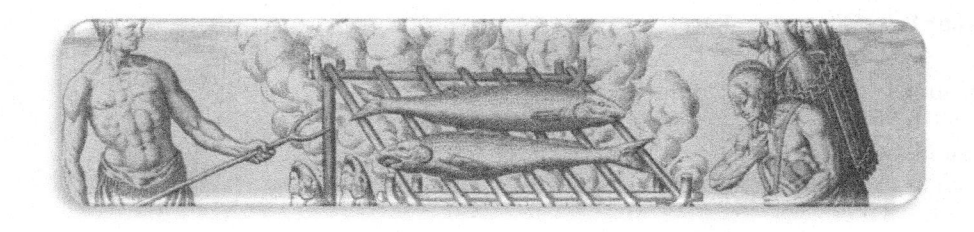

## Game Meat & Offal

*What appears to be repeats occur in this section: they are representations of different cooking approaches with the same foods.*

**Mincemeat Filling** (1890, adapted by Tammera Karr)

*Traditionally served during Christmas — often baked into pies.*
*Yields 16 pints*

3 lbs of ground elk, venison, or lamb*
1 cup rendered lard** from a humanely raised pork
7 tart winter apples sliced
2 cups dried currants
5 cups wild huckleberries or organic blueberries with juice
2 cups organic apple cider
2 cups Cognac or brandy
2 tbsp Celtic Sea salt
1 cup raw honey or organic sugar
¼ cup arrowroot powder
2 tbsp ground cinnamon
2 tbsp ground clove
1 tsp ground allspice
2 tsp ground nutmeg
1 tbsp ground ginger

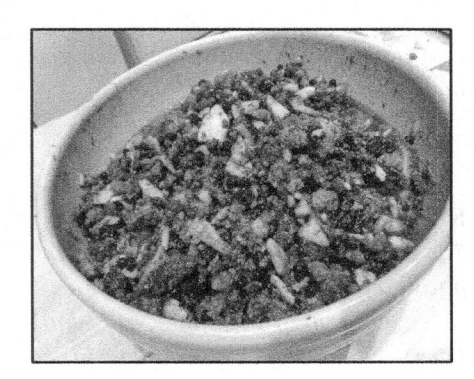

Melt lard** in a large pan, add ground meat, tossing to cook evenly on medium heat, add spices, salt, and honey or sugar. After meat is cooked and ingredients are mixed thoroughly, place in a large bowl with dried currants, apples, and huckleberries with berry juice.
Add cognac, apple cider, and arrowroot powder.

Mix well and cover with parchment paper to separate minced meat from plastic wrap used to seal bowl. Place in refrigerator for 4-6 days.

Once the mixture has stewed, it is ready to make minced pie or place in glass jars for canning.
**Palm, coconut or clarified organic butter can be used in place of lard.*
* When using lamb reduce fat by ⅓.

## Spicy Meat Bars (Tammera Karr)

1 lb of ground bison, elk, pork, or ground fowl
¼ cup olive oil
1 tsp ground turmeric
1 tbsp Italian seasoning
1 tsp red chili flakes
1 tsp smoked paprika
1 tbsp basil
1 tbsp parsley
½ large Walla Walla onion fine chopped
3-4 cloves Italian garlic minced

Mix meat together well, make a well in the center of the ground meat and add herbs and spices. Work all ingredients together until well blended. (Turmeric will stain.)

Form into small bars or patties, cook on the broiler, skillet or on a wood fire grill. Cook slowly to ensure fully cooked.

Cool and place in stainless steel or glass storage. Can be taken straight from the freezer to lunch box.


## Kidney (Elk, Moose, Deer)
*The utilization of kidneys is not new or trendy. In fact, organ foods made up a key portion of native diets. Kidney also holds a place of culinary pride on the English table. This prized food is rich in vitamin A, B vitamins, iron, and trace minerals, and kidney contains the rare amino acid L-ergothioneine. The omega-3 fatty acids in beef kidney may also increase fertility via their anti-inflammatory properties.*

Trim/pull the white lining off of the kidney
Cut the kidney into 1 inch cubes

Let the cubes soak in a mixture of cold water and lemon juice for 2 hours.
Pat cubes dry, season with salt and pepper, then coat in flour.
Heat the olive oil or ghee on high heat. Then add the cubes of kidney.

Remove the kidney from the pan once it's cooked through.
Add wild onion to the pan. Sauté, add the kidney back in, a squeeze of lemon juice.
Sizzle together for 30 seconds until coated.
Or boil the kidney; slice into strips and roll in flour, and fry in hot oil.

### Tongue (Elk, Moose, Deer)
Boil tongue until tender. Remove outer skin; slice and serve with horseradish.

### Sweetbreads (Elk, Moose, Deer)
*Despite the confusing name, sweetbreads are a type of organ meat and one of the better tasting options. Sweetbreads come from either the thymus gland or pancreas of an animal. They have a meaty-but-mild and slightly creamy taste, that is succulent and moist in comparison to other organ meats. Sweetbreads like other organ foods are rich in nutrition containing minerals, vitamin C, and B-vitamins. Sweetbreads are exceptionally high in vitamin C, providing protection from scurvy when fruits were not available.*

Cover sweetbreads with water in a bowl, refrigerate overnight and take the bowl out when you are ready to cook.

*Grill or roast sweetbreads*
Rub sweetbreads with a little butter or olive oil and place on a hot grill or in the oven.
Turn the sweetbreads to ensure they are cooked on all sides and become golden brown in color.

*Pan-fried*
Roll the sweetbreads in flour, place in a medium hot skillet and fry in olive oil or ghee with fresh herbs 6-7 minutes or until fully cooked on both sides.

### Rocky Mountain Oysters
Also known: cowboy caviar, prawn oysters, beef oscillation, Montana tenderloin, dusted nuts, bollocks, or pork chicken.

*The testicles of animals have been highly sought after for time immemorial. The testicles of buffalo, calves, lambs, roosters, turkeys, and other animals are eaten in many parts of the world under a wide variety of culinary names. In Argentina and Spain, they are called criadillas, in Turkey they are called "billur," and they are also a much quoted dish in the Chinese, Iranian and Greek gastronomy.[170] Some historical and modern cultures see testicles as aphrodisiacs, others a male energy food. In researching this food, we found the nutrition content (just like other forms of seeds) is rich in essential fats and minerals. Testicles are lean protein, low in carbohydrates, and contain zinc, phosphorous, potassium, sodium, and magnesium.*

*Rocky Mountain Oysters*: Sauteed, cooked, roasted, and are often peeled, coated with flour, salt, and pepper and fried.

Remove thin outer skins; clean well. Soak in salt water for 1 hour. Roll in flour and fry in hot oil.

**Venison or Elk Bresaola** - Charcuterie (adapted by Chef Ben Qualls)

*One of the areas Chef Ben has embraced is smoking and curing meats. This allows for a return to ancestral foods free of all additives detrimental to health. Many cured and cooked meats are often served as appetizers. Ancestral curing and fermenting techniques were used to preserve meat before refrigeration. Italy, Spain, and France are well known for their preserved meats. Bresaola is traditionally made from a lean eye of the round cut of beef, and it works equally well with game meat.*

*The eye of round cut can be found on the inside of the hind leg one quarter of the way between the top and bottom rounds. It is easily separated and is similar in shape and size to the loin, which works well for making bresaola.*

*Do not rush this recipe. Great preserved meats take several weeks to complete and is well worth the wait!*

Two 1½ lbs venison loins (backstrap) or eye of round venison cuts, trimmed of silver skin
¼ cup kosher salt
2 tbsp sugar
1 tbsp whole peppercorns
1 tbsp fresh rosemary leaves
2 tsp fresh thyme leaves
2 fresh sage leaves
4-6 juniper berries

*Preparation*
1. Weigh each piece of venison and record the weight to the closest gram or oz weight.

2. Combine all of the spices in a coffee grinder and pulse a few times to create a granular powder spice mixture. It's okay if there is just a little residue coffee flavor there.

3. Rub the spice mixture all over the meat until well coated. Place the meat in a non-reactive container, such as a glass, ceramic baking dish, or food-grade plastic storage container. Cover and refrigerate the meat for 5 days. Drain the meat. Put back in the refrigerator for another 5 days.

4. Rinse the meat with cold water to remove any remaining spices and pat dry (or you could brush all of the spices off with a wine-infused cloth). The meat will be a much darker color. Set the meat on a rack for 2-3 hours to thoroughly dry.

5. Tie the meat with butcher twine using a running butcher's knot (slip knot). Wrap the meat in a double layer of cheesecloth and hang the meat in a cool (60°F), dark location with about 60-70 percent humidity for about 2 weeks.

6. Weigh the meat. It should weigh 30% less than the beginning weight. A 24 ounce piece should weigh about 16.8 ounces. The meat should feel firm to the touch and be very uniform and smooth when sliced.

7. Serve the bresaola sliced very thin as part of an appetizer tray. It is also nice sliced thin, drizzled with olive oil and lemon and served with arugula or other mixed greens.

More: There may be a few white specks of mold on the outside of the meat after hanging, which can be wiped off with a wine-infused cloth. White mold is similar to some cheese molds and in small amounts if fine, but if there is any black mold or excessive mold, do not eat.

There should not be an offensive odor to the meat.

If the outside is dark and the inside has an appearance or texture of raw meat, then it did not dry uniformly and should not be consumed.

If the meat has lost more than 30% weight it can become hard and difficult to chew. Simply shave it very thin or even grate it to use as a topping. It is still safe to eat.

### Duck Liver Pâté

*When pâté is mentioned often, we think of rich dining or Jewish cuisine. The history is really more interesting. The practice of feeding captive geese to enlarge their livers began in 400 BC, according to archaeological information on the Egyptians. Our association with pate and royalty dates to a French chef in 1779, who was gifted twenty pistols by King Louis XVI for the excellence of his pâté.*

*In our efforts to honor the animals harvested and ancestral foods, we support the use of what might otherwise be discarded organ meat.*

*Adapted from a Jacques Pepin recipe*

3 oz duck fat or butter
1 shallot, peeled and coarsely chopped (about 2½ tbsp)
3 oz of duck liver, cut into 1 inch pieces (about 4-5 mallard size duck livers)
¼ tsp *herbes de Provence*
1 clove garlic, peeled and crushed
¼ tsp salt
¼ tsp freshly ground black pepper
1 tsp Cognac
1-2 tsp of half and half or heavy cream
16 ¼ inch thick horizontal slices from a small baguette, toasted
*milk for pre-soaking livers

*Directions*
1. Soak livers in milk, just covering them for half hour or more.

2. Drain and discard the milk off the liver. Season the livers with salt, pepper, a pinch of sugar, a few sprigs of fresh thyme for a few hours or overnight in the refrigerator. (You can add about a 1 tablespoon of Armagnac or Cognac, sweet vermouth, Madeira, port wine or sherry for added flavor.)

3. Place duck fat in a skillet, and cook over medium to high heat for 4-5 minutes, until the fat has melted and some of it has browned. If you do not have duck fat, you can melt butter or lard instead.

4. Add the shallots, and cook for about 30 seconds, stirring occasionally. Add the liver, *herbes de Provence*, and garlic, and cook over medium to high heat for about 2 minutes, stirring occasionally. Add the salt and pepper.

5. Transfer the mixture to a blender, add the Cognac and cream, and blend until liquefied. Or you can use a handheld immersion blender. If a finer textured pâté is desired, push the mixture through the holes of a strainer with a spoon. Let cool for at least 1½ hours, allowing the flavors to meld, then cover and refrigerate until serving time. Taste and adjust the seasoning to your liking.

6. Spread the pâté on the toasted baguette slices, and serve. The pâté will keep covered in the refrigerator for 3-5 days and can be frozen for up to 3 months in an airtight container.


## Hunters Stew

*Stew has its origins in antiquity and predates almost all other forms of cooked dishes and can be found in every culture worldwide. Stews can be made from any meat and vegetables available. The slow cooking and combining of flavors create the perfect freeing of nutrients for digestion.*

1½ lbs of venison, moose, elk, or caribou
Spread pieces of meat on the bottom of a clay oven-safe pot or cast iron Dutch oven. Place slices of shallots, rich yellow winter, or Spanish red onions over the top of the meat.

¼ cup red pepper, chopped
4 stalks of celery with leaves chopped
4-5 medium heirloom carrots, sliced
5-6 Roma tomatoes peeled and chopped
1 cup wild mushrooms, sliced
4-6 cloves of garlic
1½ cups stock or water
1 bouquet of herbs (sprigs of rosemary, thyme, oregano, sage)

*Optional*
1 cup Italian or Spanish red wine.
Bake at 325°F for 3 hours or until meat is fork tender.
Serve with crusty sourdough bread and a glass of table wine.


**Stuffed Heart** (Tammera Karr)

*Ancient humans prized organ meat above all other forms of animal flesh. These foods were often consumed on site and raw or minimally heated. Organ meats spoil easily and contain the highest nutrition value when raw. Humans developed traditions around the consumption of organ foods to emphasize the importance of the food. Modern nutritional analysis reveals the origins of the heart's historic reverence in part comes from the bioavailable nutrition rich in B vitamins, coenzyme Q10, essential minerals, and amino acids. Before the modern phrase of the nose to tail, native peoples utilized every part of the foods harvested.*

*Contrary to popular opinion, heart is very tender and flavorful. Heart can be ground and incorporated into many dishes. Heart is an affordable protein source, which is why organ meats returned to the dinner table during the Great Depression and WWII.*

*Following a successful hunt or beef harvest, the baked heart is a favorite dish to be found in rural areas of North America.*

1 heart from elk, venison, moose, caribou or buffalo
Using a sharp knife, carefully clean away the crown area and inner chamber of veins and valves to create an open area to stuff.
1 cup wild rice, cooked
¼ cup wild mushrooms, sliced
¼ cup berries
¼ cup sliced wild onions, shallots or onions
3 cloves garlic, minced
2 tbsp oil
½ cup stock, reserve ¼ cup for later

Sauté wild mushrooms, shallots or wild onions, fresh huckleberries or cranberries, and garlic with tallow, duck fat or olive oil. Add cooked wild rice and ¼ cup stock.

Stuff the heart with combined ingredients. Cover the crown opening with foil. Place in a Dutch oven and add ¼ cup stock to the interior and cover. Place in a hot oven.

Bake at 325°F for 45-60 minutes or when a meat thermometer reads interior temp is 130°F

Make a gravy from any juices, and serve with roasted root vegetables or crusty sourdough bread.

## Roast Wild Goose

(Stuffing is optional, if used, only fill the cavity ¾ full as the dressing will expand).
1 wild goose
1 jar spiced apples
2 tbs Irish butter or organic
¼ cup water

Clean and pluck a goose. Baste inside body cavity with 3-4 tablespoons juice from spiced apples. Brush outside with butter, salt, and pepper to taste; add water and roast at 325°F for 25 minutes per pound of goose (be sure to keep goose covered.) One-half hour before serving, remove cover and baste outside of goose with more juice from apples until glazed brown. Serve trimmed with parsley and spiced apples.

## Baked Pheasant

*Pheasants were first brought to North America in 1773 and did not begin to propagate until the early 1800s. The Chinese Ring-necked Pheasant was released in Oregon in 1881. MacFarlane Pheasants Inc is the largest pheasant farm in North America and produces approximately 1.3 million chicks per year. They are released by clubs, individuals, and government agencies to be enjoyed for sport and consumption. Restaurants and grocery stores buy meats for consumers to appreciate.*[171] *Game birds are predominately dark meat and contain higher levels of nutrients and fat.*[172]

*It should be noted game birds of all species frequent grain fields that are often seeded with GMO crops. The US Department of the Interior provided seed to farmers for developing game corridors that were suspected of being GMO seed, creating contamination of nearby non-GMO crops.*[173] *This use of GMOs and pesticides was phased out in 2016-18 in refuge systems.*[174]

1 pheasant, cut up as you would a chicken
Celtic Sea salt and pepper
1 cup organic all-purpose flour
1 cup clean lard or olive oil

Season the pheasant with salt and pepper, and roll the pieces in the flour. In a cast iron chicken frier or Dutch oven, heat oil on a medium flame; the oil should have slight ripples forming on the surface but not be smoking. Brown the pheasant pieces, lift out pieces, and drain off all but 4 tablespoons of oil. DO NOT pour down the sink drain or into glass.

Add 2 tablespoons of coating flour into the frier with the reserved oil and combine the two; slowly add filtered water to form the gravy base. Season gravy with wild mushrooms, white wine, 1 tablespoon dried or fresh minced onions, salt, and pepper. Add the pheasant into the gravy, ensuring the flesh is coated or covered with gravy.

Cover and bake at 300°F for 2 hours. Serve with potatoes, wild rice, or vegetables of choice.

## Rabbit and Gravy

1 rabbit (locally sourced and humanely harvested)
1½ pints cold water
1½ tbsp Celtic Sea salt
Soak rabbit in water and salt for 3 hours, drain, dry and cut apart for frying.
1 pinch Celtic Sea salt
1 pinch organic black pepper
1 cup organic white spelt flour
1 tsp organic garlic powder
1 tsp smoked paprika

Combine dry ingredients, and roll rabbit pieces in flour.

In a cast iron Dutch oven on medium heat brown ½ pound uncured applewood bacon. Remove bacon and use the remaining fat for frying the rabbit (there should be about ⅓ cup of fat).

Brown rabbit on all sides frequently turning to prevent burning. Cover and cook on low heat for 1½ hours. Turn rabbit during this time to ensure it does not burn on the bottom.

Add 1 cup raw or organic whole milk or broth and continue cooking on low heat for 30 minutes more. Serve rabbit and gravy straight from your casserole dish or Dutch oven with seasonal vegetables.

## Conejo Guisado - Basque Rabbit Stew (Kelsi Sitz)

1 rabbit, cut into pieces
1 cube butter
Salt
⅛ tsp clove
¼ tsp thyme
½ tsp parsley
Pinch nutmeg
1 medium onion, chopped
2 tbsp arrowroot
2 cups water
½ cup mushrooms, sliced
6 carrots, chopped
1 cup white wine
2 cloves garlic, minced
1 small bell pepper, chopped
Flour

Use a heavy pot, cut rabbit into pieces, salt and pepper it, roll in flour and fry in butter till golden brown. Remove rabbit from pan, add carrot, onion, ½ of green pepper, garlic, and sauté in butter. Add arrowroot, stir well, and gradually add wine, then rabbit and water (enough to cover rabbit), salt, herbs, and spices.

Simmer for 1½ hours. Add mushrooms and simmer for 40 minutes longer.

## Elk in Wine (Tammera Karr)

*As a rule, I prefer a simple seared piece of meat, but every once in a while, I get wild.*
Serves 6-8

2 lbs elk (1½ inch cubes)
⅓ cups organic all-purpose flour
4 medium Spanish onions
3 tbs extra virgin olive oil
¼ tsp each Celtic Sea salt and pepper
¼ tsp each marjoram and thyme
½ cup broth
½ lb wild mushrooms
1 cup red table wine

Using a skillet brown onion in oil, remove from skillet and set aside. Sauté meat in drippings, adding more oil if necessary. Combine the flour and seasonings and sprinkle over the browned meat. Add the broth and wine. Simmer slowly for three hours, stirring occasionally. Add more broth if needed. Add mushrooms and browned onions; cook one hour longer. Serve with wild rice.

## Moose Steak

½ cup shallots chopped fine
½ cup naturally fermented sour cream
1 cup chopped wild mushrooms
2 tbsp organic butter (clarified)
2 tbsp flour

Fry onions brown in butter. Sear steak on both sides in butter and browned onions. Cover and let simmer for ½ hour. When almost tender, add the mushrooms and the flour, stir into the cream. Cover and let simmer for 20 minutes.

## Buffalo Steak in Red Wine (Tammera Karr)

Serves 4

2  8 oz buffalo sirloin steaks
2 cloves garlic, crushed
½ cup chopped wild onions or shallots
½ cup wild mushrooms
1 cup hearty red wine
4 tbsp lard or olive oil
Corse grain sea salt
Corse grind black pepper

Heat cast iron skillet over fire or preheat in oven to 400°F, add oil and sear steaks on both sides. Depending on thickness and doneness preferences this will take between 5 and 10 minutes per side.

Combine wine, garlic, and shallots, pour over steak – **NOTE** if your skillet is at the right temperature, especially over an open fire, the alcohol will flame while it cooks off. Be prepared, don't panic, it only lasts a few moments.

Continue cooking for an additional 5-8 minutes after flame is out.


## Venison with Cranberry Apples Sauce (Tammera Karr)

Serves 4

2 tart winter apples
1 cup apple cider
¼ cup maple syrup
4 cups fresh cranberries
8  4 oz venison steaks
Sea salt
2-4 tbsp lard

Put apples, cider, maple syrup and cranberries in a sauce pan. Bring to a boil, reduce heat to simmer until liquid has reduced to ¼ cup, about 12 minutes.

In a heavy cast iron skillet, heat oil on medium high, sauté meat in batches, turn once, until browned about 2 minutes per side. Transfer meat to a shallow skillet or baking pan and roast in 500°F preheated oven until medium rare, about 3 minutes.

Serve with cooled apple cranberry sauce.

**Bear Fat Pie Crust**

Make it clear to your favorite hunter that every bit of precious bear fat possible is to be brought home to you. Clean fat of any meat, then render it out slowly in a heavy pan on low heat; in an oven overnight is fine. Strain and pour into clean glass containers. Store in refrigerator, root cellar or freezer. Use bear fat in your favorite pie crust recipes for a treat that cannot fail.

### *The Noble Way to Hunt* [175]

*"As you hunt, you bond with the animals, and you start to match heartbeats," my uncle Richard Sherman told me.*

*"When you do that, respect for them and the land comes naturally. You realize whatever you do has an impact.*

*For me, it's important to follow the noble way to kill an animal cleanly with one shot, so that it just drops straight down. You can't do this until you learn to know the animals."*

Sean Sherman – The Sioux Chief
*2022 Recipient of the James Beard Award*

---

[167] Li, W., Hydamaka, A.W., Lowry, L. et al. Comparison of antioxidant capacity and phenolic compounds of berries, chokecherry and seabuckthorn. cent.eur.j.biol. 4, 499–506 (2009). https://doi.org/10.2478/s11535-009-0041-1

[168] Timpsila, the "Indian Turnip": https://www.wolakotaproject.org/timpsila-the-indian-turnip/

[169] Retrieved July 2022: https://www.mexicoinmykitchen.com/purslane-recipe-steamed/#recipe

[170] https://www.lifepersona.com/testicles-of-toro-nutritional-content-and-recipes

[171] https://www.pheasant.com/facts

[172] https://www.wildharvesttable.com/pheasant-nutritional-information/

[173] https://peer.org/refuges-to-ban-genetically-engineered-crops-and-neonics/

[174] https://peer.org/wp-content/uploads/attachments/FWS_Memorandum.pdf

[175] The Sioux Chef – Sean Sherman page 119

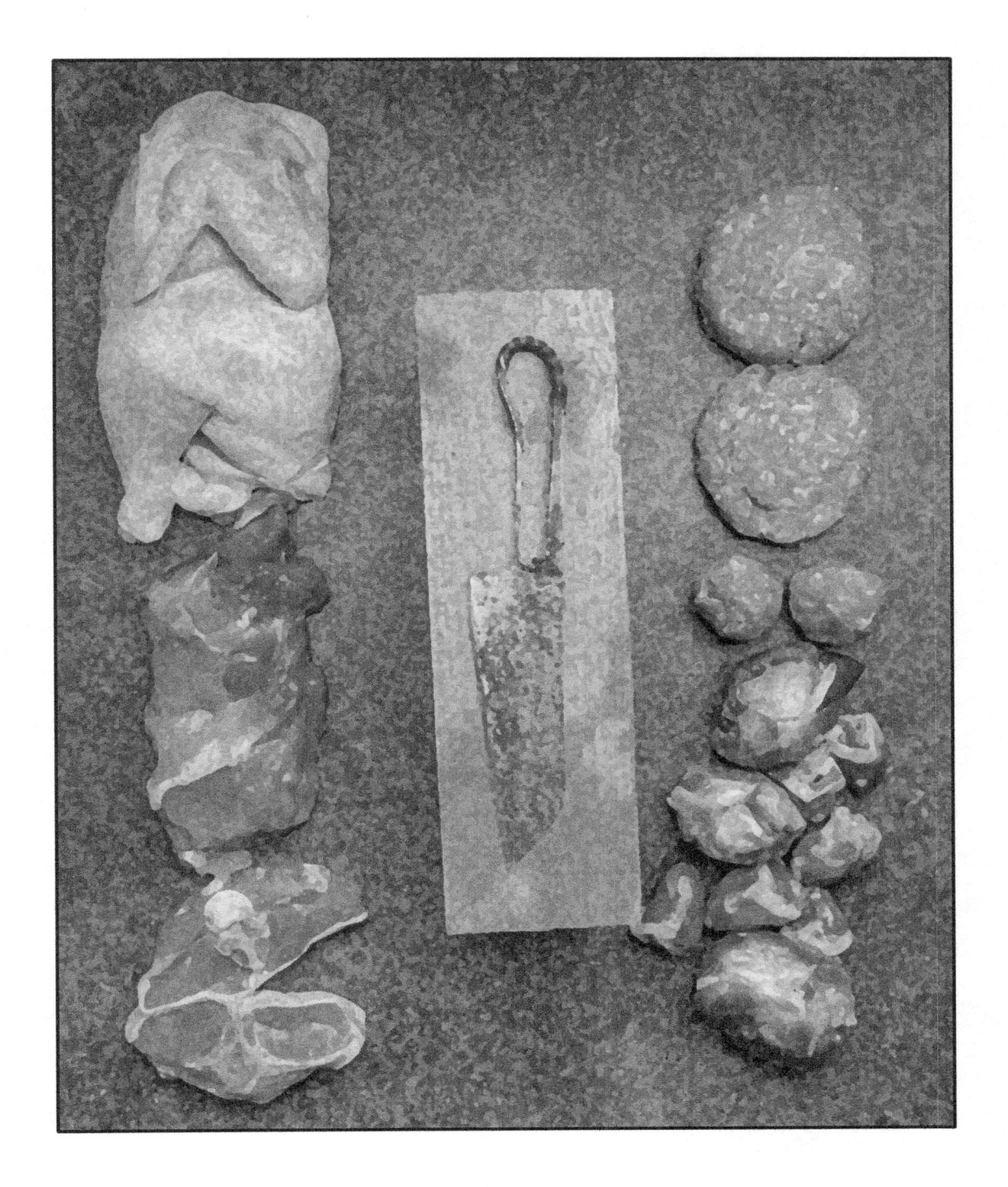

# Beef, Lamb, Pork & Poultry

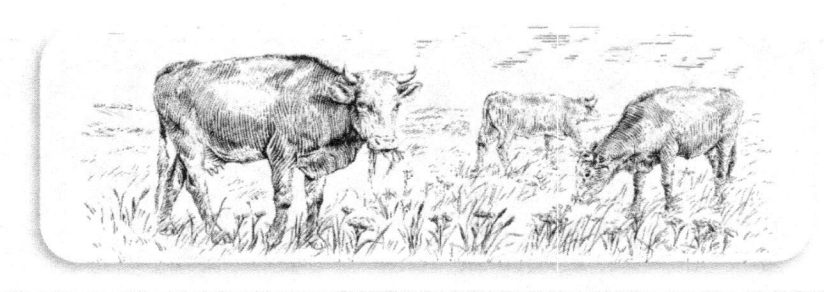

## Beef

**Filets' Con Pimentos -** Basque Tenderloin with Peppers (Kelsi Sitz)

1 lb tenderloin
1-2 clove garlic
¼ cup Spanish olive oil
½ cup bread crumbs
1 can pimentos
Salt and pepper to taste

Cut tenderloin steaks in half so the meat is not overly thick. Salt the steak. Cut garlic and spread it over the meat. Roll meat in bread crumbs and fry in hot oil for 2 minutes on each side. In a separate skillet, sauté the remaining garlic, add pimentos, and cook for 3-5 minutes. Pour over meat and serve.

**Braciole** (Lorrie Amitrano)
*I used to make this with my Grandpa Tony.*

2 beef flank steaks
Tenderize with a meat hammer, rub with extra virgin olive oil, and generously season with garlic powder, celery powder, onion powder, salt, and pepper.

Spread on each steak:
Grated Parmesan cheese
Chopped parsley
2 cloves of fresh garlic
3 hard-boiled eggs, chopped
1 small sweet onion, chopped
1 small bunch of fresh basil, chopped

Roll each flank, being careful to keep ingredients in. Snugly tie with pieces of string, tightly with square knots.

Take each roll and sear well in a pre-heated frying pan.

Place in pasta sauce over low heat and simmer all day.
Serve sliced with sauce, pasta, and salad.


### Grilled Steak with Spicy Argentinian Sauce (Chef Christine Wokowsky)
Serves 2

*Sauce*
1 cup Italian parsley, fresh chopped
1 cup watercress, fresh chopped
1 tsp red chile flakes
½ cup olive oil
¼ cup water
¼ cup red wine
1 tsp Celtic Sea salt
1 tsp black pepper
6 garlic cloves, chopped
1 tsp dried oregano
Whisk all ingredients together and set aside while making the steaks.

*Steak*
1 tbsp melted lard or olive oil
2 tsp salt
2 tsp black pepper, fresh cracked
2 New York strip steaks

Heat grill or stovetop pan to medium high heat.
Rinse off steaks and pat dry with a paper towel. Drizzle coconut oil on both sides of the steaks to coat. Add salt and pepper generously to each side of the steaks.

Once the grill or stove is hot place each steak on the hot surface and time the cooking on each side for 4-5 minutes for medium-rare depending on the thickness. Allow steak to rest for 7-10 minutes before serving.

Serve with greens, and potatoes with a generous helping of the spicy Argentinian Sauce.
Preparation time: 30 minutes. Cook time: 15 minutes.


### Hungarian Farina Dumpling Soup (Chef Ben Qualls)
*I have fond memories of this soup, called Griz Galuska. We used to call the dish "Cloud Noodle soup" because it was easier to pronounce, and the dumplings looked like little clouds floating in the broth. My Hungarian grandmother used to make this a lot during the winter when I was a boy in Michigan. She also added cooked chicken and sliced carrots to make it a bit hardier. Served with a nice crusty bread and a small green salad makes a great late fall or winter meal.*

1 egg
2 tbsp plus 2 tsp farina
¼ tsp pink Himalayan salt
1 tsp extra virgin olive oil
5 cups chicken broth

In a bowl, mix egg, farina, salt, and olive oil until well combined. Let stand 30 minutes, either in the refrigerator or at room temperature, until firm.

Place broth in a 4 quart stock pot and bring to a boil.

Using a tablespoon, scoop up the farina mixture and drop in soup. Repeat, placing as many dumplings as you can in the pot without crowding.

Lower heat to a slow, rolling boil (too strong a boil will cause dumplings to fall apart).
Cook 15-20 minutes or until a dumpling cut in half is no longer yellow on the inside. Repeat until finished with all the batter.


### **Hungarian Goulash** (Chef Benjamin Qualls)

1½ lbs flank steak, cut into cubes
2 tbsp flour
3 tbsp butter
1 large onion, chopped
2 large cloves garlic, finely chopped
2 cups water
6 oz tomato paste
½ tsp dried marjoram
½ tsp dry mustard
3 tbsp Worcestershire sauce
1 tbsp cider vinegar
1 tbsp raw sugar
Sea salt and black pepper to taste

Place the flank steak and flour in a mixing bowl; toss to coat, set aside.
Melt butter in a large stock pot over medium-high heat. Add onion, cook and stir until onion begins to soften, stir in garlic; cook for 2-3 more minutes. Stir in steak mixture and cook until browned on all sides; 5-7 minutes.

Stir in tomato paste, water, marjoram, mustard, Worcestershire sauce, cider vinegar, raw sugar. Stir well, bring just to a boil.

Reduce heat to low; cover and cook for 2-2½ hours or until beef is tender. Season with sea salt and black pepper to taste and serve with steamed potatoes or hot cooked pasta.

### Almandrongila Euskalduna Moduda - Meat Balls Basque Style (Kelsi Sitz)
Serves 8

*Meatballs*
1 lb ground veal
1 lb lean ground pork
1 large onion
½ tsp pepper
1 tbsp sugar
1¼ tsp chopped parsley
4 slices of stale bread
2 eggs
4 tbsp olive oil
4 tbsp butter
1 tsp salt approximant
Flour

Mix veal and pork in a large bowl. Add onion, salt, pepper, sugar, and parsley. Mix well. Moisten bread with milk or water, then squeeze until almost dry. Cut up and mix bread into the meat. Then add eggs and mix well. Form the meat mixture into small balls. Roll in flour and fry in oil and butter. Shake the frying pan frequently to retain small round balls. When browned, place in a large casserole or Dutch oven.

*Salsa*
2 tbsp olive oil
1 tbsp flour, heaping
1 small onion
1 chili pepper, finely chopped
2 cloves garlic, minced
1 bay leaf
¼ cup tomato sauce
2 tsp parsley, chopped
2 cups chicken broth
½ tsp paprika
2 whole cloves
4 oz canned mushrooms
⅛ tsp thyme
Salt and pepper

In a large bowl, mix all ingredients well until blended. Once the meatballs are browned and placed in a large casserole or Dutch oven and cover them with the salsa sauce.

Tacos were part of native Mexico long before the Spanish arrived. Ancient Mexicans used freshly made, soft, flat corn tortillas and fillings like fish and cooked organs. It was a staple meal that provided vital nutrients and energy to those who consumed it. These tacos didn't have hard shells or contain cheese, lettuce, sour cream, or the tomato we associate with tacos today. Glen Bell developed the everyday taco we know in the USA in 1962.

## Taco Spice Mix (Tammera Karr)

1 tbsp Ancho chili powder *(distinctive flavor and authentic to Mexican foods)*
1 tbsp turmeric
½ tbsp ground cumin
1-2 tsp Celtic Sea salt
¼ tsp Mexican oregano
½ tbsp Italian seasoning
¼ tsp jalapeno pepper powder
¼ tsp allspice
¼ tsp smoked paprika *(introduced to Europe by Columbus)*
¼ cup onion, minced or 2 tbsp dry onion
2-3 cloves garlic, minced or 1 tsp garlic powder
¼ cup fresh salsa juice

Gently warm spices in a dry skillet, add meat, mix well and brown. Add salsa juice, water, good tequila, or red wine, and let simmer for 10 minutes.

## Bobotie (Kirstin Nussgruber)

*Bobotie, a savory dish with tinges of sweet, has its origins in Cape Malay cooking. A similar dish was used in the Middle Ages in Europe during the Crusaders. They brought exotic spices, including turmeric, back to Europe. Another dish that requires long and slow cooking has many variations, using ground beef.*

Serves 6-8

2 lbs ground beef
Butter or olive oil
2 onions, peeled and diced
3 cloves garlic, peeled and crushed
1 tbsp curry powder
1 tsp ground turmeric
2 slices bread, crumbled

¼ cup milk
1 lemon, juice as well as the grated rind
1 tsp sea salt (or to taste)
1 tsp black pepper
4 oz dried apricots
1 granny smith apple, cored, peeled, and chopped
¼ cup sultanas
¼ cup slivered almonds, roasted in a dry stainless steel skillet
6 bay leaves

*Topping*
1 cup milk
2 eggs
½ tsp salt

*For a gluten-free and dairy-free version*
Replace bread slices with ¼ cup finely ground golden flax seeds.
Replace milk with dairy-free alternatives such as coconut, cashew, or almond milk.

Preheat oven to 325°F.

Grease a large casserole with butter or olive oil.
In a stainless steel pan, heat the butter or olive oil, and fry the onion until almost translucent, adding the minced garlic towards the end. Add the curry and turmeric powders, and stir until fragrant. Remove from heat.

Add the ground beef and stir.
Add the remaining ingredients except for the bay leaves, and stir well.
Add the entire mixture to the casserole, burying the bay leaves in between. Cover with foil and bake in the oven for 1-1¼ hours.

Increase the oven temperature to 400°F.

Mix the topping ingredients (depending on your size of casserole, you may need another batch), pour over the casserole and bake for another 15 minutes, uncovered, until lightly browned.

Can be served with rice or a large mixed salad.
Keeps well in the refrigerator for a few days. Delicious reheated.

*Adapted from "Rainbow Cuisine – A Culinary Journey through South Africa" by Lannice Snyman and Andrezej Sawa*

*Tongue is a delicacy in many cultures. I grew up with this being a special treat following a fall harvest of a steer (male castrated). The tongue is very tender and delicate with a rich, mildly sweet flavor.*

*You will see several versions of tongue. Some are from old cookbooks or handed down as ways to traditionally prepare. ~ Tammera Karr*

### **Beef Tongue** (Tammera Karr)

Serves 4

1 whole beef tongue, parboiled and tough skin cut or peeled away
Slice into quarter-inch pieces
½ cup spelt flour
½ tsp garlic granules or powder
1 tsp Celtic Sea salt
1 tsp parsley, dry
½ tsp fresh ground black pepper
4 tbsp olive oil
2 tbsp butter

In a large cast iron skillet, heat oil and butter on medium-high. Mix well with flour, garlic, salt, pepper and parsley in a plastic bag. Add slices of meat to a bag and toss them until they are evenly coated with the flour mixture.

Place each slice of meat in hot oil and brown both sides; approximately 2-3 minutes per side. Do not overcook.

### **Lengua or Behiki Miki** – Basque Beef Tongue

1 beef tongue parboiled and peeled
1 large egg
1 pint tomato sauce
Olive oil
Flour
Salt and pepper

After peeling tongue, slice it into ¼-½ inch pieces. Salt and pepper slices. Beat egg well, roll slices of meat in flour then dip in egg. Fry in hot oil.

In a sauce pan add 1 pint tomato sauce, 1 tablespoon olive oil, and a pinch of sugar. Heat on medium heat. Serve as a gravy with tongue.

### Liver and Onions (Tammera Karr)

*Every week this dish was served in our house and countless others in the Pacific Northwest. I never learned to like it, but I respect the nutritional value.*

1 tsp black pepper
½ tsp salt
3 tbsp extra virgin olive oil
1½ lbs beef liver, sliced
1 large onion, thinly sliced
1 cup beef broth
Spelt or gluten-free flour for dredging

Slice liver and dredge in flour seasoned with salt and pepper.
Place olive oil in a large skillet and brown both sides of the liver over medium-high heat. Do not overcook.

Place sliced onions in the skillet with the liver. Pour beef broth on top of liver and onions. Cover and simmer until onions are tender and broth forms a nice gravy.


### Scottish Haggis

*A savory pudding is traditionally made from sheep. Haggis means chopped or minced bits of animal parts. In the 1800s, Scotsmen roamed the hills, valleys, and shores of the Pacific Northwest. The founding father of Oregon is John McLaughlin, who served as an agent of the Hudson Bay Company and aided pioneers wanting to settle in the Oregon territory.*

*The roots of Scotland run deep in the Pacific Northwest and the crew at Holistic Nutrition for the Whole You. In celebration of those who survived to tell the tale, we offer up this ancestral dish. In his poem Address to a Haggis, Robert Burns immortalized the haggis, which starts "Fair fa' your honest, sonsie face, Great chieftain o' the pudding race!"*

NOTE: Read this recipe all the way through before attempting to cook – this will allow for doing the steps in the proper order.

½ lb liver
¼ lb suet (ideally from the kidney)
2 yellow onions
1 cup thick cut oatmeal (grind in a food processor)
1 cup brae (reserved water from cooking the liver)
Salt and pepper
Beef honeycomb tripe

Place whole liver and onions into a pan of cold water and bring to a boil for 40 minutes. Lift liver from the water and place it on a platter to cool. Reserve 1 cup of liver water. When cool, grate or mince the liver. Chop the onions fine.

Toast the oatmeal in a dry cast iron skillet until browned; add liver, suet, onions and seasonings. Moisten with the brae.

*The Bag:* Thoroughly wash the beef honeycomb tripe. Boil for 15 minutes, then scrape and clean the inside (not the honeycomb side) as much as possible. Let soak in cold water overnight. Fold the tripe over to make a bag, and sew the side with cotton kitchen twine; do not make stitches too small and tight or they will not hold during the expansion of cooking. Leave a space open to insert the liver and oats; do not overfill as the mix will expand during cooking. Finish sewing the opening shut. Prick with a toothpick here and there.

Place the haggis in a pan of hot water, bring to a soft boil, and cook for 3 hours. Place haggis on a platter and allow to cool slightly. With a sharp knife and a Robert Burns flourish, cut a slit in the haggis for all to have access to the filling. Serve with mashed turnips.

## Marrow Bones

Marrow bones should be cut into 2 inch pieces for serving. Wash and scrape sides. Place in hot oven for 6 minutes or until cooked through. Salt and serve on organic sourdough rounds with minced fresh parsley and watercress.

## Oxtail Casserole

Oxtails cut into 2 inch pieces
Lard for browning
1 small onion
1 carrot
1 stalk celery
2 small bay leaf
3 cloves Italian garlic
1 cup stewed tomatoes
1 cup hot water
2 tbsp spelt flour or gluten-free flour mix
Salt and pepper

Brown oxtails in hot lard.

Add the onion, carrot, and celery (minced) and allow these to brown.
Sprinkle with flour and seasoning. Place in a buttered casserole dish, add tomatoes and water, and let cook in a moderate 350°F oven until done; about two hours.[176]

## Broths/Bouillon/Stocks (Chef Christine Wokowsky)

Basically, in the words of James Beard, one of the most decorated chefs and food writer of all time, broth, bouillon, and stock are *"all the same thing."* However, there are distinctions that separate one from another. For example, a broth is typically cooked over many hours, especially bone broth. A stock usually has a shorter cook time.

When I worked in the restaurant industry, there was always a stock sitting on the back burner, simmering away. It was birthed with roasted bones to give a richer, more complex taste and color. Scraps were contributed throughout the day of leeks, carrots, parsley stems, and the like.

To make a vegetable stock and get the most from the nutrients, don't let it simmer more than 1 hour. If you want to be creative and frugal, dehydrate the rendered veggies and/or use them in the garden. Instead of just tossing them in the trash, think of creative ways you can use up these veggies.

Bone broth that has simmered for 12-24 hours has many health benefits, including restoring a leaky gut. It makes a terrific base for soups, stews, bean dishes, or just plain sipping on a cold night.

*Tip*: What prevents broth from gelatinizing: 1. too much water, 2. cook at too low a temperature, 3. cooked at too high a temperature, 4. not enough connective tissue or joints, 5. cooked to short of a time.


## Thick Pickle with Pearl Barley & Beef Ribs (Anastasiya Terentyeva)

*Pearl barley is widespread in Ukraine cuisine. Since the 1930s, it has been produced on an industrial scale. This soup was very popular in childcare facilities in our USSR during my childhood, so our childhood flavors are here! In Ukraine and parts of Russia, they used porridge in catering: to military personnel, prisoners, schoolchildren, and students. So, this famous soup will keep you full for a long time, provide lots of health benefits, and, most importantly, it's delicious!*

600 g beef ribs
1 cup barley
200 g cucumbers (salted pickles)
3 medium potatoes
1 carrot
1 onion
2 cloves garlic
2 tbsp virgin olive oil
3 black peppercorns
Salt to taste
2½ liter water (filtered)
2 green onions (for serving)

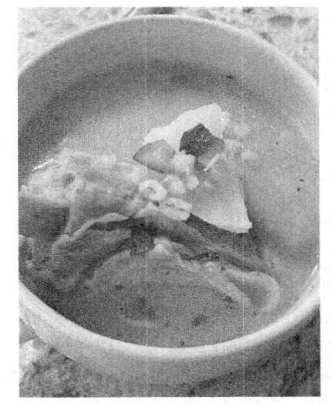

Rinse the beef ribs, peel off the films, cut and place in a sauce
pan. Add washed barley, black peppercorns, and water. Cook for 1 hour over low heat.

Finely chop cucumbers, peeled potatoes, and onions. Grate carrots. Fry the onion with carrots in oil until golden brown. Add the onion and carrot mix, potatoes, and cucumbers to the pan with the meat. Continue cooking for another 10 minutes.

Add salt and minced garlic. Turn off the heat after 2 minutes.

Serve with pickles and chopped green onions.

Add any of your favorite herbs. I like it with chopped dill and parsley.

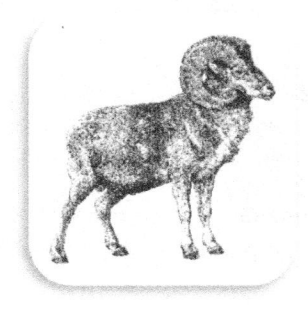

## *Lamb*

**Pierna De Cordero Asada** -Basque Roast Leg of Lamb (BeeBee Sitz)

5-7 lbs leg of lamb
Garlic
Salt and pepper

Peel and sliver garlic. Cut tiny slits in the meat and place slivers of garlic in each slit. Rub with a generous amount of salt and pepper, and place on a rack in a roasting pan. Roast at 375°F for 30 minutes per pound. You can add tomatoes, carrots and green peppers to the drippings and cook. Do this about 1 hour before the meat is done.

**Going Greek** (Tammera Karr)

½ lb ground lamb formed into small meatballs
2 red chili peppers, thinly sliced
½ bunch fresh basil, chopped
4 precooked red potatoes, sliced into small pieces
3 cloves garlic, chopped or minced
1 tbsp extra virgin olive oil

Fresh ground black pepper
Celtic Sea salt

In cast iron skillet, warm oil; add chilies and garlic, then basil. Sauté for 5 minutes on medium heat and add lamb; brown the lamb then add potatoes. Cover for 10 minutes, then add ground pepper and stir until mixed. Cook for 5 minutes more. Salt to taste and serve.


**Lamb and Potatoes** (Michael Karr)
Serves 4

1 lb ground lamb
4 large red potatoes, quartered and cut into thin slices
1 medium hot chile, minced
3 cloves garlic, minced
½ medium yellow onion, minced
2 tsp Italian seasoning
Celtic Sea salt to taste
½ fresh lime

Brown lamb in a skillet. Add and toss garlic, onion, chile and Italian seasoning. Sauté until onion is translucent. Add potatoes, combine well and cover. Cook on low heat till potatoes are tender.

Add fresh squeezed lime after serving onto plates, salt to taste.


**Roasted Cauliflower and Cabbage with Lamb Burger** (Chef Christine Wokowsky)

2 tbsp extra virgin olive oil, divided
½ head cauliflower cut into florets
1 cup cabbage roughly chopped
1 carrot peeled and cut in rounds on the diagonal
½ tsp paprika
½ tsp fennel seeds
1 tsp fresh rosemary minced, or ½ tsp dried
½ tsp freshly ground black pepper
½ tsp sea salt
8 oz ground lamb
¼ tsp fennel seeds
1 tsp fresh rosemary or ½ tsp dried
1 tsp fresh chopped minutest or ½ tsp dried
¼ tsp paprika
¼ tsp ground ginger
¼ tsp ground or fresh garlic
1 tsp dried minced onion or fresh

Salt and pepper to taste

Preheat oven to 400°F.

In a bowl toss cauliflower, cabbage, carrot, and first five spices. Place on baking sheet and bake until done or they begin to get lightly browned.

Mix ground lamb with all the remaining spices, garlic, and onion. Form two patties.

Heat olive oil to medium temperature in a skillet and add lamb patties. Sauté until done. You can also grill the patties on medium flame.

Serve with a side of probiotic rich fermented veggies. Kimchi would be great with this.

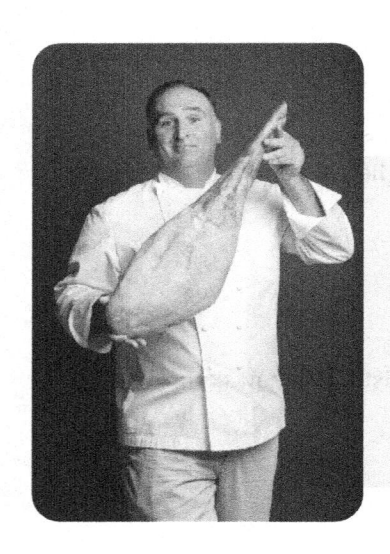

*"I realized very early the power of food to evoke memory, to bring people together, to transport you to other places, and I wanted to be a part of that."*

~ José Andrés Puerta

### Tripe (Yonnie Travis at *Give it Forth*)

What is tripe? Tripe is the edible lining of an animal's stomach and comes from cows, pigs, goats, or sheep. When I think of tripe, I think of the "honeycomb" tripe that comes from a cow's stomach. In fact, the honeycomb is only one of four different kinds of tripe found.

Plain tripe is the lining of a cow's first stomach (rumen) and appears flat and smooth. Honeycomb tripe is the second form in the lower part of a cow's second stomach (the reticulum). Book tripe or Bible tripe, from the omasum, contains many folds giving it the appearance of a book. The fourth kind, called reed tripe, is found in the cow's fourth stomach, the abomasum.

Lamb tripe is smaller and thinner than the more usual beef tripe. Straight from the stomach, it is olive green in color and requires meticulous cleaning and some bleaching to become the pale color we are familiar with.

The tripe has a very mild, almost neutral flavor, likened to a taste between the liver and heart because it adopts the flavor of the surrounding organs. It is the texture that makes it unique. It should be chewy, soft enough to bite through, and buttery when properly cooked.

*Retrieved August 2022: Yonnie Travis, Food Historian, Blogger, Historic Cook:*
*https://giveitforth.wixsite.com/giveitforth/post/harleian-ms-279-ab-1430-trype-de-motoun-ix-lx-trype-of-turbut-or-of-codlyng?fbclid=IwAR1KpGiqswSLvoJkJ3knmCT6sPuJX3S0IkWIfLXccVmbOop7YgR3-hfxaEY*

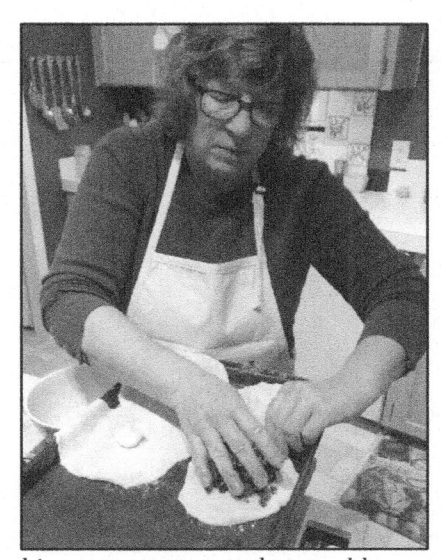

Tammera making savory meat and vegetable pastries for lunch.

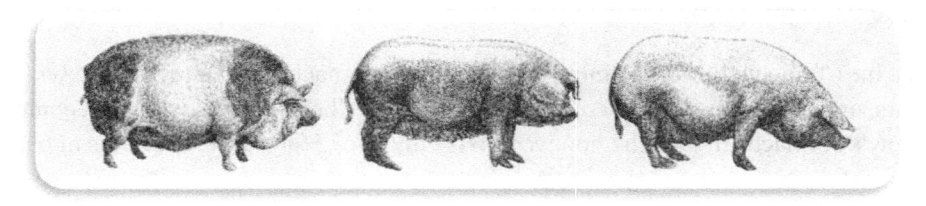

## Pork

A word of warning from the Farmers Bulletin NO.1186, 1938

> **COOK PORK THOROUGHLY**
>
> Man may become infected with a very serious disease called trichinosis through the eating of raw pork. This disease is caused by parasites called trichinae, which are too small to be seen by the naked eye but may be present in the lean meat of hogs. The danger of trichinosis may be entirely avoided by cooking pork thoroughly.
>
> Trichinosis may be contracted from tasting sausage during its preparation to determine when seasoning is satisfactory, from hastily cooked hamburgers that contain some pork, from imperfectly cooked fresh pork, and sausage, smoked hams, bacon, and shoulders, and from improperly prepared ready-to-eat products such as Bologna-style sausage, boneless loins, capocollo, coppa, dry or summer sausage, and Italian-style ham. When these latter products are eaten without further cooking in the home, one must be sure that they have been made in a plant where competent official inspection has insured a treatment of the pork muscle that will destroy possible live trichinae.

### **Wienerschnitzel** (Chef Benjamin Qualls)

1½ lbs veal or pork cutlets
½ cup flour
3 tbsp grated Parmesan cheese
2 eggs
1 tsp minced parsley
½ tsp each sea salt and black pepper
Pinch of nutmeg
2 tbsp milk
1 cup dry breadcrumbs
6 tbsp butter
Lemon slices

Place each cutlet between two pieces of plastic wrap and pound flat until about ¼ of an inch thick. Dredge with flour to coat.

In a medium bowl, stir together the Parmesan cheese, eggs, parsley, salt, pepper, nutmeg, and milk. Place breadcrumbs on a plate.

Dip each cutlet into the egg mixture, then press in bread crumbs to coat. Place coated cutlets on a plate and refrigerate for 1 hour or overnight.

Melt butter in a large cast iron skillet over medium heat. Add cutlets and cook until browned on each side; 3-5 minutes per side.
Remove cutlets to a platter and pour pan juices over them. Garnish with lemon slices.


**Basque Chorizo**
*This is a version of the dried Spanish Chorizo.*
Yields 3 lbs of sausage

1½ lbs lean boneless pork
12 oz fresh pork fat
½ lb ground beef or venison
6 large cloves Italian garlic, minced
4 tbsp crushed red pepper flakes (grind these a bit to make powder)
1 tbsp smoked paprika
1 tbsp Celtic Sea salt
1 tbsp cumin seed
1 tbsp dried oregano
½ tbsp organic sugar
½ tbsp fresh ground black pepper
¼ cup good red wine
¼ cup balsamic vinegar

With a meat grinder, grind meat and fat to medium-course texture. Mix meat with wine, vinegar, and seasonings in a large bowl. Chill mixture for 4-6 hours.

Stuff into natural casings (order through a quality butcher), tie off at 4 inch lengths. Let sausages air dry in a cool room overnight (uncovered in the refrigerator).

*To cook*: Prick sausage in several places and place in a cast iron skillet with ¼ inch water. Cover and simmer 10 minutes; drain. Add olive oil or lard to a skillet and brown on all sides over low heat until well done.

**Fall Foods Breakfast Sausage**  (Michael Karr & Chef Ben Qualls)
Yields 16–4 inch patties

2 lbs lean ground pork
3 small tart winter apples
1 cup dried cranberries
1 small yellow onion
4 large cloves garlic
1 tbsp chile flakes
¼ cup extra virgin olive oil
1 tbsp parsley
1½ tsp coarse sea salt
1 tsp cinnamon
2 tsp turmeric
½ tsp nutmeg
¼ tsp clove
Black pepper

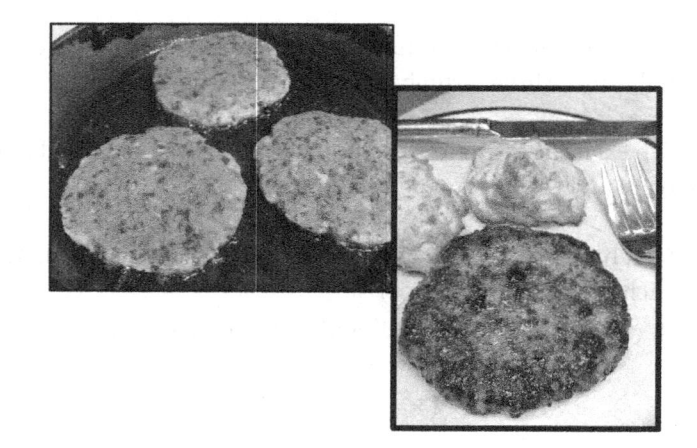

Blend oil, herbs, and spices into ground meat. Chop apple, onion, and garlic so it will fit into a meat grinder hopper.

With a meat grinder, grind all ingredients and mix well.
Form into patties on a cookie sheet lined with parchment paper and freeze. Once frozen, transfer to freezer containers.

Cook on medium heat in olive oil or lard. Because of the fruit, caramelizing or burning can happen quickly. Ensure you have ample oil to act as a medium between the skillet and the patties.

Ground turkey or chicken can be substantiated for pork.


**Pork & Fennel** (Tammera Karr)

4 organic pork loin steaks, trimmed of fat
¼ cup fresh fennel top, finely chopped
¼ cup sweet onion, thinly sliced
¼ cup fresh sweet basil, chopped
2 tbsp extra virgin olive oil

Warm oil in a cast iron skillet. Lightly brown pork loin and cover with the rest of the ingredients. Cover with a lid and cook on medium low heat until pork is done. Do not overcook the pork. Serve with rice, pasta or sweet potatoes and sliced apples.

## Smoked Sausage (Chef Ben Qualls)

4 lbs pork trimmings
5 tsp salt
4 tsp sage, ground
2 tsp black pepper, ground
½ tsp ground cloves
1 tsp nutmeg, ground
1 tsp sugar

Grind the trimmings and mix all the seasonings into the ground meat thoroughly.
Using an attachment for casings on a meat grinder or Kitchen Aid®, fill natural casings immediately after grinding, which allows for a tight fill without the need for water. Allow to cure in the refrigerator for 24 hours. Smoke and dry at a temperature of 70-90°F for a day or two until a dark mahogany color is reached.

## Creamy Cabbage-Potato & Pork Soup (Chef Ben Qualls)

¼ cup olive oil
1½ lbs pork loin, cut into ½ inch cubes
1 small head of green cabbage, sliced
1 medium sweet onion, cut in half and sliced
2 cloves garlic, crushed
6 cups chicken stock or vegetable stock
1½ lbs potatoes, washed, peeled and chopped
3 medium carrots, chopped
1 tsp pink Himalayan salt
2 tbsp white wine vinegar
¾ cup sour cream
Pink Himalayan salt and cracked black pepper to taste
1 tbsp chopped fresh dill or 1 tsp dried
1 tsp smoked paprika

Heat oil in a large stock pot over medium high heat. Add diced pork and cook until lightly browned. Add cabbage and onion, and season with Himalayan salt and pepper. Cook and stir until cabbage and onion begin to wilt and brown slightly, 8-10 minutes. Add garlic and cook another couple of minutes. Add stock. Bring to a boil. Reduce heat to medium low and simmer, covering for 30-45 or until pork is tender.

Add potatoes and carrots, and return to a boil. Reduce heat to medium low and continue to cook until potatoes and carrots are tender. About 20 minutes.

Remove pot from heat. Stir in vinegar and sour cream. Season with Himalayan salt and pepper. Sprinkle with dill and paprika.

## Pork Steak Grill with Spicy Sauce (Chef Ben Qualls)

1 thick pork steak
Lard
3 fresh tomatoes
1 head cauliflower
Salt and pepper
2 tbsp flour
½ cup minced onion
2 tbsp cider vinegar
1 tsp dry mustard
¾ cup hot water
½ tsp organic coconut sugar

Brown pork steak on both sides. Cover; cook slowly for thirty minutes. Arrange steak on a fire or oven-proof platter. Around the edge place the tomato halves and buttered cauliflower flowerets. Place in the broiler to broil tomatoes and brown cauliflower. Make a sauce by browning flour in drippings, and add dry mustard, salt, and pepper. Cook until thick and pour over pork – serve hot.


## Pork Loin with Fruit (Tammera Karr)

2 lean pork loin steaks: Brown both sides in a skillet with
1 tablespoon extra virgin olive oil on medium heat.

Drizzle 2-4 tablespoons of zesty Italian dressing over each browned loin, and cover for 10 minutes. Remove the lid and cover both pork loins with 2 cups of frozen or fresh berries, including cherries, raspberries, marionberries, and or blackberries.

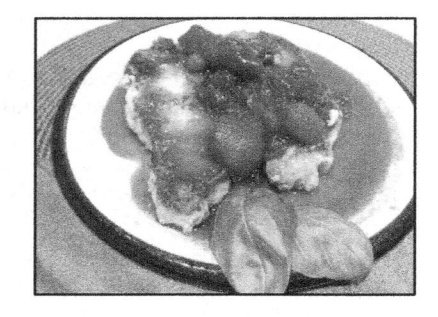

Cover and turn heat to low, let slow cook for 30 minutes. Remove the lid, turn the heat back to medium-low, and let the liquid evaporate for another 15 minutes. Serve with salad, cauliflower, or wild grains.


## Pork with Mulberry Chutney

2 boneless pork loins or chicken breasts
2 shallots, minced
2 cloves garlic, minced
1 bulb of fennel, thinly sliced
¼ cup dried mulberries

¼ cup dried cranberries
½ cup hot water
1 tsp apple cider vinegar
Fresh ground black pepper
Celtic Sea salt
2 tbsp extra virgin olive oil
1 knob Irish butter (1-2 tbsp)

Add hot water and vinegar to dried fruit in a glass bowl, and let sit while browning meat and sautéing vegetables.

Brown chicken breast or pork loin on medium heat in olive oil.

*Chutney*
Sauté shallots and garlic in butter on medium heat until they are transparent and beginning to brown. Add thin slices of fennel. Toss to coat evenly with oil, and cook until tender. Add dried fruit with water, stir and allow moisture to cook out on medium low heat. Stir to keep from sticking; about 10 minutes.

Cover meat with chutney, turn heat to low, and cover for 20 minutes.
Serve hot with steamed vegetables.

## Dad's Bacon Curls (Tammera Karr)

*Breakfast always was and is the husband's job in my family. Growing up, my dad used side bacon whenever he could. After slicing off bacon, he would then deftly cut the rind into thin strips that he would fry in the bacon grease. I would stand transfixed as the strips curled, bubbled and browned to crunchy perfection.*

½ lb uncured bacon with rind

With a sharp knife, slice the rind into thin strips.

In a medium heat cast iron skillet add a few strips of uncured bacon and the strips of bacon rind, and fry until crispy. The rind can be curled with a fork while frying to form curls. Great crispy, chewy treat for kids of all ages.

## Sausage Spezzatino (Cynthia Edmunds)

*This is a recipe that was handed down to me from my mother and my aunt (her sister). It is a family recipe that made its way over when my grandmother immigrated from Italy. We always just called it "spezza." This was served at family gatherings or celebrations, but now I like to make it whenever.*

*It can be served over pasta, but we always ate it as is. Top it with a little freshly grated Parmesan cheese and you're good to go!*

- 6-8 Italian sausage links, cut into quarters (can be hot or sweet sausage, depending on preference)
- 1 large onion, cut into slices
- 2 bell peppers, any color, cut into slices
- 4 cloves garlic, chopped
- 28 oz can stewed tomatoes (do not drain!)
- 1 cup water
- ½ cup red wine
- 1 tsp dried basil
- 1 tsp dried oregano
- 1 tsp dried rosemary
- Salt and pepper to taste
- Olive oil

Heat a large deep skillet or stock pot over medium high heat, adding about 1 tablespoon olive oil when hot (not searing). Add the onion and sausage, cooking until browned and the sausage is cooked through about 8-10 minutes. Add peppers and garlic, cooking for 2-3 minutes more.

Add the water and red wine, then add the stewed tomatoes. I crush the tomatoes as I add them to the pot so they are bite sized. Add the herbs, salt, and pepper, and cover. Turn the heat down and simmer for about 30 minutes.

Can be served over pasta or eaten as a stew. Top with freshly grated Parmesan, if desired.

### Sausage & Brussels Sprouts Soup (Tammera Karr)

*To date this soup is the only way I can get my husband to get near Brussels sprouts. He loves the broth.*

- 1 lb Italian sausage
- 1 large yellow onion, sliced
- 1 cup chopped celery
- 1 cup heirloom cherry tomato
- 4 garlic cloves, minced
- 1 tsp red chile flakes
- 2 tbsp organic extra virgin olive oil
- 3 red potatoes, yams or sweet potatoes
- 2 lbs Brussels sprouts (or a large head of cabbage)
- 2 15 oz cans of white beans (cannellini, great northern, garbanzo or navy), drained
- 1 tsp Italian herb seasoning
- 8 cups bone broth (2 qts)
- Salt and pepper to taste

Trim ends off Brussels sprouts, remove any damaged external leaves and cut in half lengthwise. Set aside.

Wash potatoes and cut them into roughly ½ inch pieces. Add 1 cup of broth, potatoes, and brussels sprouts. Stir for about 3 minutes.

Add the rest of the broth and bring it to a boil. Add white beans. Reduce heat to low or medium low to maintain a steady simmer. Cook soup until potatoes and Brussels sprouts are tender, about 15-25 minutes.

**Stuffed Delicata Squash with Sausage, Greens, & Garlic** (Tammera Karr)
*This recipe combines the squash's natural sweetness with savory elements like sage, garlic, and Italian sausage.*
Serves 8

4 medium delicata squash
A knob of ghee or other cooking fat
1 medium yellow onion, diced small
2 tbsp garlic minced
1 lb sweet Italian sausage, or lamb, pork, or buffalo
1½ tsp sage for rub
⅛ tsp grated nutmeg
Pinch red chile flakes or more to taste
½ tsp Celtic Sea salt, fine
Fresh ground black pepper
6 cups rainbow chard, chopped leaves, stems removed *(See Recipe Notes)*
⅔ cup Parmesan cheese, finely grated,
1 tbsp nutritional yeast
⅓ cup pine nuts, toasted (optional)

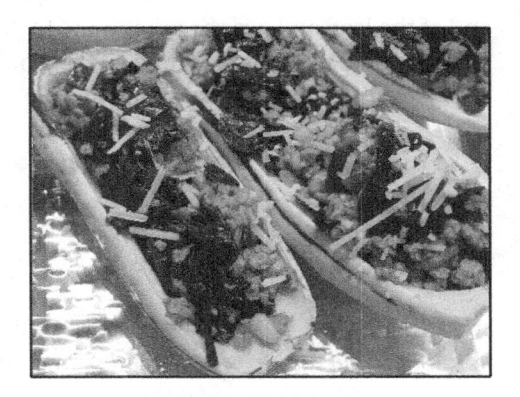

Preheat oven to 350°F. Wash the squash and cut lengthwise through the middle. Use a spoon to scrape the seeds and stringy flesh from the squash halves. Place the squash halves cut side down onto a parchment lined baking sheet and place in the oven for 25-30 minutes or until the squash gives a little when pressed.

While the squash is baking, heat the ghee in a large, high sided skillet over medium high heat. Choose a pot big and deep enough to accommodate the greens. Add diced onion and sauté 3 minutes or until softened. Add minced garlic and sauté another 2 minutes.

Add sausage, herbs, and seasonings and cook, stirring until meat has browned. Add greens to the pot and stir until they begin to wilt. You may need to add about ¼ cup water or broth to the pot (for steam) if the mixture is too dry, but the meat and greens should release some liquid as they cook. Reduce heat to medium low, cover pot, and cook until greens are tender, stirring occasionally. Taste for doneness.

Remove from heat and stir in half of the Parmesan cheese and nutritional yeast. Taste filling and adjust seasonings. It should be robust, so add salt to taste if necessary.

When squash is tender, remove from oven and arrange cut side up on baking sheet (you can use the same parchment sheet). Divide the filling evenly among the halves. Top with remaining cheese.

Return to oven for 20-30 minutes or until cheese is melted and everything is heated through (this will take longer if they've been refrigerated overnight). Top with toasted pine nuts and enjoy!

*Recipe Notes*
Remove the tender leaves from the tough stems of hearty greens: With one hand, grasp the stem end of the leaf, and use the other hand to grasp the leaf at the base. Pull upwards along the central rib. The tender part of the leaf should come right off, ready to be chopped and cooked up. This works well with both chard and kale.

> "The English have always been poultry fanciers. Not just chalk white eggs, which are tough and tasteless, but light brown, dark brown, speckled and all the shades of buff. The poultry yard and dairy were traditionally run by the mistress of the house, and the farmer's wife obtained her "pin money" from her profits on selling surplus eggs, butter and cheese at market."
>
> *The Cookery of England*
> ~ Elisabeth Ayrton 1975

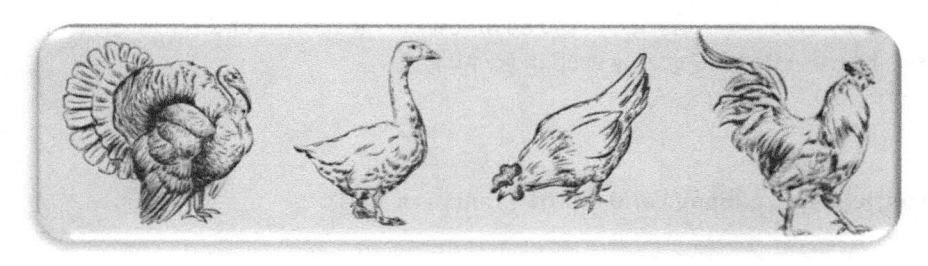

## Poultry

### Tammera's Whole Chicken Routine

I usually roast a whole chicken 2-4 times per month. I may make broth from one chicken, eat a portion roasted, shredded, stewed, ground, and stir-fried. One good sized, free range bird can produce a surprising number of meals, which accounts for its popularity in so many countries and as a staple in poor regions.

- Cook or roast a whole chicken for supper one evening and eat it with veggies, sweet or red potatoes, pasta, or grains.

- Pull all leftover meat from the bones, trim away fat and gristle, and dice it

- Pop the carcass with skin, fat, giblets (gold mines of vitamins, minerals, and essential fats), neck, gristle, and bones in the Instant Pot® or slow cooker to make a gallon or so of chicken broth. Plan on this taking about 1-2 hours. You do not want to overcook poultry broth, or it can become bitter.

- Use the leftover meat in the soup, pot pie, stir fries, pizza topping, shredded for tacos, nachos, or a chicken skillet meal the following night, and use the broth throughout the next 1-2 weeks.

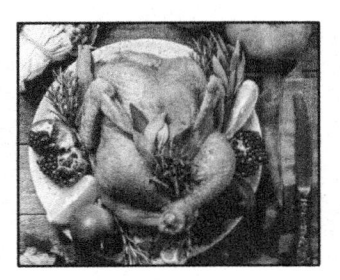

- Cook pasta, grains, vegetables, and potatoes in broth. This adds flavor dynamics and synergistic nutrient release for digestion.

- Savor the chicken fat, if free range and organic chickens are used. Enjoy the fat; it adds to mouth feel and essential saturated fats for nerve and brain health. Research studies have shown chicken fat contains nutrients that support healthy immune function.

I generally ignore directions in recipes that specifically list breast meat, any chicken meat works. Often, dark meat has a richer flavor and is tender and moist, unlike breast meat. The modern trend to use only breast meat is due to the no or low-fat movement of the 1980s. Prior to that, the whole bird was interchangeably used in cooking.

## Chicken with Purple Cabbage and Chard (Tammera Karr)
Serves 4

1 cup shredded purple cabbage
1 cup chopped rainbow chard
½ cup thinly sliced sweet onion
3 medium cloves garlic, minced
1 whole boneless, skinless chicken breast, cut into ½ inch cubes
5 tbsp avocado oil
1 tbsp Celtic Sea salt, course
½ tsp coarse grind black pepper

In a large bowl, combine cubed chicken, 1 tablespoon oil, coarse salt, and pepper. Thoroughly mix until meat is covered with oil and seasoning.

Preheat carbon steel or cast iron pan, add remaining oil, and chicken. Brown all sides. Add garlic and onion, toss, then turn heat to medium and cover for 5 minutes. Remove lid and cover the chicken with chopped chard and cabbage. Continue cooking on medium low for 15-20 minutes. Turn off the heat and let rest the last 5 minutes of cook time.
Serve with rice or as is.

## Burrito in Turmeric Buttermilk (Soneil and Leena Guptha)

6 medium corn tortillas
500 ml buttermilk
500 g of minced protein (plant-base, Chicken, Turkey, Lamb, or Beef)
¼ tsp cumin
¼ tsp coarse ground coriander seeds
¼ tsp coarse ground black pepper
½ tsp turmeric powder
1 pinch of saffron threads
⅔ cup shaved almonds
2 tbsp olive oil
Onion, garlic, and ginger, if you like the taste, minced

*Preparation*
1. In a pot or pan, heat olive oil on high heat; add cumin, coriander and black pepper and fry till you smell the aroma of the spices (1 minute). Add garlic, ginger, onion, and cook till soft and light brown.

2. Reduce heat to medium and add minced protein and mix until cooked. Add small quantities of water periodically if needed, to prevent minced (protein and spices) from burning. Constant stirring may be needed.

3. Once the mince is cooked, add salt to taste, stir, and set aside.

*Preparation of buttermilk sauce or gravy*
1. In another pan add buttermilk and bring to a boil.

2. Lower heat to simmer and add turmeric and almonds, simmer for 5 minutes.

*Preparation of burrito rolls*
1. Distribute the cooked mince in the 6 tortillas and roll the tortilla tight.

2. Immerse the rolled, stuffed tortilla in the turmeric buttermilk.

3. Put the mixed food on simmering heat and prepare Tadka.

*Tadka*
1½ tbsp ghee
½ tsp cumin
½ tsp mustard seed (black)
1 tbsp dried fenugreek leaves (Kasuri Methi)
Spice mix (¼ tsp chile powder, chile flakes, ¼ tsp garlic, finely chopped
Salt to taste
Coriander or parsley leaves to garnish

*Preparation of Tadka*
1. In pan heat ghee on medium.

2. Lower heat to simmer and add remaining cumin, mustard seed, dried fenugreek leaves, and chile.

3. Cook for ½ to 1 minute (make sure that the Tadka does not go brown or black).

4. Add pinch of saffron, stir and pour over rolled up burritos in turmeric buttermilk.

5. Garish with coriander and parsley leaves.

Serve over boiled rice and with a side salad of your choice (we prefer Greek with feta cheese) or roasted veggies (capsicum, courgettes*, onions, shitake mushrooms).

*The zucchini courgette or baby marrow is a summer squash fruit harvested when its immature seeds and epicarp (rind) are still soft and edible.*

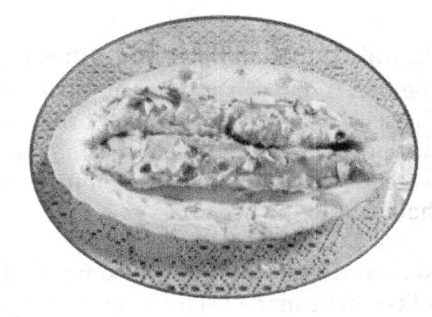

**Eggs** (*Century Cook Book* by Mary Ronald 1897, pg 261)

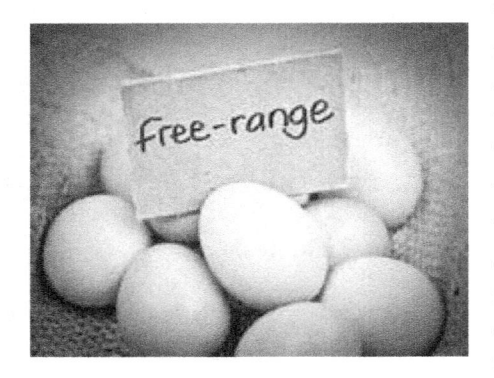

The variety of purposes which eggs serve, the many ways of cooking them, their value as a highly concentrated, nutritious, and easily digested food, make them one of the most useful articles of food. To have them fresh and rightly cooked is within the power of the simplest household. They hold the principal place as a breakfast dish, and although the original methods of cooking them may be limited to boiling, baking, poaching, etc, each one of these can be varied in an indefinite number of ways, given a menu of eggs unlimited in extent, and thus securing always a new way of presenting them, if desired. Urbain Dubois has recently published a book giving 300 ways of preparing eggs. The varieties are attained mostly by sauces and garnishings. It is not generally understood that sauces can be served with poached, hard-boiled, and scrambled eggs, and also with omelets.

A fresh egg should feel heavy, sink in water, and when held to a bright light show a clear round yolk. If old, a part of the substance will have evaporated through the pores of the shell, leaving a space filled with air, which will cause it to float on water. It will also contain dark specks.

**Should You Wash Eggs, and Other Egg Information**
The USA is one of a small handful of areas where eggs are washed and stored in refrigeration. The scrubbing with disinfectant removes the protective wax coating provided by nature. In Europe, hens are routinely vaccinated, so it's best not to wash the egg to preserve its natural protective coating. In many countries, washing eggs is unnecessary; you will find them on the shelf next to the bread.

**Look at that Color**: The chicken's food plays a role in determining the hue of the egg's yolk. Egg yolks can be made brighter by feeding the hen bugs, worms, stinging nettles, alfalfa, peas, or millet.

**Wise Tales**: It's a common misconception that pregnant women who consume eggs can inadvertently introduce their unborn babies to a lifelong allergy to the food. It may very well help babies develop antibodies to aid in preventing allergies.

**Bigger is Better**: If chicken eggs are not to your liking, try duck, geese, and turkey eggs. Duck eggs have a creamier texture and are slightly richer in flavor than chicken eggs. They are a nice alternative to chicken and more digestible for many.

## Migas (Mely Martinez)

Serves 2

4 tbsp vegetable oil
4 corn tortillas
⅓ cup white onion, chopped
1 serrano pepper, diced or ½ jalapeño pepper
1 cup tomato, chopped; about 2 large plum tomatoes
4 large eggs
Salt to season

*To serve*
Black beans, either just cooked or refried
Queso fresco
Avocado slices, optional
Green onions sliced, optional

Cut the corn tortillas into small squares, about 1½ inch wide. You can use a knife or a pair of kitchen scissors to cut them.

Heat the oil in a large frying pan. Once it is hot, place the tortilla pieces in the oil and fry them until they are golden brown. Make sure to use a frying pan that is large enough in order to not overcrowd the pan. Stir and turn the tortilla pieces as needed until they acquire a golden brown color. This step will take about 6 minutes. Set tortilla pieces aside.

Return the frying pan to the stove and place it over medium heat. Add the chopped white onion and lightly fry it for a few seconds, then stir in the chopped serrano pepper. Keep cooking for about 2 minutes.

Add the chopped tomato and cook for about 3 more minutes, then add the eggs. Let the eggs start to cook without stirring them yet.

Once the egg whites start to look cooked around the edges, gently stir the eggs. Once you see the egg yolks start to cook, stir in the tortilla chips, season with salt, and gently mix them with the eggs. Remove the frying pan from the heat when the eggs are cooked to your liking. The tortillas should still be crispy by the time you serve your migas. Do not wait until the eggs are cooked to add the tortilla chips. Remember that the eggs will keep cooking even after you remove the frying pan from the heat.

*What to serve with migas*
Like many Mexican breakfasts, migas are traditionally served with refried beans or plain cooked beans topped with crumbled queso fresco and avocado slices on the side. Some people also place a spicy salsa on the table for those who want to add more heat to their migas.
From Mexico in My Kitchen: https://www.mexicoinmykitchen.com/migas-recipe/#recipe

**Eggs and Sausage** (Chris Smith *The Cookery of England 1977*)
Serves 4

8 eggs
A little grated cheese
Butter
3 pork sausages, skinned and cut into rings
1 onion, cut very fine
2 tomatoes, skinned and quartered
A little-cooked celery and carrots in small pieces
A few olives or sliced gherkins
A few cubes of cooked vegetable marrow* or cucumber
Some chives and parsley, finely chopped
A little thyme, finely chopped
Salt and pepper

Fry the sausages, vegetables, and herbs gently in butter or oil. Transfer to a large flat, fireproof dish, sprinkle with salt and pepper and flatten the surface. Carefully break 2 eggs per person on top of the mixture so that it is covered with eggs. Sprinkle with grated cheese and knobs of butter. Put in a hot oven (450°F, gas mark 8) until the eggs are just set. Finish them under the grill if the tops seem slow to set.

* Vegetable marrow is a general term used to refer to several summer squash varieties.


**Sausage and Wild Grains** (Tammera Karr)

1 lb natural smoked or Adel's® apple chicken sausage, chopped
1 red sweet pepper, chopped into chunks
½ sweet onion, chopped
2 cloves garlic, chopped
1 small zucchini or summer squash, thick slices
1 cup broccoli flowerets
2 cups cooked organic wild rice, quinoa blend (recommend the use of a rice cooker for this)
1 tbsp extra virgin olive oil

In a cast iron skillet over medium heat add olive oil, garlic and meat, and sauté until meat is heated through. Add remaining vegetables, stir into meat, and cover with lid for 10 minutes or until broccoli changes color to a bright green. Cover with the pre-cooked grain, gently mix and serve.

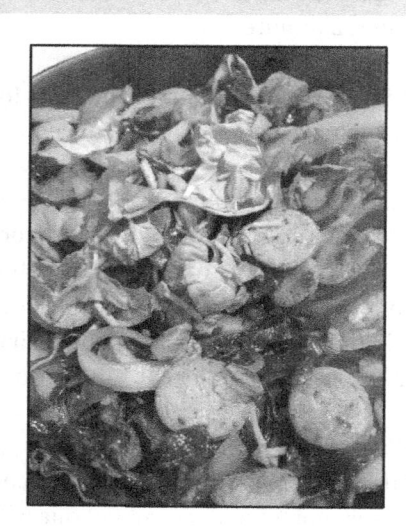

**Tam's Anytime Tortillas -** Basque Frattata
Serves 4

4 large eggs, beaten
2 organic sweet chicken Italian sausages, sliced into medallions
1 small sweet onion, chopped
2 cloves garlic, minced
2 small Roma tomatoes, chopped
½ cup rainbow chard, chopped (use crisp stems also)
1 mild red chile, seeded and minced
1 small red sweet pepper, chopped
2 small parboiled red potatoes, peeled and cut into small chunks
4 tbsp extra virgin olive oil

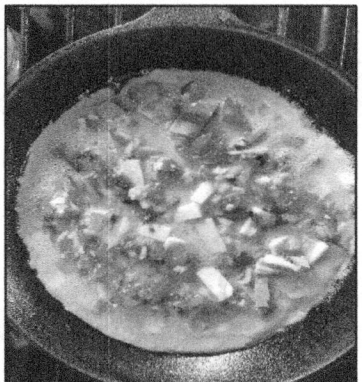

In a large cast iron skillet, heat oil and brown sausage. Add garlic and onion and cook until transparent. Add chard and peppers and sauté until soft. About 5 minutes.

Add cooked potatoes, mix well so oil coats vegetables.

Slowly pour beaten eggs around and over vegetables and sausage with the heat still at medium-high. Sprinkle with coarse Celtic Sea salt and fresh ground black pepper. Cover and turn heat to low. Let cook for 10-15 minutes.

The more vegetables, the longer it takes to cook the egg. The egg may have liquid on top, that is, vegetable juice. Sprinkle top with freshly grated Parmesan cheese and serve. Good cold also.


**White Chicken Chili** (Nicole Hammond)
*I am an artist at heart, and this especially comes out in the food that I create. As an Italian we rarely measure anything. However, for recipes that I share there is certainty in the deliciousness in the measurements provided. As an adult and wife and mother, I have enjoyed venturing outside of my Italian background, yet always go back to it somewhere in my mind and in my approach.*

1 onion
4 cloves garlic
2 tomatoes chopped
¼ cup olive oil
½ cup chopped jalapeño
2 cooked and shredded chicken breasts
2 cups corn
2 tbsp whole wheat flour
1 qt chicken stock
16 oz cannellini beans

½ cup shredded Parmesan or mozzarella
1 tsp sea salt
1 tsp black pepper
1 tsp curry powder
1 tsp cumin
1 tsp paprika
1 tbs parsley

Sauté onions, garlic, one tomato, corn, flour, olive oil, and seasonings. Add chicken breasts, cannellini beans, chicken stock, and half of the chopped jalapeño.

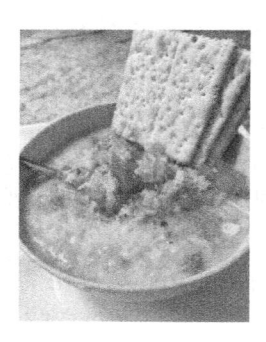

Simmer for 30 minutes, then top with shredded Parmesan or mozzarella, tomato, and jalapeño.


### **Duck, Date and Rutabaga Pot Pie** (Vivian Howard of Chef & the Farmer)

*Filling*
3 duck leg quarters 10-12 oz each
1 tbsp salt, divided
1½ tsp black pepper, divided
1 tbsp (14 g) duck fat
2 large onions, diced
2 medium carrots, peeled and diced
2 ribs celery, diced
3 garlic cloves, smashed
2 cups (454 g) red wine
2 cups (454 g) chicken or mushroom stock
4 cups (680 g) rutabaga, diced into 1 inch cubes
⅔ cup (99 g) dried dates, cut into eighths
4 sprigs rosemary
4 sprigs thyme
2 bay leaves
3 pieces star anise
¼ tsp nutmeg
2 tbsp (28 g) ghee
2 tbsp (14 g) organic all-purpose flour

*Crust*
1¼ cup (150 g) organic all-purpose flour
2 tsp baking powder
¾ tsp salt, divided
¼ cup (57 g) duck fat or lard
½ cup (113 g) buttermilk

Season the duck with 2 teaspoons salt and 1 teaspoon black pepper.

In a 4-6 quart Dutch oven, heat the vegetable oil over medium low heat and brown the duck legs, skin-side down, for 7-10 minutes. Do this slowly so that you render out as much fat as possible.

When nicely browned, flip the legs over and brown them on the other side. Remove them from the pan, pour off and reserve all but 1 tablespoon of the rendered fat, then add the onion, carrot, celery, garlic, and the remaining 1 teaspoon salt and ½ teaspoon black pepper. Raise the heat to medium and cook, occasionally stirring, for about 15 minutes, until the vegetables begin to brown.

Once the vegetables are browned, add the wine. Bring to a boil and cook for 2-3 minutes. Stir in the stock, rutabagas, dates, herbs, bay leaves, star anise, and nutmeg.

Add the duck legs and any juices that accumulated while they were resting, and bring to a simmer. The liquid should come about ¾ of the way up the sides of the duck legs; they shouldn't be submerged. Adjust the liquid level with stock or water if needed. Lower the heat, cover, and cook over medium-low heat for 1 hour at a brisk simmer.

After an hour, uncover and cook for 10 minutes more. Remove the pan from the heat and let the duck rest in the braising liquid for 20 minutes.

Transfer the duck to a plate. Once it's cool enough to handle, pull the meat off the bone in small, bite-sized pieces. Meanwhile, strain the braising liquid. Reserve the vegetables and discard the herbs and spices. Skim any fat you can from the top of the braising liquid. If you have time, chill the liquid so all the fat floats to the top, and scoop it off.

In a 10 inch cast iron skillet, melt 2 tablespoons butter over medium heat until foaming. Whisk in the flour and cook for 1-2 minutes. Whisk in 2½ cups of the reserved braising liquid, and bring to a boil. It should thicken and coat the back of a spoon. Stir in the reserved duck and vegetables.

*To make the crust*: Sift the flour, baking powder, and ½ teaspoon of the salt into the bottom of a large bowl and make a deep, wide well in the center. Add the duck fat followed by the buttermilk, taking care to keep both contained in the well for now. Using your fingers, rub the mixture together, making as much of a homogenous mixture as possible without incorporating too much flour.

Start moving the wet mixture back and forth in the flour with your fingers. Keep turning it over and introducing more flour with each movement. Try using a gentle motion like a one handed knead, using your thumb as if it were on the other hand. Continue introducing flour until the dough is very soft and tender but not sticky. You'll have about 2 tablespoons of flour left in the bowl. Lay a 10 inch square of parchment or waxed paper on the counter and turn the dough onto it. Form it into a ball and roll it ¼ inch thick.

To assemble and bake: Preheat the oven to 375°F. Make sure the filling is warm. It doesn't need to be hot, but it shouldn't be cold.

Pick up the parchment by the edges and gently flip the pastry on top of the skillet. Trim the edges with a knife or crimp as you like. Cut a 1 inch slit on top of the pastry and sprinkle with ¼ teaspoon salt.

Put the skillet on a baking sheet, slide it onto the middle rack of your oven, and bake for 30 minutes. The crust should be golden brown, and the filling should have started to bubble up the sides. Serve warm.

## Chicken Kabob (Nicole Hodson)

½ cup fresh lime juice
2 tbsp avocado oil
1 large onion peeled and thinly sliced
½ tbsp ground Persian saffron, dissolved in 1 tbsp hot water
1 tbsp Himalayan pink salt
1 tsp freshly ground pepper
1 broiling chicken cut into pieces

*Baste*
Juice of 1 lime
¼ cup butter, melted
½ tsp ground Persian saffron, dissolved in 1 tbsp hot water
½ tsp salt
½ tsp freshly ground pepper

In a large bowl, combine the lime juice, avocado oil, onions, saffron, salt, and pepper. Beat well with a fork and add the pieces of chicken.

Toss to coat. Cover and marinate in the refrigerator for at least 6 hours and up to 2 days. Turn the chicken twice during this period.

Preheat a gas grill to medium (350°F-400°F) on one side or push hot coals to one side of a charcoal grill.

Combine the basting ingredients just before grilling the chicken and set aside.

Place chicken skin side down on oiled grates over the lit side of the grill. Grill until skin is well marked and crispy, 5-6 minutes.

Turn pieces over, and transfer to the unlit side of the grill. Grill until a thermometer registers 165°F when inserted into thickest part of a chicken thigh, 20-25 minutes. Turn frequently and baste occasionally. The chicken is done when the juice that runs out is yellow rather than pink.

Serve with basmati rice, plain full fat yogurt, and a Greek salad.

*Note: For best results, skewer the chicken pieces using <u>flat skewers.</u>*

### **Aunt Pari's Picnic Cutlets** (Nicole Hodson)

*Spending my childhood in pre-revolution Tehran provided ample opportunities for summertime outdoor activities. Tehran is a rather vertical city since most dwellings are apartment buildings with little to no backyard space. For access to the great outdoors, my folks joined a country club with swimming pools, a golf course, tennis courts, etc. The best weekends of those summers included a visit to the country club where I would spend the entire day in the pool splashing about with my cousins. The whole family would join in, everyone bringing their signature, picnic-friendly fare. My favorite dish of all was my Aunt Pari's ground chicken cutlets. Crisp and golden on the outside, light and juicy on the inside, I couldn't wait to dig in. I hope you'll enjoy these little gems as much as I do! Nushe-joon!*

2 large russet potatoes
1 lb ground chicken meat, preferably dark meat for extra flavor and moisture
1 small onion, grated
1 egg
1 clove garlic, minced
1 ½ tsp salt
¼ tsp freshly ground pepper
1 cup fine breadcrumbs
3 tbsp avocado oil
1 tbsp butter

Boil potatoes with skin on until fork tender. Let cool, then peel.

Place chicken meat in a large bowl.

Grate the potatoes and onion into the chicken, then add the garlic, egg, salt, and pepper. Mix gently with your hands and form into oval shaped patties. Be careful not to over mix.

Heat a large pan over medium heat. Add the oil and butter.

Roll each patty in the breadcrumbs, and brown until golden brown.

This dish is especially delicious with a light salad of diced cucumber, tomato, and onion, with olive oil, lemon juice, salt, and pepper.

**Chicken Pie** (Tammera Karr)

1 organic or free range chicken
½ medium onion
2 cloves garlic, minced
1 small carrot, minced
1 stalk celery, minced
1 tbsp fresh parsley
1 small bay leaf
Celtic Sea salt
⅛ tsp pepper
¼ cup spelt flour or gluten-free flour mix
Libby's Baking Mix (or gluten-free version)

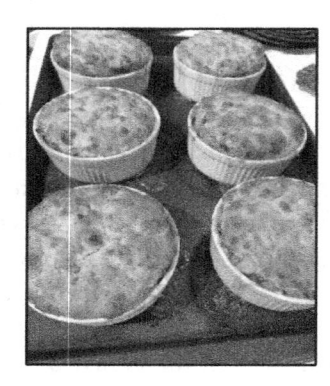

Cut up chicken. Put into a stew pot with onion, garlic, celery, carrot, parsley, bay leaf, salt, and pepper. Cover with boiling water, and cook slowly until tender; debone chicken.

Thicken stock with flour (potato starch if gluten-free); should pour easily. Cover the chicken mixture with biscuit mix crust; leave air vents.

Bake in a moderate oven 350°F, until crust, is risen and browned.


**Fricase De Pollo** (Jennifer Grafiada)
*Cuban chicken stew by Maria Grafiada (my paternal grandmother)*

4 half chicken breasts
3 cloves of garlic, minced
4 cans of tomato sauce
8 cups water
1 small onion, chopped
½ green pepper, chopped
4 red potatoes, peeled and cut in half
3 carrots, chopped
1 tbsp cumin
1 tsp salt
1 tsp turmeric for color
¼ cup olive oil, plus 2 tbsp
½ cup white wine

Cut the four pieces of chicken into eight, mash the chicken, and dry with paper towels. Put about ¼ cup of oil into a heavy sauce pan. Add the chicken and brown on both sides.

In a skillet add 2 tablespoons olive oil, bring to medium heat, and sauté garlic, onion, and green pepper. Add cumin, salt, and turmeric. Mix well.

In pan with chicken, add sautéed vegetables, spices, carrots, tomato sauce, and water. Fill each can with water and add that plus ½ cup white wine. Cover and simmer on medium heat for about 30 minutes. Add potatoes and simmer 20-30 minutes more until potatoes are tender.

Serve it with white rice and sliced avocados.


## Shredded Spicy Chicken (Michael Karr)

4 boneless skinless chicken breasts
16 oz container salsa or all natural hot green or red chile sauce
2 tbsp extra virgin olive oil

Warm olive oil and place chicken breasts (can be frozen) in a skillet. Cover and cook on medium heat for 10 minutes. Pour chile sauce over the top of the chicken. Cover and let slow cook for 30 minutes; chicken should be cooked through.

Shred the chicken into the remaining sauce and use for tacos, salsa salad or sliced chicken. Serve on a bed of brown rice or quinoa with beans and blue corn chips.


> *"Food is everything we are. It's an extension of nationalist feeling, ethnic feeling, your personal history, your province, your region, your tribe, your grandma. It's inseparable from those from the get-go."*
>
> ~ Anthony Bourdain


## Traditional South African Potjiekos – Cape Malay Chicken Curry Potjie (Kirstin Nussgruber)
Serves 6-8

*This dish is an amalgamation of two South African heritages, the Afrikaners, or Boers (Farmers) who originated from German and Dutch settlers to South Africa from the mid 1600s, as well as the Cape Malay culture, a collective group of inhabitants of mainly the Cape region, who originated from slavery utilized by the Dutch settlers when Cape Town served as a trade and refreshment port for the Dutch East India Company. Cape Malays have their roots from East and West Africa, Madagascar, Indonesia, Malaysia, and the Philippines. A potjie is the Afrikaans name for "small pot" and refers to a cast iron, 3-legged pot that was traditionally placed over a hearth or outdoor fire.*

*Today, potjies are still used outdoors over coal fires, gas cylinders or even indoors over a gas stove. If you do not have a potjie pot, use a cast iron pot and cook over the stove and in the oven.*

*Making a potjie is supposed to be a very social event. The most important part is not to rush the cooking, using the time to sit and chat. This dish owes its deep flavor to hours of gentle, stir-free cooking and the fusion of piquant spices. This can serve as a one-pot meal with a light side salad.*

Ghee or olive oil for cooking
4½ pounds (2 kg) of skinless chicken thighs
5 medium onions, chopped
5 garlic cloves, minced
1 tsp freshly grated peeled ginger
1 medium green chili, seeded and sliced fine
6 carrots, peeled and sliced
6 red potatoes, unpeeled and cubed
1½ cups frozen peas
½ head of cauliflower as smaller florets
4 zucchinis, diced
2 cups mushrooms, halved (button, bella or shiitake)
28 oz can crushed tomatoes (or 4 large fresh tomatoes, skinned and chopped)
1 can (13½ oz or 398 ml) coconut milk

*Spices*
2-3 tsp sea salt
2 sticks cinnamon
2 tsp ground turmeric
1½ tsp ground cumin
1½ tsp ground coriander
1 tsp ground cardamom
1 tbsp Roasted Masala Spice (see below)

*Roasted masala spice blend*
Makes about 7 oz

2½ oz coriander seeds
2 oz cumin seeds
1½ oz dried red chilies
½ oz black peppercorns
1 tsp whole cloves
2 cinnamon sticks, broken into small pieces
1 tbsp cardamom pods, lightly crushed
1½ oz ground turmeric
1½ oz ground ginger

Mix all spices except turmeric and ginger and roast in a dry stainless steel skillet until the aroma begins to infuse your kitchen. Stir frequently to prevent burning. Allow to cool and grind, using either a pestle and mortar or a coffee grinder. Store in a glass jar away from sunlight.

Heat ghee in potjie and fry the chicken pieces, a few at a time; don't crowd the pot until a little browned. Remove and keep aside.

Fry the onion and chili until the onion is almost translucent, then add the minced garlic for 2 minutes. Return the chicken to the pot.

Arrange the vegetables in layers on top of the meat, starting in the order as listed.
In a medium bowl, add all spices to the coconut milk and crushed tomatoes. Pour over the ingredients. If the mixture is too thick, add a little water. Cover with a lid and slowly simmer on ultra-low heat, for 60-75 minutes. The flavors need to infuse with the meat and vegetables; the meat needs to be so tender as to fall apart.

Keeps well in the refrigerator for a few days. Delicious reheated.
*Inspired by "Potjiekos" by Marlene Hamman*


### Chicken Livers and Mushrooms

4 organic chicken livers cut into 4 pieces each
6 mushrooms, diced
2 slices uncured applewood bacon, cut into small pieces
1 tsp arrowroot powder
¼ cup organic raw cream
Organic rye toast

Fry bacon in skillet, add livers and mushrooms, season with salt and pepper, let cook 4 minutes. Stir arrowroot powder into the cream. When smooth, add to liver and mushrooms, let thicken, stirring to keep from scorching. Serve on toast.


### Restorative Pâté (Tammera Karr)

*This pâté was developed for a critically ill Crohn's patient after returning home following 4 weeks in the hospital on parenteral nutrition (PN). Unable to hold down more than a few ounces of food at a time and anemic, the client started with 1 tablespoon. Within three days, they could eat ¼ cup and had significantly improved mental clarity, digestion, and physical energy. Each ingredient is high in iron and digestives, and the cooking method created a synergistic healing food.*

1 lb organic chicken livers
1 lb chicken hearts
½ tsp garlic powder
¼ tsp black pepper
¼ tsp cayenne pepper
¼ tsp cumin
2 tbsp olive oil
1 fennel bulb, medium large, sliced; reserve the feathery top for later

2 large shallots
6 cloves garlic
½ tsp Celtic Sea salt
2 cups water

Place liver, heart, garlic powder, spices, shallots, and fennel in a sauce pan with water and simmer until fennel is tender. About 15 minutes.

Place garlic cloves, olive oil and ¼ cup of tender feathery fennel tops in food processor with ¼ cup of broth from a sauce pan; chop finely while blending. Gradually add the cooked liver, shallots, and fennel; adding reserved liquid from the meat until pâté is smooth and creamy in texture.

Use 1 teaspoon on gluten-free rice crackers or toast.

### Poultry Stock (Tammera Karr)

*While making stock is time-consuming, it isn't hard and is well worth doing. Once you get used to having this versatile staple in your refrigerator, freezer or canned in glass jars, you will wonder how you ever got by without it. This versatile stock can be used almost anywhere stock is required. Using just bones is fine, but many birds' bones are hollow. To compensate for this lack of marrow, meaty pieces like wings, backs, and necks are usually added to poultry stock. You can mix and match the bones of different birds. The finished stock is the foundation for hundreds of soups.*
Makes 7-8 cups

4 lbs poultry bones and backs, cut into 2-3 inch pieces (or any other kind of marrow bone)
2 medium carrots or yams, sliced
2 celery or lovage stalks, sliced
1 yellow onion, unpeeled, cut into wedges
2 leeks or scallions, trimmed and quartered lengthwise
6 flat leaf parsley or watercress stems
3-4 mashed garlic cloves
1 large thyme sprig
1 large rosemary sprig
1 bay leaf
¼ tsp ground turmeric
¼ tsp black peppercorns
Celtic Sea salt, to taste

Rinse the bones and backs under cold water, then place them in a large stock pot, along with the herbs and vegetables. Pour in enough cold water to cover the bones, about 12 cups, and bring slowly to a boil. As soon as the stock begins to boil, reduce the heat so it simmers. Using a soup ladle, skim off any scum that has risen to the surface (rotate the bowl of the ladle on the surface of the stock to make ripples; this will carry the scum to the edges of the pot, and you can then use the ladle to lift it off). Add turmeric and peppercorns and simmer uncovered for 5 hours, skimming from time to time.

Strain the stock through a sieve into a large bowl. Discard the debris left in the sieve and cool the stock quickly by placing the bowl in a larger bowl or sink filled with ice water; occasionally stir as it cools. If you are not reducing the stock, add about 1 teaspoon salt.

Refrigerate the stock for 6 hours or overnight to allow the fat to rise to the top and the debris to sink to the bottom. Remove the fat before using, if desired (and discard the debris at the bottom of the bowl). Divide into 1 cup quantities and refrigerate for up to 3 days or freeze for up to 6 months.

## Chicken Liver Sautéed

4 chicken or goose livers
2 shallots, chopped fine
1 garlic clove, minced
½ cup fennel bulb, chopped
½ tsp Celtic Sea salt
⅛ tsp paprika
¼ tsp ground cumin
⅛ tsp ground cayenne pepper
¼ tsp ground turmeric
½ cup strong soup stock
1 tbsp organic butter or olive oil

Cut livers into 4 pieces each. Combine salt, pepper, spices, and gluten-free oat or buckwheat flour. Dredge liver (cover with a coating) well. Fry shallots, garlic and chopped fennel bulb in oil until light brown. Add liver and shake skillet over heat to sear all sides. Add soup stock. Allow to boil up once. Serve immediately on organic rye toast or as a side.

## Easy Chicken Parmesan (Tammera Karr)

4 boneless, skinless organic chicken breasts
1 qt organic marinara sauce
1 tbsp extra virgin olive oil
1 cup grated organic Parmesan cheese
¼ cup chopped black olives
¼ cup finely chopped organic parsley

Split chicken breast meat in half (butterfly cut through the center).
Coat the bottom of a skillet or glass baking dish with oil. Place chicken in a skillet or baking dish and cover with marinara sauce.

Cover skillet with a lid or baking dish with foil and cook for 20 minutes at 350°F. Remove from oven or burner, uncover, and garnish top with grated cheese.

### Turkey Stir Fry (Chef Christine Wokowsky)

2 tbsp extra virgin olive oil or coconut oil, or a mixture of both
1 lb turkey breast cut into strips or tenders cut into bite sized pieces
1 cup broccoli florets
1 cup mushrooms, shiitakes preferably
1 onion cut in half and sliced
3-4 garlic cloves, sliced (after slicing wait 5 minutes before using)
1-inch piece ginger, cut into rounds then matchsticks
1 red bell pepper, sliced
⅛ cup Braggs liquid aminos or coconut aminos
⅛ tsp arrowroot powder plus 1 tbsp water mixed together
½ cup cooked brown rice or quinoa
Salt and pepper

Season the turkey generously with sea salt and freshly ground black or white pepper. If you have any organic, gluten-free Asian seasonings feel free to use this on the turkey as well. Of course, omit the sea salt if salt is present in the seasoning mix. In a wok or large frying pan heat oil. Add the turkey and cook just until it no longer is opaque. Remove from the wok and set on a plate.

Add onions, garlic, and ginger followed by all other vegetables. Cook until crisp-tender.

Add turkey and any collected juices.
Re-stir the arrowroot and water. Add liquid aminos or coconut aminos to pan. Turn up heat and stir until thickened.

Add 1-2 tablespoons of fermented veggies. Serve with brown rice or quinoa.

### Zing'n Hot and Saucy Turkey Meatballs (Karen Langston)

*Turkey Meatballs Ingredients*

1 lb ground pasture-raised turkey
1 pasture raised egg, beaten (can omit if you have a sensitivity or allergy)
2 sprigs scallion, finely chopped
1 celery stalk, finely diced
1 tbsp almond or coconut flour
1 tbsp Paleo mayonnaise (or Primal Garlic Aioli Mayo-oh ya)
1 tsp organic onion powder
1 tsp organic garlic granules

1 tsp Celtic Sea salt
1 tsp organic ground black pepper

*Cilantro Lime Riced Cauliflower Ingredients*

I prefer ricing cauliflower myself over using frozen riced cauliflower. If you are lucky enough to find it fresh, you can use this too. If you are going to use frozen, please read the package; many of them have unnecessary ingredients. I love cilantro! Well, obsessed, really, so I use the entire bunch which is usually more than ½ cup. If you are not into cilantro the way I am then just go for the ½ cup. If you want to save time on the garlic, use a fine cheese grater and shred the garlic; it will look like purée but is just as effective.

1 bunch fresh organic cilantro, chopped
1 medium organic cauliflower
1 organic lime, zest and juice
2 tbsp coconut oil
2 sprigs scallion, finely chopped

Zing'n Hot Sauce

4 tbsp organic butter from pasture-raised cows
3 cloves organic garlic, minced
¼ tsp organic paprika
¼ cup hot sauce, I use Cholula hot sauce
¼ tsp Celtic Sea salt

Change the oven rack to the upper top of the oven. Preheat the oven to 400°F.
Lightly grease a cookie pan with coconut oil or ghee, and set aside.

Using fresh cauliflower, cut into pieces and place in a food processor. Chop until it resembles grains. Bigger grains work better than small; they will become smaller once cooked. Set aside.

Finely chop cilantro leaves and stems, and set aside.
Finely chop 2-3 sprigs of scallion, and set aside.

Wash lime and dry. Using a fine cheese grater or parmesan grater zest lime, and set aside. Gently cut the lime in half, squeeze the juice into a small bowl, and set aside.

In a large bowl, combine all turkey meatballs ingredients and mix well. The mixture will be quite sticky and that is OK.

Use your hands to form 2 inch balls. You can add some almond flour to coat your hands, however, do not go overboard or you will end up with grainy, dry meatballs. Place meatballs on lightly oiled cookie sheet pan. Bake in oven for 15 minutes.

While the meatballs are cooking, let's get the riced cauliflower going. Add 2 tablespoons of coconut oil to a medium sized skillet over medium heat, add riced cauliflower, and sauté for 2-3 minutes stirring to coat cauliflower with oil; add a little more oil if needed.

Now get your Zing'n Hot Sauce going while the cauliflower is sautéing. Add butter, minced garlic, paprika, and sea salt in a small pot. Melt over medium heat, stir well, then add in hot sauce. Turn the heat to low and stir occasionally.

When ready, take the meatballs out of the oven and set aside. Back to your cauliflower rice. Add the cilantro and lime zest; stir well, place lid on the pan, and turn to low heat for 2-3 minutes while you prepare the rest of the dish.

And now for the presentation. Take the lid off the cauliflower, add lime juice, and stir well. Add to serving plate, and sprinkle with salt. Add turkey meatballs on top of cilantro lime riced cauliflower. Give the zing'n hot sauce a good stir and pour over meatballs and riced cauliflower. Sprinkle with scallions and serve. Bon appétit!

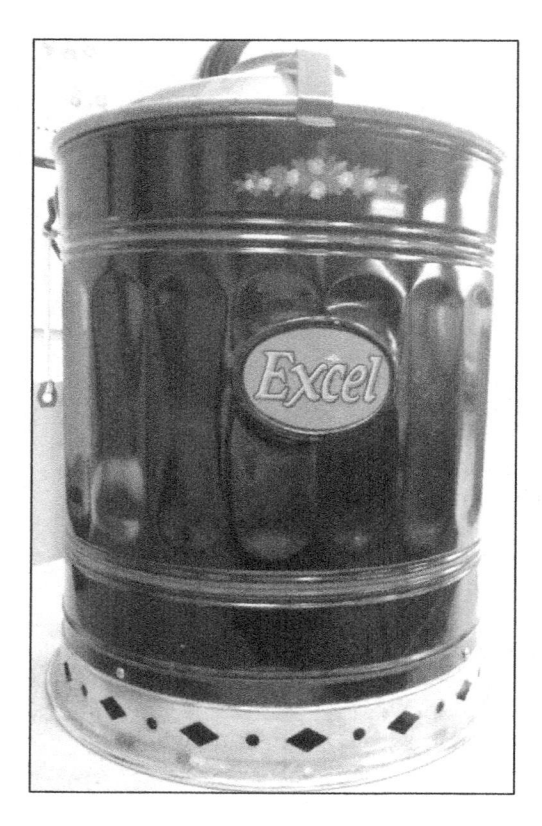

**Meet the Excel Crockpot**

This pristine electric crockpot, never used, was a wedding gift. The newlyweds would not have electricity for almost 60 years!

Wedding gift to R. M. Templeton and Effie Hoover January 13, 1892. It resides at the Bowman Museum, Prineville, Oregon.

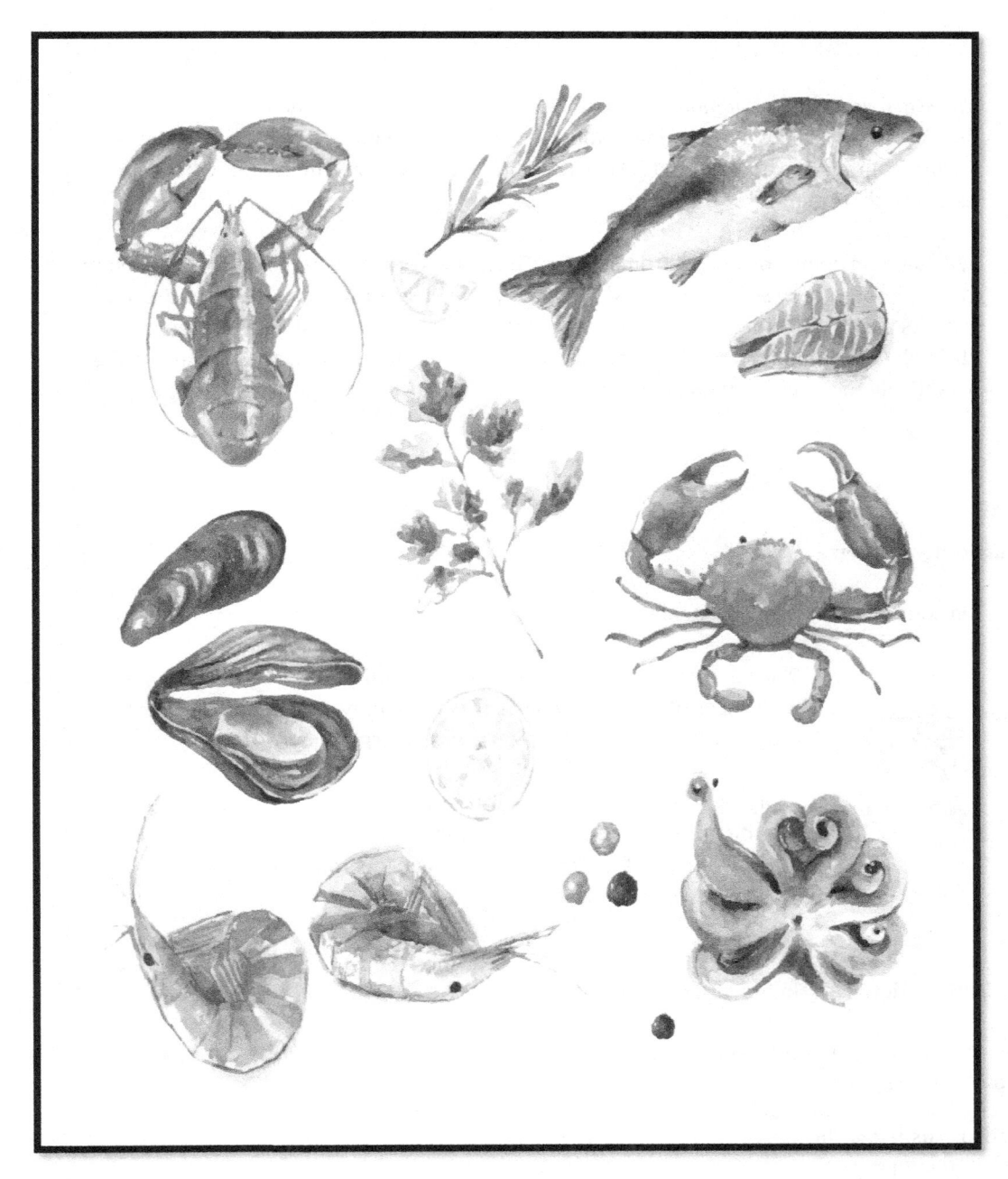

**Crustaceans, Fish & Mollusk**

*There are two types of salmon*: the Atlantic, an ocean going trout, and the type found in fish farms. This is not a true salmon and often contains higher levels of heavy metals. Farmed salmon (an apex predator) are fed GMO grains and soy, neither of which are native to their diet.

Wild salmon comes primarily from Alaska. These fish return from the ocean to spawning grounds once every seven years and can be any one of several subspecies; coho, sockeye with its pronounced deep red flesh, dog, humpback (popular in Asian countries) and chinook or king salmon, the largest and most abundant of the Pacific salmon and is the least likely to be found in fish markets.

## Alaskan Summer

2-4 Alaskan salmon or halibut steaks

Place fish steaks on individual heavy aluminum foil sections. Top each steak with slices of summer squash, fresh tomatoes, sweet onion, fresh basil, chopped garlic, and 1 tablespoon extra virgin olive oil.

Wrap tightly and place on grill at low heat 300°F, If the fish is thawed, cooking time will be about 15 minutes; 25 minutes if frozen or pieces are thick. When fish flakes but is still moist, it is ready to serve.

## Halibut with Green Beans and Quinoa

7-9 oz halibut fillet (cod or rockfish can be used)
2 oz sesame seeds
¼ cup extra virgin olive oil
1 tbsp crushed garlic
Salt and pepper
4-5 oz fresh green beans
4-5 oz quinoa
5 dried apricots
¼ cup mulberries
1 small red onion
2 cinnamon sticks
1 tbsp coconut sugar

Combine garlic, salt, and pepper with half the olive oil and marinate the fish for a couple of hours in a bowl or shallow glass dish. When ready to cook encrust with sesame seeds and grill or pan sear the fish.

In an Instant Pot®, rice cooker or sauce pan, heat 1 cup of water with 1 teaspoon olive oil to boiling, add quinoa and cover. Turn the heat to low and simmer for 20 minutes.

Thoroughly wash green beans and sauté in a pan with olive oil, garlic, and a pinch of salt.

Dice apricots, shave half of the onion, and put mulberries all together in a small pot with half a cup of water. Boil over medium heat. Add cinnamon sticks and 1 tablespoon of coconut sugar. Reduce heat, stir occasionally, and let it thicken.

## Warm Salmon and Asparagus Salad
Serves 2-4

12 young asparagus spears, trimmed
½ cup extra virgin olive oil
6 oz cremini mushrooms
1 clove garlic, minced
10 oz center cut salmon, cut in 2½ inch strips
Celtic Sea salt and fresh ground black pepper
2 tbsp apple cider vinegar
2 tbsp fresh lemon juice
3 scallions, minced
4 cups mixed salad greens

Blanch asparagus in salted water for about 5 minutes. Rinse with cold water and pat dry. Heat 2 tablespoons oil in a skillet over medium heat. Add mushrooms and garlic. Cook, frequently stirring, until wilted, about 2 minutes.

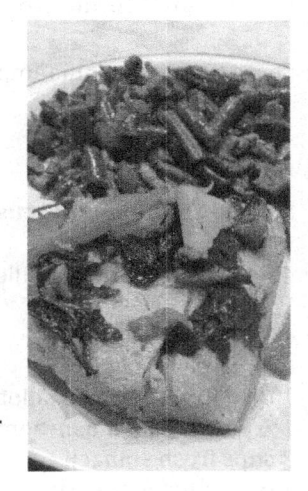

Season salmon with salt and pepper. Heat 2 tablespoons oil in a skillet over medium heat. Cook the salmon for about 5 minutes, turning to sear evenly. Remove from heat.

Whisk together ½ cup oil, vinegar, lemon juice, scallions, salt, and pepper in a small bowl. Pour all but 2 tablespoons of dressing over salad greens in a bowl. Toss to coat greens evenly.

Divide greens onto plates, top with salmon, arrange mushrooms on one side and asparagus on the other side, and drizzle the remaining dressing over the mushrooms, asparagus, and salmon.

## Salmon Kabobs

Serves 4

10 oz skinless salmon fillet, cut into 1 inch cubes
4 small zucchinis, trimmed, skin on, cut in ½ inch slices
20 cherry tomatoes, stemmed
¾ cup olive oil
6 tbsp fresh lemon juice
5 sprigs of fresh rosemary leaves, chopped
Celtic Sea salt and pepper
Cold Libby's mayonnaise for dipping

Thread 8 skewers with alternating chunks of salmon and vegetables. Whisk together olive oil, lemon juice, rosemary, salt and pepper in a large glass bowl or ceramic dish. Add skewers, turn to coat evenly, and marinate in the refrigerator for ½ hour.

Preheat the grill or broiler and rub the grate with oil to help prevent sticking.
Remove skewers from the marinade and evenly season with salt and pepper. Grill or broil for 5-6 minutes total, turning frequently and brushing with marinade.

Serve hot or at room temperature with mayonnaise for dipping.


## Seared Salmon with Mushrooms and Spinach

4 6 oz Alaskan salmon fillets (about 1 inch thick)
½ tsp salt
¼ tsp black pepper
1 tsp organic olive oil
1 tbsp thinly sliced shallots
1½ cups sliced mushrooms
2 cups fresh spinach
1 tsp grated lemon rind
1 tsp fresh lemon juice

Add oil to a hot cast iron skillet. Immediately place the flesh side of the salmon fillet in a skillet to sear (side without skin) for about 3 minutes or until golden brown. Turn fillets onto the skin side with browned flesh up. Turn heat to medium, add shallots and mushrooms, cover, and let cook for 10 minutes.

Remove the lid and toss mushrooms and shallots with a wooden spoon to ensure even cooking. Add spinach and lemon rind. Cover and let steam on medium low heat for 10 minutes more.

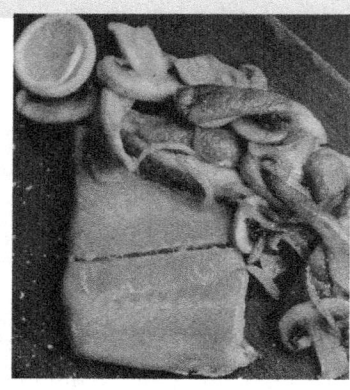

Slide spinach to the side of the fish, and check for doneness (it should easily flake apart); the skin should slip easily off as you lift the fillet out. Place fillets on a dish, arrange vegetables on the side, squeeze fresh lemon juice over all, and sprinkle with medium coarse Celtic Sea salt and black pepper.


**Bacalo A La Vizcaina** - Basque Cod Biscayne

1 lb codfish
1 small onion
Olive oil
12 Spanish red dry peppers

Soak codfish overnight, changing water several times. Soak peppers overnight, changing the water until they lighten in color. Strain peppers in a sieve to get the pulp out. Add pulp to oil and onion and boil for 10 minutes. Pour over codfish. Cover and simmer for 10 minutes. Cut in pieces and place in a shallow pan. Sauté onion in olive oil.

### Basque Cuisine

Basque Cuisine is a local cuisine, and traditional recipes are passed from generation to generation. The most typical dish, which also shares the same colors as the regional flag, is "Piperade," a mix of tomatoes, onions, and green or red peppers spiced with *Espelette* pepper. It is paired with meat or fish dishes such as chicken, lamb, or tuna. It can also be consumed as a main dish with scrambled eggs or Bayonne ham. Many typical Basque dishes are based on fish: the cod cooked "*a la biscaye*" with tomatoes and peppers; the *ttoro*, fish soup specialty of Saint Jean de Luz or the *chipirons* (small squids), which are cooked with the ink or "*à la plancha*" complemented with garlic and parsley, make a delicious meal with a glass of *Irouleguy* white wine, as well as *txangurro*, a stuffed crab.

In the countryside, recipes based on meat are favored. Pork, lamb, and veal are cooked *à l'ancienne*, most often in a stew, like *axoa*, a lamb and veal dish, paired with rice or jacket potatoes. Close to the rivers, trout, and rainbow trout, pan-fried with butter, make great starters. During the hunting season, game is featured, including a delicious wood pigeon salami.

**Bacalao Con Tomates Y Pimiento** - Basque Cod with Tomatoes and Peppers (BeeBee Sitz)

1 lb codfish
1 small onion
1 qt stewed tomatoes
1 can red pimentos
Flour
2-4 cloves garlic, chopped
Pinch of sugar
Olive oil

Roll fish pieces in flour and fry in olive oil. Sauté onions. Add tomatoes and a pinch of sugar. Cook until thickens, making sauce. Sauté garlic, add red peppers and cook for 10 minutes; add to tomatoes and fish.

Simmer for ½ hour.

> **Principle 22:** *Let Go ~ stop trying so hard, and allow your generational intuition to guide you. The best way to get the flavors of the past is to use your senses versus precision measurements.*

**Paella** - Basque Shellfish and Rice (BeeBee Sitz)
Serves 8-10

¼ cup olive oil
2 chorizos, crumbled (Basque chorizos are in a casing and dryer than that found in Mexico)
1 yellow onion finely chopped
4 cloves garlic, minced
1 green pepper, finely chopped
½ cup chopped pimiento
1 large tomato, peeled, seeded, and finely diced
2 cups long grain rice
3½ cups clam juice
1 cup white port
1 pinch saffron
Salt and pepper to taste
10 whole clams in shells, well-scrubbed
12 large shrimp, peeled and deveined
½ lb crab meat
½ lb chicken, cooked and cubed
9 oz artichoke hearts (frozen is ok)
½ cup peas

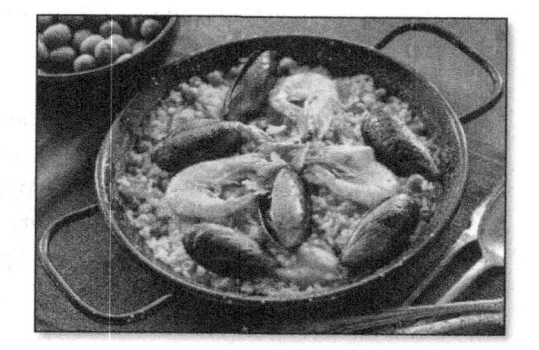

In a 4 quart sauce pan heat olive oil. Add chorizo, cook while stirring for about 3 minutes. Add onion, garlic, and green pepper, then add pimiento, tomato, and sauté gently until most of the liquid evaporates and the onion is tender.

Preheat oven to 350°F.
Stir rice, clam juice, port, saffron, salt and pepper into the chorizo mixture. Bring to a boil.

As soon as the mixture boils, transfer to a large paella pan* or 4 quart casserole. Bake, covered, for 40 minutes. Stir in whole clams, shrimp, crab, chicken, artichokes, and peas. Cover and bake for 10 minutes.

*Crafted in Valencia, Spain, the birthplace of paella, this pan showcases the traditional Valencian style. The wide, shallow carbon steel cooking surface is designed to sauté meats and vegetables prior to adding rice.

### Marmitako -Basque Tuna and Potato Soup
*Marmitako means "from the pot." It is a rustic, filling soup that began as a meal local tuna fishermen would make during long fishing routes on their boats. Traditionally, locals crack the potatoes with a partial cut, then break off ragged chunks to toss into and add starchiness to the potato soup. Adding the tuna right at the end keeps the fish moist and tender, just as the soup is removed from the heat.*

1 lb raw tuna, cut into ½ inch cubes
Kosher salt
1 tbsp extra virgin olive oil
1 green bell pepper, coarsely chopped
1 yellow onion, coarsely chopped
1 lb yellow potatoes, peeled and coarsely chopped
1 garlic clove, finely chopped
1 tsp pimentón (smoked paprika)
Coarsely chopped Italian parsley leaves, for garnish

In a medium bowl, season the tuna lightly with salt and toss to coat. Set aside.

To a large pot set over medium heat, add the oil. When the oil is hot, add the bell pepper and onion and cook, occasionally stirring, until the onion is softened and translucent; 8-10 minutes. Add the potatoes and garlic, season with salt, and continue cooking until vegetables are softened but not colored; 3-5 minutes.

Add the pimentón and 3 cups of water, and bring to a simmer. Cook until the vegetables are tender; 13-15 minutes. Turn off the heat, add the tuna, and immediately cover the pan. Set aside until the fish is just barely cooked through; 3-5 minutes.

### Basque Pasta (Tammera Karr)

1 lb Mexican shrimp or prawns (scallops or chicken can be substituted)
4 tbsp organic butter
4 tbsp extra virgin olive oil
3 cloves garlic, minced
½ bunch fresh parsley, chopped
½ cup organic cream
¼ cup grated Parmesan cheese
Fresh ground black pepper
Pinch Celtic Sea salt (at table)

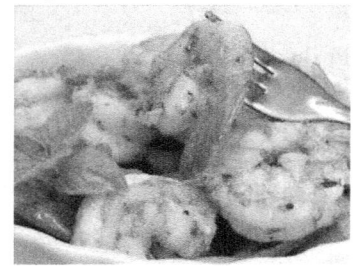

Add butter and oil to the skillet, and warm. Add garlic and parsley. Stir or toss for 5 minutes on medium heat; don't smoke your oil.

Add shrimp or scallops and cream. Cook until shrimp are pink but still tender (about 8 minutes). Serve over gluten-free pasta. Top with cheese and black pepper and garnish with chopped tomato.

### Shrimp & Broccoli (Tammera Karr)

15-20 medium prawns, peeled and deveined
2 cloves garlic, minced
2 tbsp organic butter
2 tbsp extra virgin olive oil
2 broccoli spears, whole or tops

Warm butter and oil in a skillet, add garlic and shrimp. Toss over medium heat until shrimp turn bright salmon color. Cover with broccoli, then cover with lid for 5-10 minutes on medium-low heat until broccoli turns bright green. Toss together and place on plates as is or serve with rice pasta topped with a sprinkle of Parmesan cheese.

Prep time 15-20 minutes, cook time 15-20 minutes; total time 35-40 minutes.

### Tomato Basil and Shrimp Soup (Tammera Karr)
Serves 2

1½ pints fresh tomato sauce
1-2 cloves Italian garlic, minced
¼ cup fresh basil, minced
¼ cup shallot, minced
3 tbsp extra virgin olive oil

¼ lb of shrimp
¼ cup grated fresh Parmesan cheese
Fresh ground black pepper
½ tsp Celtic Sea salt
¼ tsp Italian seasoning

Combine everything but the cheese in a sauce pan and cook on medium heat until the shrimp are cooked (place them in frozen for a little more time).
Put a drizzle of grated cheese on the bottom of the soup bowl.

Add shrimp and tomato soup, sprinkle with more cheese and black pepper.
Garnish with fresh basil.
Cook time 15 minutes.

## Southern Rockefeller

24 Lowcountry cups, shucked and heeled (separate the oyster from the back of the shell)
2 tbsp bacon fat or olive oil
½ cup red onion, diced
½ cup bell pepper, diced
½ cup celery diced
½ cup bacon lardons cooked (1 cup of bacon cut into ¼ inch strips, cooked and drained)
1 cups spinach, chopped
2 cups pimento cheese (store bought or homemade)
Salt and pepper to taste
2 cups bread crumbs
¼ cup brown butter

Sauté vegetables in fat with a pinch of salt until soft. Add spinach and wilt. Add bacon and pimento cheese. Stir over medium low heat until all cheese is melted. Cool immediately.

*Cook's tip:* Make the bread crumb filling the day before.
2 cups toasted bread crumbs with brown butter.

Preheat the oven to 325°F. Brown ¼ cup butter in a sauté pan and remove from heat. In a mixing bowl, add bread crumbs and stir in butter. Bake crumbs on a sheet pan for 25 minutes or until golden brown.

*For the dish:* Preheat the oven to 400°F (350°F with convection). Place about 1½ tablespoons of filling on top of each oyster and top with bread crumbs. Place oysters on a sheet pan and bake with a layer of rock salt in the oven for 3 minutes until the cheese is melted. Remove from oven and top with some extra bread crumbs. Serve on a plate with a layer of rock salt to keep oysters from falling over.

*Tip:* Place rock salt on the bottom of your sheet pan or whatever you are baking your oysters on. It keeps the oysters from falling over.

> *Note: The following two recipes from an antique cookbook are verbatim, except for measurement abbreviations. (The Century Cook Book by Mary Ronald, 1897, pg 248)*

## Gumbo File

50 oysters
1 fowl cut into pieces
½ lb of veal cut into pieces
½ lb of ham cut into pieces
3 tbsp of tomato
1 tbsp of drippings
2 onions
½ tsp of salt
¼ tsp pepper
¼ tsp powdered thyme
¼ tsp of marjoram
Dash of cayenne
2 tbsp of sassafras powder

Wash well the outside of the fowl and cut into pieces. Cut the veal and the ham into small pieces, and dredge all of them well with flour.

Put onions, sliced into a pot or large sauce pan with one tablespoon of fat or drippings, and fry until brown; then add the pieces of chicken and ham. Turn them often, so all will brown evenly; this will take about twenty minutes. When the meat is browned, add two quarts of hot-water; cover the pot, and let simmer for two hours. After the first hour add the salt, pepper, thyme, marjoram, and tomatoes. At the end of two hours, if the meat is tender, add the oysters and the oyster juice, and let remain on the fire long enough to ruffle the gills of the oysters. Take from the fire, and add two tablespoonfuls of sassafras powder, and stir until a little thickened (do not add the sassafras until the pot is removed from the fire).

Serve in a meat dish with a border of boiled rice. This is a dish much used in the South. It may be served as a chowder, with the meat and liquor together, or may be served separately, using the liquor as a soup.

Powdered sassafras leaves may be obtained at the grocers.

### Southern way of Cooking Rice

Wash the rice thoroughly through several waters, using the hand. Put it into a sauce pan with a pint of water and a half teaspoon of salt to each cupful of rice. Let it boil covered until the water has boiled away; then draw it to the side of the range, open the cover a little, and let it steam until thoroughly dry. Do not touch the rice while it is cooking. This recipe is by a Southern negro cook.

> *As a mother and African American, I loved reading the recipe from a white woman who gave credit to the "negro" for the recipe in 1897. Women back in the 1800s were seldom able to be published under their own name, let alone give credit to a person of color. To read the words she used to describes the recipe and where it came from made me proud. Learning about and preserving history is essential, and this book does just that.*
>
> ~ Sharena Graves
> Decedent of Chef James Hemings

### Fish with Green Peppers and Clams (Kelsi Sitz)

⅓ cup extra virgin olive oil
2 cloves garlic, finely chopped
1 tbsp all-purpose flour
½ cup dry white wine
2 cups fish stock or clam broth
¾ tsp salt, plus more to taste
3½ cups assorted mild green peppers, cut into ¼ inch strips
1 medium Spanish onion, thinly sliced
2 tbsp coarsely chopped Italian parsley, plus more for garnish
2 lbs skin on, hake fillets cut into 8 equal portions
12 small, fresh clams, scrubbed
1-2 tsp piment d'Espelette (optional)

In a large skillet, heat the olive oil over medium high heat. Add the garlic and cook, occasionally stirring, until just beginning to brown; about 1 minute. Sprinkle the flour over the garlic and stir to combine. Add the wine and cook, stirring rapidly, until the mixture thickens and reduces slightly; about 2 minutes. Add the fish stock and salt, then bring the mixture back to a boil. Add the peppers, onion, and parsley, and spread into an even layer on the bottom of the pan. Raise the heat to high, cover the pan, and simmer until the vegetables are softened; about 5 minutes.

Uncover the pan and place the hake pieces skin-side up in a single layer atop the vegetables. Nestle the clams between the fillets and season the fish with salt to taste. Cover and cook until the fillets are opaque at the center and the clams have opened for 5-7 minutes. (Discard unopened clams.)

On a deep serving platter, scatter the vegetables, then place the fish and clams on top. Spoon the remaining broth over the fish and garnish with chopped parsley and d'Espelette pepper, if using; serve immediately.

**Mussels in White Wine** (Chef Christine Wokowsky)

⅓ cup olive oil
3 large shallots, chopped
6 large garlic cloves, chopped
1 tomato, diced
½ tsp salt
1 cup dry white wine
3 quarter inch thick lemon slices
½ cup chopped fresh parsley
2½ lbs fresh mussels, scrubbed, and debearded

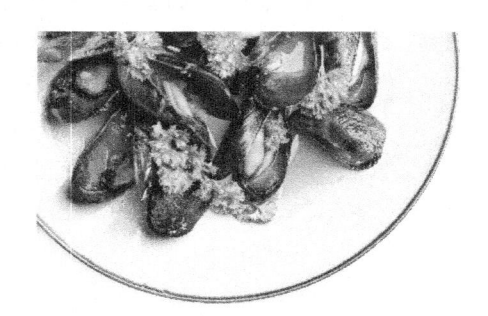

Serve with a side salad or lightly sautéed cabbage.

Most mussels you buy from the supermarket are clean already; unless there are noticeable threads on the shells, there's no need to scrub. Fresh mussels can be stored in the refrigerator, covered with a damp cloth, for one to two days; do not store them submerged in water or they will drown.

Heat oil in a large heavy sauté pan over medium heat. Add shallot, garlic, crushed red pepper and salt; sauté until shallot is light brown; about 4 minutes.

Add wine, tomatoes, lemon slices and ¼ cup parsley; bring to boil.
Add mussels. Cover pot and cook until mussel shells open, stirring once to rearrange mussels; about 4-5 minutes. Discard any mussels that do not open. Serve immediately.

Add in 1-2 tablespoons of fermented veggies.

**Silver-Wrapped Fish with Tangerine Peel** (Yuan Wang, *Ancient Wisdom Modern Kitchen*, pg 146)

4 g dried tangerine peel or 1tbsp fresh, shredded
1 lb white fish or hake, halibut, or bottom fish
1 tbsp kudzu, powdered or arrowroot
2-3 tbsp cold water
¼ tsp salt
¼ tsp pepper
2 tbsp soy or tamari sauce
1 tbsp olive oil
1 inch piece of fresh ginger
1 medium sized green onion, chopped into ¼ inch pieces

Preheat oven to 350°F
1. Soak dried tangerine peel in warm water until soft.
2. Place each piece of fish on a separate sheet of foil.
3. In a small bowl or cup combine kudzu with cold water and blend until smooth. Then brush mixture over the fish. Season the fish with salt, pepper, soy sauce and olive oil.
4. Place the ginger shreds, green onion, and tangerine peel on fish, evenly distributing it.
5. Seal the foil around and over the fish, forming a packet to steam the fish.
6. Place packets on a baking sheet or grill and bake for 15 minutes at 350°F.
7. Remove the packets and allow them to continue cooking while you prepare side dish of vegetables and rice.


**A Note on Fish Broth** (Chef Christine Wokowsky)

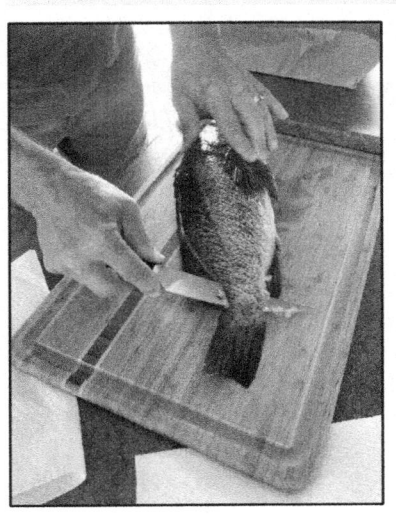

Do not overcook!
Fish and shellfish stocks require just 1 hour to 1½ hour on simmer; longer will make the flavor bitter.

Additionally, roasting the shells and lobster carcasses in a high oven, will enhance the flavor your broth. This brings out a rich, smooth flavor and vibrant color. Collect shrimp, lobster shells and fish heads and bodies in a Ziplock® bag in the refrigerator freezer for this very purpose.

### Citrus Poached White Fish (Tammera Karr)

Serves 4

2 tbsp Spanish olive oil
1 large ripe lemon, sliced
1 large lime, sliced
4 cod, hake, or rockfish filets
1 tsp garlic, minced
Fresh rosemary
1 tsp coarse Celtic Sea salt

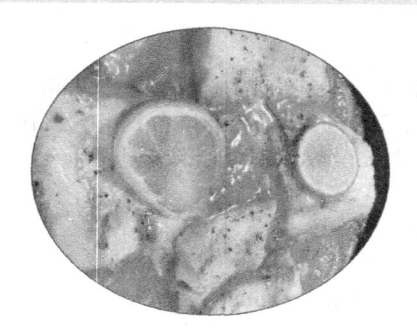

Warm oil on medium-low heat in a large cast iron skillet. Place lime and lemon slices around the bottom (citrus rind can add bitterness if cooked too long), let the oil heat, and infuse the citrus for 1-2 minutes. Add about 10-20 fresh rosemary needles, sprinkle garlic and allow time to heat about 1 minute.

Place fish on top of citrus and herbs sprinkle coarse salt, and crushed black pepper, 1 slice lemon and 1 of lime with a small sprig of rosemary. Cover and allow the fish to poach until the fillets flake easily with a fork but are not overcooked. If the filets are fresh, this only takes 5-10 minutes.

One of the biggest mistakes folks make is overcooking fish. It is better to take the fish off the heat when slightly underdone and allow it to rest and finish cooking with the reserved heat from the pan. Overcooking white fish makes it dry and a tad bitter.

Reserve the fish and lemon broth for a lemon zest soup or rice or use in a stir fry.

*"Good Eating brings happiness two ways. First, there is the joy and satisfaction of eating delicious, well-prepared food. Then there's the buoyant health, vitality, and joy of living that comes from a wise choice of foods. Both are important to good nutrition."*

Betty Crocker
*the Betty Crocker Picture Cook Book* 1952

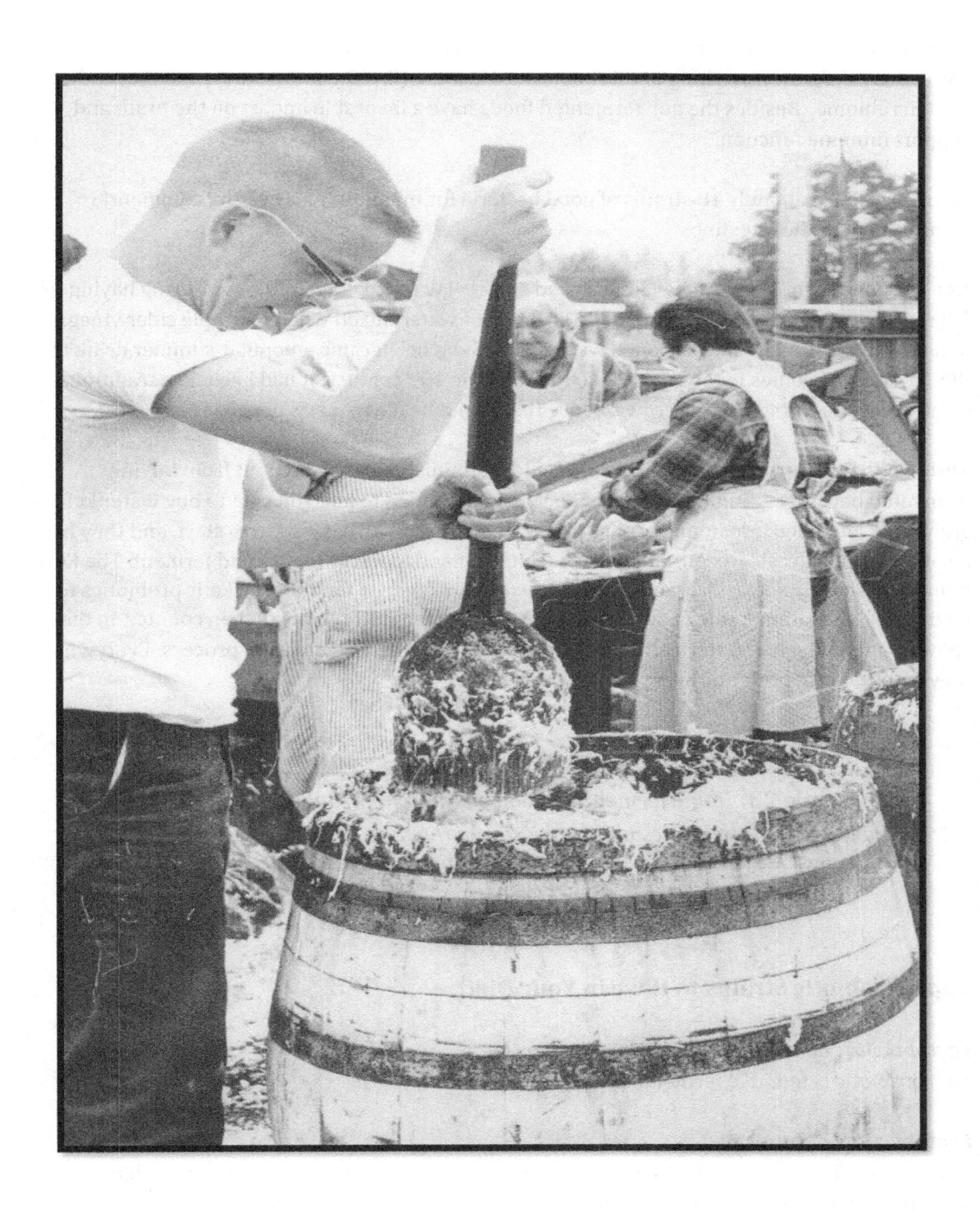

# Fermented Foods

Fermented foods have received much fanfare in the last ten years as research on the microbiome has escalated. As of the writing of this book, PubMed has 47,469 clinical studies on the study of the microbiome. Besides the gut, fermented foods have a favorable impact on the brain and support immune function.

There are approximately 18 strains of good bacteria for maintaining a healthy commensal environment in the intestines.

As a kid in eastern Oregon, a beverage called switchel was provided for crews during haying or fall round up. Switchel is a fermented drink made of water mixed with raw apple cider vinegar, honey, or brown sugar and seasoned with ginger. Switchel became a popular summer drink in the American Colonies in the late 17th century. By the 19th century, it had become a traditional drink served to thirsty haying crews, hence the nickname haymaker's punch.

Through the encouragement of a colleague and a diminishing bank account from buying fermented beverages, Tammera's husband, Michael, headed to amazon.com to buy water kefir grains and launched into home fermenting. Water kefir was an easy place to start, and they had an abundance of fresh, frozen, and canned fruits on hand to flavor the second ferment. The Karrs found their locally sourced organic blueberries were a favorite food for the kefir probiotics to feed on. By midsummer, they had half-gallon jars of water kefir on the kitchen counter, in the RV shower, and in the home refrigerator in various stages of the fermentation process. Everywhere they went, a jar of probiotic brew went with them.

> **Principle 23:** *Home fermenting is an easy and affordable way to preserve food and add prebiotics and probiotics to the diet.*

## Top 5 Probiotic Strains to Have in Your Diet

### *Lactobacillus acidophilus* DDS-1
This probiotic is found in fermented milk products.

### *Lactobacillus plantarum*
This is a very beneficial probiotic strain found in fermented vegetables and products like kimchi and sauerkraut. A product that is good for most people as it helps support the health and integrity of the stomach lining.

### *Lactobacillus brevis*
This strain occurs naturally in the body and is found in human breast milk. Fermented vegetables are a perfect source as well. It supports digestion and immune health.

### *Bifidobacterium lactis*
This bacteria is considered a good "basic" bacteria, occurs in the intestinal tract and is found in healthy breastfed babies. It helps your body absorb vitamins and minerals and has been shown to promote regular bowel movements.

### *Bifidobacterium longum*
Bifidobacterium longum is possibly the most significant probiotic strain to support a healthy digestive tract. It can be acquired in sauerkraut and fermented vegetables.

> **Principle 24:** *Too much of a good thing can lead to digestive health challenges for some individuals. <u>Not everyone can tolerate fermented foods</u> due to imbalances in the gut microbiome.*

### What is Water Kefir?

Water kefir, like kombucha, is first cultured by introducing a SCOBY (symbiotic culture of bacteria and yeasts) into sugar water. The beneficial bacteria and yeasts present in the water kefir grains metabolize the sugar, turning it into an array of beneficial acids and infusing it with beneficial microorganisms, additional B vitamins, and food enzymes.

Water kefir grains are small, translucent, gelatinous structures that are comprised of various bacteria, including *lactobacillus hilgardii*, which gives them their characteristic crystal like appearance. They produce an excellent probiotic-rich beverage when properly cared for and regularly cultured. They will continue to grow and reproduce indefinitely.

~~~~

Tammera learned that placing the fruit for flavoring in a jelly bag for the second fermentation eliminated fruit pulp and straining from the process. Water kefir is picky about metal, so all containers, utensils, and strainers must be glass, wood, nylon, or cloth. A jelly strainer bag made a clear pulp-free effervescent beverage. Next, a conversation with Sarica Cernohous, DACM, L.Ac, emphasized the need to use unrefined organic sugar over turbinado, honey, coconut, or other low glycemic sweeteners. Sarica reminded Tammera that probiotics need sucrose for food and the purpose of fermenting was to break down sugars, leaving a low glycemic, almost sugar-free beverage. Water kefir makes a terrific electrolyte drink for the hot summer days and a way to keep your gut healthy.

By spring 2018, the Karrs were confident enough to tackle kombucha. For some reason, this looked like the more difficult of the two fermented beverages. It turned out to be far less temperamental than water kefir.

**What is Kombucha?**

Kombucha has a history dating back 2,000 years and originated in China, where it was prized for its energizing qualities. The fermented drink found its way into Russia and then Germany. In the 1960s, Swiss researchers reported that drinking kombucha was just as beneficial as eating yogurt. From there, kombucha boomed into a popular health drink. The basic ingredients include water, black or green tea leaves, sugar, and the probiotic colony of bacteria and yeast referred to as a SCOBY.

During fermentation, glycolysis (the chemical breakdown of glucose and lactic acid) produces ethanol. The bacteria in the SCOBY use ethanol to produce vinegar. That's why you get an initial citrusy-sour smell and taste. Fermentation is the breakdown of a substance by bacteria, yeast, or other microorganisms. Kombucha is brewed (or fermented) over 10-14 days.

**How to Make Kombucha**

First, like kefir water, you need a starter SCOBY, purchased at natural food stores, online, or from a friend. Your kombucha begins with fresh brewed organic black sweet tea. After the tea has reached room temperature, place it in a clean glass wide-mouth gallon jar and add the SCOBY. Test the *pH*. You may need to add a teaspoon of raw organic apple cider vinegar (refer to information that came with your SCOBY or kit). Cover the mouth of the jar with a muslin fabric square and a rubber band to allow air circulation. Set the jar in a well-ventilated warm area for nine to 12 days. We suggest affixing a thermometer on the outside of the jar to monitor the temperature. Fermentation increases when ambient temperatures exceed 75°F.

Once the first round of fermentation is completed, carefully reserve one cup of liquid to rest your SCOBY. At the same time, you pour the kombucha into brown glass growlers for the flavoring and carbonation, which takes about three days. The carbonation happens best in a narrow-necked growler jug. Now is when you add flavoring; lemon balm or hibiscus tea, slices of ginger root, tangerine, or lemon juice. The growler should be left at room temperature for up to six hours to increase its effervescent properties. Your beverage should swish and fizz when you open the sealed growlers. This indicates your water kefir or kombucha underwent a normal fermentation process.

**Tools Water Kefir and Kombucha**

Purchase a Kombucha Shop Starter Kit from Amazon; it includes a jar, muslin topper cloth, *pH* papers, SCOBY, organic black tea, a cloth tea bag, organic sugar, and a stick-on thermometer. A step-by-step laminated guide with clear instructions is also included.

Next, we read the *Funky Kitchen* by Sarica Cernohous, DACM, L.Ac, and *Delicious Probiotic Drinks: 75 Recipes for Kombucha, Kefir, Ginger Beer, and Other Naturally Fermented Drinks* by Julia Mueller, which filled in the gaps, answered questions, showed images, provided a selection of flavoring ideas and tips. Buy bulk organic black tea for making each brew from Stash Tea, Portland, Oregon, or Mountain Rose Herbs.

The Karrs had two SCOBYs in the gallon jar in about four months. Tammera separated the SCOBYs into two one-gallon jars and invested in two Propagate Pro 10 inch round fermentation heating pads. This allowed for moving the brew jars out of the kitchen to an open pantry away from the heat and kept the kombucha brew stations warm during cool to colder weather.

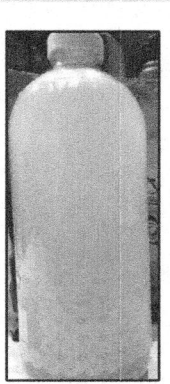

~~~

**Lacto-fermentation or lactic acid fermentation**, in contrast to ethanol fermentation in which alcohol is created, is the fermentation process used in making a wide variety of foods, including fermented vegetable dishes such as sauerkraut and beet kvass and cultured dairy products like yogurt and kefir. These bacteria are responsible for gobbling up carbohydrates naturally in cucumbers and turning them into sour pickles. Since the bacteria responsible for lactic acid fermentation exist on your skin, food, and countertops, it is not necessary to inoculate your foods with a starter culture. They will ferment without a starter and do so successfully, safely, and often with better-tasting results.

Sarica Cernohous, DACM, L.Ac, instructor on *Traditional Food Preparation Methods via The Funky Kitchen*, is our fermenting mentor. Sarica has graciously contributed many of the recipes and information for this chapter. For more fermented recipes from Sarica, go to Naturally Living Today at https://naturallylivingtoday.com/category/recipes/.

### Lemon Ginger Water Kefir

3½ cups water kefir
1 tbsp lemon juice
1 inch piece of fresh ginger, peeled and sliced into sticks

Pour the water kefir into an airtight bottle (we use brown glass ½ gallon growlers). Add lemon juice and ginger root.

Cap the bottle and ferment for 1-3 days, depending on the desired level of carbonation. Place the bottles of flavored water kefir in the refrigerator and serve chilled.

## Finnish Sima Spring Mead

*This recipe was shared by one of Tammera's clients.*
*A lightly fermented lemonade from Finland. It is fine to serve kids if you drink this sparkling beverage as soon as the raisins float. But be warned—Sima transforms from being slightly bubbly to being very bubbly and somewhat intoxicating the longer it ferments.*

1¼ gallons of water (5 liters)
2 lemons
½ cup brown sugar
½ cup white sugar plus sugar for the bottles
¼ tsp dry yeast
25 raisins

Peel lemons with a potato peeler, taking off just the rind. Remove the white pulp layer and toss it. Slice the lemon and rind. Place lemon and sugar in a large, NON METAL bowl. Bring the water to a boil, and pour it over the lemons and sugar. Let the mixture cool until lukewarm. Dissolve the yeast in a small amount of its own lukewarm water for a few minutes. Add the dissolved yeast to the lukewarm water, lemon, and sugar mixture. Stir it briefly.

Let the mixture ferment at room temperature overnight. (I cover mine with a lid.) In the morning, pour the mixture into a sieve and bottle it. Put 4-5 raisins and a teaspoon of sugar into each bottle before closing. Keep bottles at room temperature for a few hours, then store them upright in a cool place like a pantry for a couple of days. Place it in the refrigerator to store. The drink is ready to serve in a few days but is best in a week. Raisins float to the top when it is ready to taste.

The earlier you use it, the more you can taste the lemon. We like it at least seven days old; it becomes transparent and more like cider. Be sure to open the bottle over the sink if you hold it long because it can come out of the bottle like champagne. Use glass bottles, please.


## Dandelion and Hibiscus Kombucha

2 tbsp unflavored organic black tea
1 cup organic cane sugar
1-2 cups kombucha starter liquid
1 kombucha SCOBY
2-4 tbsp dried dandelion root
3 tbsp dried hibiscus flowers
12 cups of filtered water

1. Bring water to a boil in a stainless steel or glass stock pot, turn off the heat, and add the black tea. Let steep for 20-30 minutes, and strain the tea leaves.

2. Add the sugar to the tea and stir until it is completely dissolved.

Transfer the tea to a glass wide-mouth gallon jar when it is completely cooled to room temperature. Add the kombucha starter liquid, and float the SCOBY on top. Don't worry if it sinks.

3. Cover the jar with a clean tea towel or cheesecloth secured with a rubber band, and place it in a warm, dark place for about 10-14 days. When it has reached your desired sweetness, it is time to bottle.

4. Remove the SCOBY (and any new ones that may have formed) and 1-2 cups of kombucha. Set aside and reserve for use in making your next batch.

5. Put the dandelion and hibiscus into a stock pot with 1-2 quarts of filtered water and bring to a boil for 3-5 minutes. Let cool to room temperature and strain.

6. Combine the dandelion and hibiscus tea with the finished kombucha. At this stage, especially if your kombucha is less sweet, you can add 1-2 tablespoons of sugar.

7. Pour the mixture into a growler half-gallon jug and cap tightly. Let rest for 24-48 hours in a cool area. Look out; you will want to open the jug over a sink or outside as it could fountain out the top when the pressure is released.

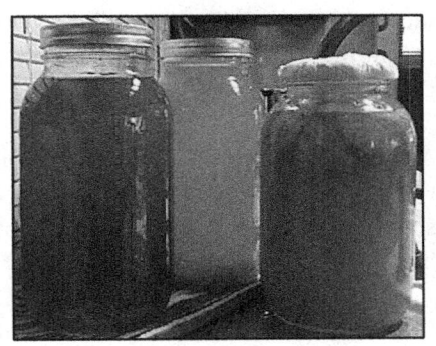

## Fermented Cranberry Apple Relish (Sarica Cernohous & Chef Amy Mirate)

1 lb cranberries, roughly chopped*
10 oz (2) apples, finely chopped
1 orange, juiced and zested
½ cup water kefir**
⅓ cup raw honey
1 tbsp cinnamon
1 inch piece of fresh ginger, julienned
½ tsp sea salt

*Chop cranberries by pulsing in a blender or food processor
**Whey may be substituted for water kefir

*Procedure*
1. Place all ingredients into a large non-metal mixing bowl and mix to combine thoroughly.
2. Once all ingredients have been combined, pack tightly into a mason jar or crock, submerging the mixture under the liquid completely.
3. Cover loosely and allow to sit at room temperature for at least 3 days before refrigerating.

## Homemade Dairy Yogurt Instructions for Pasteurized Milk (Sarica Cernohous)

Using a food thermometer, bring 1 quart of pasteurized milk to the proper temperature (160°F for most thermophilic cultures). You can set the thermometer in a pan with the milk and slowly heat it to its correct temperature. Allow the milk to cool to its proper culturing temperature (105-110°F for thermophilic; 72-78°F for mesophilic). Although this milk has been pasteurized previously, simply bringing it to the proper culturing temperature is tempting fate. Because the milk lacks its naturally occurring beneficial bacteria and enzymes, it is a sugary substrate for potentially pathogenic bacteria to proliferate in warm conditions. Better to first re-sterilize it and then allow it to cool to culturing temperature.

Remove from heat and pour into a glass quart jar. Add your cultures and stir well to incorporate them into the milk. Cover with a paper towel and cinch with a rubber band. Place the jar in an incubator, oven, yogurt maker, or on the counter that works best for the type of culture you are using.

After about six hours, check your yogurt to see if it has "set." You will know because it will all move as one unit away from the sides of the jar when tilted. It will also take on a lovely tart smell. If not, allow it to culture for another hour or two; longer if necessary, checking every hour.

(*Note*: If yogurt goes too long at the culturing temperature, it will become liquid whey and milk curds. If this happens, you can strain off the whey and use it for drinking, as a base for a smoothie, or as a wonderful soaking medium for grains, legumes, and meat marinades. The milk curds can be enjoyed as a thicker type of yogurt or yogurt cheese on top of a salad. I have had some success using yogurt that has differentiated like this to start a new batch of yogurt, though sometimes it is best just to start over. You will just have to experiment for yourself.) Once your yogurt has set, enjoy it immediately or refrigerate it to halt the culturing process.

Whenever you make yogurt, always reserve about ½-1 cup as the starter for your next batch. Follow the same instructions as above by bringing your milk to the proper temperature, pouring it into a new glass jar, adding your existing yogurt (starter), stirring, and setting it at the culturing temperature for 6-7 hours.

## Coconut Milk Yogurt

2 cans of organic Aroy-D coconut milk (carrageenan-free)
2 probiotic nutritional supplement capsules
1 tsp real vanilla extract (optional)
3 tbsp organic honey (optional)
3-4 tbsp organic coconut oil (optional for added thickness)
1 qt glass jar

Blend coconut milk with the contents of probiotic capsules. Transfer to a 1 quart glass jar with a tight-fitting lid. (If you have an immersion blender, place all ingredients in the jar and blend it right there.)

Store somewhere warm in your house, like on a window sill. After 24-48 hours, it should smell yogurt-y. It may be runny, more like kefir than yogurt. If you prefer, leave it out longer. After 48-72 hours, it should be thick and have a tangy flavor.

Store in the refrigerator for up to 7 days.
Add fresh or frozen berries or homemade jams for flavors.

Yogurt adds zest to salads, smoothies, granola, and other foods. If you are Scandinavian, congratulations on reconnecting with an important aspect of your food history. It was the Scandinavians who invented many of these healthy fermented dairy foods. [177]

**Pre-Biotic Onion Bread** (Chef Christine Wokowsky)

3 large purple onions or 2 large purple onions and one leek, white part only
¾ cup ground golden flaxseeds
½ cup coconut aminos
1 tbsp coconut vinegar (or any vinegar)
⅓ cup softened coconut oil
¼ cup nutritional yeast

Soak the flax seeds overnight. Rinse well.
Peel and chop the onions and leeks in a food processor using the slicing attachment. Place onions in a large mixing bowl.

Put the seeds in the food processor with the bottom blade inserted. Add all other ingredients except the onions. Process until smooth. Scoop this mixture into the large bowl with the onions and mix well. Spread batter on dehydrator trays lined with parchment paper. You can make them into small cracker sizes or large flatbread sizes, or a combination of the two for different eating options.  The batter should be about a ¼ inch in thickness.

Dehydrate at 105°F for approximately 10-12 hours.  Flip them over and continue dehydrating for another 1-2 hours until they are firm but slightly moist.
Store in the refrigerator in a glass container.

> **Principle 25:** *Fermentation reduces carbohydrate content and naturally occurring toxins in plant foods.*

### Fermented Potato Chips (*Modern Stone Age Kitchen* & Dr. Bill Schindler)

Potatoes, despite their prevalence in our modern diets, are toxic. They contain glycoalkaloids ($\alpha$-solanine and $\alpha$-chaconine), and when they are improperly stored, they can become even more toxic. Essential tips for implementing immediately. These go for all potatoes and all types of cooking applications:

- Store potatoes in a cool, dry, dark place.
- If they begin to turn green or sprout, DO NOT EAT. They are not fit for human consumption at this point and should be composted.
- The peels contain a higher level of toxin. Potatoes SHOULD ALWAYS BE PEELED and the peels composted. I realize this is the opposite from what we have been told our whole lives. Whatever nutrition the peels may contain is not worth the dangers the toxins pose to our health.
- Do not use a zero-waste approach to potatoes and attempt to find dietary uses for discarded potatoes or their peels. They are not fit for human consumption. They should not be considered food.
- NEVER EAT A POTATO RAW! Cooking does help some with detoxification. Potatoes should always be cooked before consumption.

Potatoes (such as Russets) or sweet potatoes
Water
Salt
High-quality lard or tallow

1. Fill a large bowl full of water. Peel the potatoes. Once each potato is peeled, place it in a bowl of water so that the peeled potatoes do not oxidize while you peel the rest. Once all the potatoes are peeled, use a food processor, mandolin, or knife to slice thinly. Place a large glass jar on a scale, make sure it is set to grams, and tare to zero.

2. Place the sliced potatoes in the jar and fill with room temperature water to cover the potato slices. The number on the scale should represent the combined weight of the potatoes and water (NOT including the jar). Multiply the combined weight of the potatoes and water by 0.025 (2.5%) and weigh that amount out in salt. Add the salt to the container and stir gently to combine. Cover the container with a cloth or lid not screwed on too tightly and set aside at room temperature to ferment for a few days. Ensure that the water level is no less than an inch from the top of the vessel or it will overflow during fermentation.

3. Fermentation should begin in a day or two. I usually let the fermentation continue for 3-5 days depending on temperature (less time if warmer, more time if cooler) and on the desired flavor.

4. Heat high-quality animal fat to 300°F or 150°C for 5-7 minutes or until the desired crispiness is achieved.

5. Transfer to a drain rack, crumbled-up brown paper, or paper towels, and immediately sprinkle with salt. Cool and enjoy immediately or store in a sealed container. These are an excellent addition to my kids' lunch boxes.

*NOTES:*
The longer the potatoes ferment, the more acidic they become due to the build-up of lactic acid. A 5 plus-day ferment will result in a "salt and vinegar" flavor that my kids love!

300°F or 150°C is the ideal temperature for potato chips because the lower temperature works to drive off the remaining moisture in the chip before it finishes cooking, resulting in a crispier, well, crisp!

These chips will not brown like "normal" potato chips; most of the starch that causes browning during the *Maillard Reaction* (which produces acrylamides) is gone due to fermentation. Don't worry – they will still crisp up the same way despite the lack of color!

6. Check out Dr. Bills Blog for more information:
https://eatlikeahuman.com/?s=ferminted+potato+chips

## Sourdough Bread ~ *embracing simple*

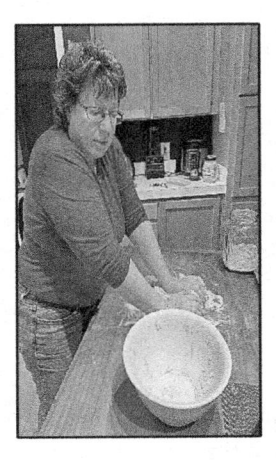

In the summer of 2022, Tammera took on a personal challenge of consistently making a good loaf of sourdough bread. She wasn't expecting this to be a journey of learning bread from an older, simpler perspective or one that would show her she had been doing everything wrong for 40 years. She wrote on her blog. "I made a lot of bread using the "milk or Amish" yeast bread approach. I used spelt flour for years, and if the bread fell or was claggy, I took that to mean I needed more yeast, longer rise time, and higher heat. I was wrong. I didn't need more yeast. I needed less yeast because I was over fermenting the dough. I didn't need more rise time and dryer dough. I needed a young and energetic dough that rose once and then rose again in a hot pan like a lava dome on a volcano. The dough texture is now soft and youthful, not dry, and tough. Most of all, I needed to uncomplicate this ancient food".

Part of the original goal was to make fresh bread from the 3 year old sourdough starter at elevations above 3,000 feet that looked, felt and had the texture of the artisanal bread from Stone

Age Kitchen. The second part of the plan was to make bread without an expensive and cumbersome wood fired bread, convection, or conventional oven, but instead in a cast iron Dutch oven on a barbecue. The ability to bake a nice loaf or three of bread while camping, RVing, or when the power goes out; brings this ancient food closer and moves it from the mythical realm to daily life.

As a history buff, Tammera looked at old cookbooks dating back to the 1860s, when a wood cookstove dominated the kitchen.

Tammera searched the internet and modern cookbooks for solutions that fell short. She realized her antique cookbook collection provided a simple answer. The introduction to the chapter on bread read so close to modern versions written by bakers in New Mexico and Colorado that it was as if they had copied it from the page. The prevailing difference with the contemporary versions was complicated directions like folding the dough in half every 20 minutes from 90 degree opposing angles for 1 hour. The antique versions contained simple efficiency, understanding the day was full of enough chores without adding more. Now her dough is soft and more like batter bread than heavy handed kneaded bread. She may fold the dough once during a 2 hour rise period, and she can see where at higher elevations, 2-3 times may increase the loft of rising.

### *The Century Cook Book*, 1897

Chapter XV Bread

*Yeast is a minute plant, and like other plants, must have the right conditions of heat, moisture, and nourishment in order to live or to flourish……therefore, as we depend upon the growth of little plant for raising our bread, we must give its requirements as much care as we do our geraniums or roses.*

*General Directions for Making Bread, page 340.*

*Bread is often mixed the night before it is to be baked and left to rise from eight to ten hours. But the whole process of bread-making, from the mixing to the serving, can be done in two and a half hours if a fresh, lively starter is used. In hot weather, it is desirable to complete the work in a short time in order to prevent fermentation or souring, which occurs if left too long a time.*

Another change was forgetting what she had always been told to let the dough rise until it has doubled in size, punch the air out, shape it into loaves, and let it rise a second time. Place bread gently into a 350-375°F oven for 40 minutes. Tammera found when it comes to wild yeast sourdough at elevations above 2,500 feet, this process leads to over fermentation and collapsed underdone loaves.

What worked best was to form the rounds after the first rise, place them on parchment paper, and put them in the refrigerator for 30-60 minutes. Heat the oven and cast iron to 400°F, then set parchment paper and the soft round in the Dutch oven and cover. The cooler the dough, the better the loaves' rise and signature ears (edges of dough at the cuts)

The next step was to ensure the process held from 7,000 to 4,300 to 2,800 feet using a basic RV gas oven, a small Weber barbecue, and an electric range at home. The challenges with the gas RV oven were small size, adequate heat, and burned bottom. These same challenges on the barbecue resulted in foil blankets to stop heat loss from wind and puzzling over heat diffusing to reduce burning. Using what was on hand, two cast iron trivets and foil, bread without burned or overcooked bottoms finally materialized. Thankfully the home oven required none of the challenges of the other cooking appliances. And crispy browning on the top was achieved with a few minutes under the broiler.

**Use a Thermometer**

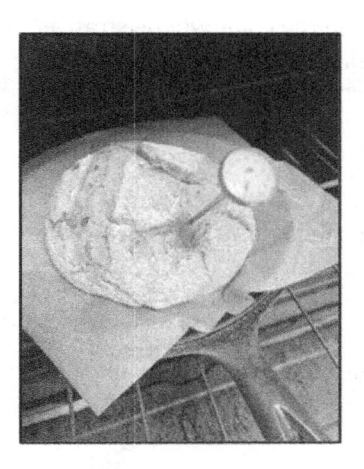

The following understanding came after gauging doneness with a thermometer instead of a timer. When baking at elevation, heat, moisture, and time adjustments may need to be made daily for the bread to be done inside; not claggy, sticky, or raw. The best baking temperature ranges fall between 375°F and 400°F for 30-45 minutes based on internal temperature. Your bread is done when the interior temperature lands between 175°F and 200°F (based on elevation and additives to the dough like dried fruit or herbs). Barometric pressure also affects how fast your dough rises and cooks. The higher the barometric pressure, the lower the atmosphere, affecting dryness and air pocket development (signature holes) in sourdough bread. The simple solution is to bake when the weather is nice versus a hurricane.

This process took almost precisely what the *Century Cook Book* described; 4-4½ hours from start to finish, with the sourdough starter made 18-24 hours earlier. The starter should be bubbly and active.

Here's the equipment for baking from an RV during a power outage or to impress neighbors.

Weber Q barbecue with a thermometer. 2 cast iron heat-defusing trivets (Lodge)

4 quart cast iron Dutch oven with lid (The cast iron disperses the heat evenly, and the lid holds the steam, allowing the bread to cook correctly.)

Meat thermometer or probe thermometer

Unbleached compostable parchment paper

Aluminum foil

**Sourdough Starter:** made from grape water (Michael Karr)
*The sourdough starter that has outperformed and remained the hardiest is the one we still use years later, made with organic concord grapes.*

2 cups organic all-purpose flour
2½ cups filtered chlorine free water
½ lb unwashed organic stemmed red grapes

Combine the flour and water. Wrap the grapes in well washed cheesecloth, tying the corners to form a bag; lightly crush them with a rolling pin or hands (to release the sugar to mix with the natural yeast on the skins; just like making wine!) and immerse them in the flour water mix. Cover tightly with a lid or plastic wrap secured with a rubber band. Leave at room temperature for 6 days, stirring once or twice daily.

The bag of grapes will eventually appear inflated, and the liquid will begin to separate from the flour base. The mixture will begin to taste and smell slightly fruity, and the color will be strange. That is as it should be. By the sixth day, the bag of grapes will have deflated, the color will be yellow, and the taste pleasantly sour; the fermentation is complete. The starter is living but weak, and it needs to be fed.

Remove the grapes and squeeze their juices back into the starter. Stir it up thoroughly and transfer it to a clean container. (Although you can use it after just one feeding, the starter will be stronger and healthier with the full treatment.) You can refrigerate it until you're ready to proceed.

Three days before you plan to use it, stir 1 cup flour and 1 cup water into the container, blending well. Let stand uncovered at room temperature until it bubbles up; 3-4 hours, then cover and refrigerate. Repeat this the second and third day.

Store the starter tightly covered in the refrigerator, where it will keep for 4-6 months, after which it's a good idea to pour off all but 2 cups and give it another feeding. Before using the stored starter for bread, give it the full 3 day feeding schedule once again to restore it and tone down excess sourness.

**Easy Sourdough Starter** (Tammera Karr)
*Sourdough is the oldest form of grain fermenting next to brewing beer and ales. Humans have been making some form of sourdough bread for over 10,000 years. Over the years, I have made and discarded countless sourdough starters. Some were experiments and others were death by neglect. There have also been times when our diets rejected bread due to inflammation and gluten sensitivities. It wasn't until I read Jill Winger's Prairie Homestead Cookbook that an aha moment happened.*

½ cup organic whole spelt flour
½ cup organic white spelt flour
2 cups filtered warm water
6 cup ceramic canister with a loose-fitting lid or ½ gallon wide mouth Ball jar

*Day 1*: Mix ½ cup whole spelt flour with 1 cup water. Stir vigorously, loosely cover, and let rest in a draft-free area for 24 hours. Do not seal the top; air needs to get into the jar for wild yeasts to populate. If your air is dry, add slightly more water to the starter.

*Day 2*: Add ¼ cup white spelt flour and ½ cup water to starter jar and stir vigorously. Your starter should have the consistency of thick pancake batter; if too thick, add water to thin it. Loosely cover, and rest for 24 hours out of direct sunlight. You should begin seeing bubbles form by day 3; if not, don't give up.

Day 4: Stir the starter until well incorporated, then pour off ½ of the starter (the discard). You can use the discarded starter for English muffins or add them to compost. Next, feed the remaining starter with ½ cup white spelt flour and ¼ cup filtered water. Stir, cover, and let sit for 24 hours. Keep repeating until the starter doubles within 4-6 hours after feeding.

*Tip:* Weather and barometric pressure will affect the length of time fermentation requires. The Number One Rule for sourdough is patience. If you still aren't seeing any bubbles after several days of this process, it's probably best to dump it out and start over.

Once the starter is bubbly, active, and doubling consistently after each daily feeding, it's ready to use. The key to successful sourdough bread is using the starter when the cultures are the most active. The starter that has separated and has liquid on top will perform poorly. The starter will perform best between 24 and 36 hours, depending on ambient temperature.

*TIP:* Keep your sourdough starter about 2 feet away from other cultures (kefir, kombucha, fermenting vegetables, or sauerkraut) to avoid cross contamination.

*TIP:* The older the sourdough starter, the more pronounced the sour flavor. However, the stronger the sour flavor, the longer it will take for the dough to rise. If you find your starter is very slow to rise, even on nice days, discard all but 3 tablespoons of the starter before feeding.

*TIP:* Open and sprinkle in 1 probiotic capsule every three months to your starter.

*TIP:* Once or twice a year, add 1 teaspoon of blackstrap molasses to the starter for added minerals.

*TIP*: For intermittent use, store in the refrigerator. This will prevent daily feedings (and ultimately use a lot of flour). To transfer a starter to the refrigerator, feed it, then let it rest for one hour. Next, place it in the refrigerator, covered and away from the coldest area. It's best to continue to feed it weekly. Strong-smelling foods like onions will affect your starter.

To wake up a dormant sourdough starter, remove it from the refrigerator 24 hours before baking. Discard 1 and feed the rest in a 1:1:1 ratio; 1 part starter to 1 part water to 1 part flour. Repeat every 12 hours or until the sourdough starter becomes active and bubbles within 4-6 hours of feeding.

## English Muffins (Michael Karr & Chef Ben Qualls)

*On average, this makes about 12-18 muffins depending on the cutter size. Our favorite has dried cranberries and spice or caramelized onions and cheese. We use onion and cheese for hamburger buns.*

½ cup (290 g) active sourdough starter
1 tbsp (25 g) honey, sugar, or maple syrup
1 cup (240 g) milk
3 cups (500 g) spelt flour
1 tsp (6 g) baking soda
1 tsp (6 g) fine sea salt
¼ cup (40 g) cornmeal or oat bran for sprinkling

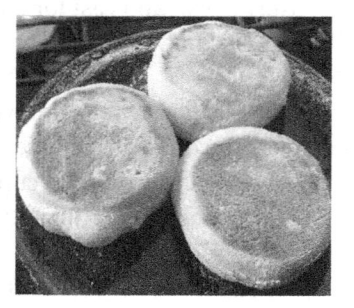

*Make the Dough*
1. Place all ingredients EXCEPT corn meal into a large bowl, and use your hands to mix until well combined. Cover and let rest 30-60 minutes.

2. Turn the dough out onto a floured surface (now is the time to add dried currants, cranberries or cheese and onion) and knead the dough by hand for 5 minutes. (A stand mixer with a dough hook attachment can be used on the lowest speed.)

3. Place the dough back into the bowl, cover it, and let ferment on the counter at room temperature for 2 hours or until double in size. (Room temperature is 65-70°F.)

*Cut and Cook*
1. Turn the dough onto a floured surface, flour the top, and press it out using your fingertips until it is ½ inch in thickness.
2. Use a 3½-4 inch biscuit cutter to cut rounds and place them on a parchment lined baking sheet. Sprinkle the tops with cornmeal or oat bran, cover with a tea towel and allow to rise for 20-30 minutes at room temperature.
3. Preheat your dry skillet or griddle over LOW heat. Place 4 muffins into the skillet spaced 2 inches apart, and cook the first side for 4 minutes. Turn the muffins over and cook for an additional 4 minutes. (When done, the center of a muffin should register about 200°F on an instant-read thermometer.)

*Notes*
*Spice Blend*: 1 teaspoon of ginger and cinnamon with ¼ teaspoon of clove (40g total)

*Dried fruit*: 1 cup dried cranberries, blueberries, or fruit of choice. (149 g)
Caramelized onion and ½ cup sharp cheese can also be added for a savory flavor.

Use the scoop and level technique to measure your flour if you do not have a kitchen scale. To do this, use a spoon to fluff the flour in the bag. Use a spoon to scoop the flour into a measuring cup until it is heaped on top. Take a butterknife and level off the top. This should give you the most accurate measurement for flour.

You may need to adjust the recipe if you live in a very warm or humid environment. I recommend reducing the milk by 2 tablespoons and using granulated sugar instead of honey to help prevent the dough from being too sticky to work with. Add more liquid if the dough is too stiff.

Store at room temperature for up to 5 days in a container or freeze for up to 3 months.

## Sourdough Apple Oat Muffins

3 cups oats
3 cups milk
1½ cups sourdough starter
½ cup oil
½ cup applesauce
3 eggs, beaten
4½ cups flour
1½ tsp cinnamon
1½ tbsp baking powder
¾ tsp baking soda
1½ tsp salt
1 cup brown sugar
1½ cups unsweetened coconut (optional)
½ pint jam, any flavor

Preheat the oven to 400°F. Combine oats and milk and set aside to soak. Place liners in muffin pans; they make clean-up easier as the jam make things sticky.

Stir sourdough starter, applesauce, oil, and eggs into the oatmeal mix and set aside. Combine flour, cinnamon, baking powder, baking soda, salt, brown sugar, and coconut in a large bowl.

Add in the oat mixture and stir until just combined. Fill liners halfway with the batter. Add 1 teaspoonful of jam to each, then fill with the remaining batter. Bake for 20-25 minutes or until golden brown.

**Sourdough Pizza Crust** (Tammera Karr)

1 cup (227 g) sourdough starter, unfed discard
½-¾ cup (141 g to 170 g) filtered water, lukewarm
2½ cups (300 g) bread flour
1 tsp salt
4 teaspoonfuls of pizza herbs; combine 2 teaspoonfuls of Italian seasoning herbs, 3 teaspoons of garlic granules, and 1 tsp red chili flakes

Stir any liquid on top of your refrigerated starter back into it before measuring out 1 cup (227 g) into a large mixing bowl. Note: This is a good opportunity to feed the remainder of your starter, if necessary.

*To make the dough*: Weigh your flour; measure it into a cup, then sweep off any excess. Add water, flour, salt, and pizza dough flavor.

Mix to combine, adding the remaining water 1 tablespoon at a time if the dough looks dry. Knead for about 7 minutes using a stand mixer with its dough hook until the dough wraps itself around the hook and cleans the sides of the bowl.

Cover with plastic wrap and let rise until almost doubled in bulk. Depending on the vitality of your starter, this will take between 1-2 hours. For a faster rise, place the dough in a warm spot.

For two thin crust pizzas: Divide the dough in half and shape each into a flattened disk. Place crusts on unbleached parchment paper, lightly cover with organic tomato sauce, add toppings, drizzle with Spanish olive oil, and let rest for 5-10 minutes.

**Barbecue Grill or Conventional Oven**: Preheat the grill with a cast iron skillet or griddle on the rack to 450°F. The temperature will drop when you open the lid on the grill; maintain a 400°F grill.

Slide the parchment paper and pizza onto the cast iron griddle, (recommend placing the pizza and paper on a wooden cutting board or pizza board for transferring) and bake for approximately 10 minutes.

When cooked, use a metal turner to slide the paper and pizza off the cast iron griddle onto the wooden cutting board. Slip the paper out from under the pizza and slice.

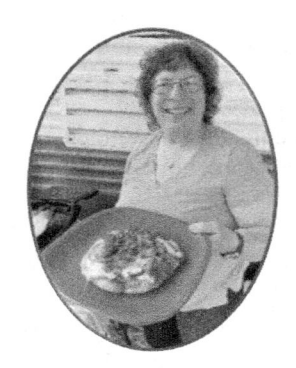

If the bottom of the pizza burns before the toppings are fully heated, place a heat diffuser between the grill rack and the griddle; adjust heat down 25°F.

> **Archaeobotanical Evidence Reveals Origins of Bread 14,400 Years Ago**
>
> In the Near East in an area known as the Black Desert, where the wild ancestors of domesticated crops such as wheat and barley occur naturally, hunter gatherers of the Upper Paleolithic period were already producing flour from wild grasses, and possibly inventing brewing and use of groats, porridge, and unleavened bread, as early as the late Epipaleolithic or Natufian period 9,500 to 12,000 BC. Archaeologists discovered two big fireplaces in an old structure; one of which contained different kinds of flours. They cataloged 24 bread-like types of remains. They found mainly crucifers, legumes, barley, oat, and einkorn wheat.[178]

### Sprouted and Cultured Spelt Pancakes (Sarica Cernohous)

Makes approximately 16, 5 inch pancakes

2½ cups sprouted spelt flour
1-1½ cups warm, filtered water (105°F range)
½ cup fresh water kefir
1½ cups whole milk, preferably raw
2 eggs, beaten
¼ cup ghee (clarified butter) or coconut oil
3 tbsp raw sugar or coconut crystals
1 tsp sea salt
¾ tsp baking soda
1 tbsp real vanilla extract
Fat or oil for the griddle (pastured lard, coconut oil, pastured tallow, ghee)

The evening before you plan to make your pancakes, add warm water, and water kefir to the flour in a large glass mixing bowl. Mix all ingredients well, then cover with a lid and set in a warm environment. I use my yogurt maker, plugged in, with the dome lid removed and the bowl resting in the top of the maker. You could also use a dehydrator with the trays removed and set to 100°F. If you don't have either of these, use a microwave (turned off!), oven (turned off!), or ice chest. You need an incubation chamber, which should have at least a couple of bottles filled with hot water to keep the air temperature warm.

(The beneficial bacteria and yeast in the water kefir like a warm temperature to function and thrive, so keeping the air warm will allow for more breakdown of the complex carbohydrates into simpler, easier to digest sugars.) Plan to keep your flour soaking and fermenting in the range of 6-10 hours.

When you've finished the first stage of soaking and fermenting, you will likely notice a tart, lively smell as you remove the lid and see that the batter has risen that is *lacto-fermentation*! In a separate bowl, combine all the remaining dry ingredients and mix well. In another bowl, add all the remaining wet ingredients and mix well. Add the dry to the wet ingredients, mix well and incorporate them into the soaked flour. You will likely notice the batter rising substantially as the baking soda comes into contact with the fermented grains.

Heat a griddle or frying pan to low medium heat. Add your choice of oil or fat to coat the cooking surface. Once a drop of batter bubbles on the oil, add a ladle of batter, letting it cook until bubbles appear throughout the pancake, then flip it over. These pancakes will be moister than those made with dry flour, so be sure the heat isn't too high so that the pancakes can cook through on both sides without burning.

Top immediately with butter and any other accompaniments of your choice. Maple syrup, yogurt, yacón syrup*, molasses, and fresh fruit are great choices. Or, if you'd like to save the pancakes to reheat later, simply stack them on a plate with a piece of parchment paper between each to keep them from sticking to one another. Store covered in the refrigerator, and enjoy within a few days' time.

* Yacón syrup is extracted from the tuberous roots of the yacón plant indigenous to the Andes mountains. The syrup contains up to 50% fructooligosaccharides.

## Injera - Ethiopian Flatbread (Kimberly Killebrew)
Serves 6

2 cups teff flour, brown or ivory, or substitute a portion of it with some barley or wheat flour

*Note*: If you're new to making injera, I recommend combining teff and barley or wheat, as 100% teff is more challenging to work with.

3 cups water

*NOTE:* Using mostly or all teff (which is the traditional Ethiopian way) will NOT produce the spongy, fluffy injera served in most restaurants has been adapted to the western palate and uses mostly wheat, sometimes a little barley, and occasionally a little teff added in.

In a large mixing bowl, combine the flour and water. Loosely place some plastic wrap on the bowl, punch holes in the wrap with a toothpick so air can circulate. Let the mixture sit undisturbed at room temperature for 4-5 days (the longer it ferments, the deeper the flavor). Depending on what kind of flour you're using, you may need to add a little more water if the mixture becomes dry. The mixture will be fizzy, and the color will be very dark, and, depending on the humidity, a layer of aerobic yeast will form on the top. Aerobic yeast is a normal result of fermentation. If your batter forms mold on it, it will need to be discarded. Pour off the aerobic yeast and as much of the liquid as possible. A clay-like batter will remain. Give it a good stir.

In a small sauce pan, bring 1 cup of water to a boil. Stir in ½ cup of the injera batter, whisking constantly until it is thickened. This will happen quickly. Then stir the cooked and thickened batter back into the original fermented batter. Add some water to the batter to thin it out to the consistency of crepe batter. Added about ⅔ cup of water, varying from batch to batch. The batter will have a sweet-soured nutty smell.

Heat a non-stick skillet over medium heat. Depending on how good your non-stick pan is, you may need to lightly spray it with oil. Spread the bottom of the skillet with the injera batter, not as thin as crepes but not as thick as traditional pancakes. Allow the injera to bubble and let the bubbles pop. Once the bubbles have popped, place a lid on top of the pan and turn off the heat. Let the injera steam cook for a couple or so more minutes until cooked through. Be careful not to overcook the injera or it will become gummy and soggy. Remove the injera with a spatula and repeat.

*IMPORTANT NOTE:* Both the texture and color of the injera will vary greatly depending on what kind of teff you use (dark or ivory) and whether you're combining it with other flours. Gluten-based flours (e.g., wheat and barley) will yield a much different texture than 100% teff.

### Parmesan Polenta with Bacon and Greens (Sarica Cernohous)
Serves 6 as an entrée

*To prepare polenta*
1½ cup corn grits (polenta)
1½ tsp sea salt
2 cups warm, filtered, dechlorinated water (approximately 105°F)
1 cup fresh water kefir

Combine all ingredients in a glass or ceramic bowl and stir well to incorporate. There should be about ⅛ inch to ¼ inch of the water kefir over the top of the polenta. Cover and store in a warm spot. (I set mine on top of the yogurt maker–turned on–to help maintain a gentle, warm heat to encourage mild fermentation of the grain. You could also set the bowl in a dehydrator set around 100°F or in an ice chest or an oven turned off; with a couple of bottles filled with hot water.) Allow to rest undisturbed for at least 8 hours until you see the little bubbles of fermentation and there is a mild tart scent. When this point has been reached, begin preparing the rest of the recipe.

For the remainder of the recipe, you will need the following:

4-5 cups Swiss chard, sliced in ½ inch strips
5-6 slices of pastured beef or pork bacon, cut in ½ inch slices
3 cups chicken broth, plus 1 additional cup, heated
1 cup freshly grated Parmesan cheese
½ cup field garlic, chopped in ½ inch pieces, or 4 scallions, chopped in ½ inch pieces with 3-4 cloves garlic, minced finely
Sea salt and black pepper to taste
Cherry or plum tomatoes, sliced, for garnish
Freshly chopped basil leaves and lemon wedges for garnish

In a 5-6 quart pot, combine soaked polenta with 3 cups of chicken broth over medium heat. Bring to a mild simmer, constantly stirring from the bottom. In about five minutes, you will notice the grits have firmed up substantially, and the grain has softened. Stir for another 5 minutes or so and turn off the heat.

Start cooking the bacon in a separate, large pan over medium heat. Once it has begun to release its fat into the pan, add the field garlic or scallions or garlic, occasionally stirring to keep all ingredients from burning. After a few minutes, once the garlic or onions have softened, add the Swiss chard, and incorporate well into the mix. Keep cooking and stirring periodically until most of the moisture has evaporated and the chard has softened. Turn off heat and return to the polenta.

Resume a low heat under the polenta, which will have stiffened while cooling. Add the Parmesan cheese and pour in an additional cup of hot chicken broth. Stir all ingredients well to incorporate and to soften the polenta. Spoon in the bacon and greens mixture and mix well into the polenta. Remove from the heat and serve immediately with a garnish of fresh, sliced tomatoes, a sprinkling of basil leaves, and a healthy squirt of lemon juice.

Store any remaining in a covered glass or ceramic bowl for up to 3 days in the refrigerator.

## **Turkey and Fermented Quinoa Patties** (Sarica Cernohous)
Makes approximately 28-30 patties

4 cups cooked quinoa (soak quinoa in water and water kefir overnight before cooking); I like to cook mine with bone broth for added flavor and nutrition.
2 lbs ground dark turkey
5 pastured eggs
1 cup freshly shredded raw Parmesan cheese
2 tsp organic poultry herb blend
1-2 tsp of sea salt
1 cup frozen, organic spinach
Ghee, coconut oil, or grass fed beef tallow for the pan
12 inch fry pan

Combine all ingredients into a glass or stainless bowl and mix well.

Melt a tablespoon of oil in the frying pan over low medium heat.

Using an ice cream scoop or serving spoon, make 3 or 4 inch patties about ⅓ inch in thickness. In a 12 inch pan, you should be able to fit 3 patties easily. Cook for about 4 minutes on the first side or until golden brown, and then flip. Allow another 3-4 minutes of cooking, then transfer to a non-plastic plate or dish.

Continue re-oiling your pan with each batch.

Patties store well in the refrigerator for 3 days or in the freezer for 3 months for reheating in the toaster oven or in a pan. Wrap separately in parchment paper and use heavy duty aluminum foil or a freezer safe container for storage.

> *Traditional cooking techniques truly do become an art once you understand some of the basic ground rules....and from that point on, the terroir of your cooking environment, encompassing the ingredients you choose to work with, combined with the inherent bacteria and fungal spores in the air, the level of humidity in your cooking space, the seasonings you will select and any derivations on the theme you make to make it your own....all of these pieces will make your kraut different from your neighbor's and mine.*
>
> Sarica Cernohous, DACM, L.Ac
> The Funky Kitchen

## Fermented Fruits

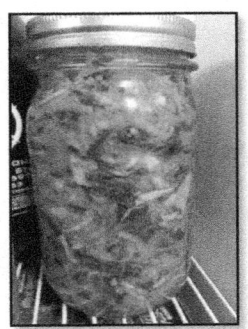

Any fruit can be lacto fermented, but some produce better results than others. Lacto fermented plums are typical of Asian cultures. Also known as *umeboshi plums*, they are used to season rice and numerous dishes. Most stone fruit (peaches, cherries, apricots, etc.), blueberries, gooseberries, currents, and citrus are also great picks for fermentation.

The basic principles for fermenting fruit are the same as for fermenting vegetables:

1. Mix the fruit with salt. Because fruit is delicate, blending fruit with salt will result in mush. The simplest solution is to use brine to submerge the fruit.
2. Put in a jar.
3. Let them ferment for a few days at room temperature.
4. Refrigerate.
5. To prevent yeast from attacking your fruit, make sure you add salt equivalent to 2% of the weight of the fruit.

There are many great sources for fermenting on the Internet and in print. So have fun and enjoy the ease of preserving fruit and veggies through fermentation.

**Easy Fermented Kraut or Veggie Slaw**  (Tammera and Michael Karr)

1 small organic cabbage
1-2 organic carrots, grated
3-6 cloves of garlic, minced
1-2 tsp minced fresh ginger
1 small purple or sweet onion
1-2 mild-hot chiles, sliced into thin rings. Seeds add to the heat, remove if you want a mild heat.
1 red or orange sweet pepper, sliced into thin strips about the thickness of a spaghetti noodle.
2 tbsp coarse salt
½ cup Bubbies Naturally Fermented Kraut with juice, starter
1-2 cups filtered water

Place washed veggies on a towel to absorb water while you begin thin slicing (shredding or julienning) vegetables. It is easier to cut a cabbage, onions, radishes, turnips, and beets in half, then do thin slices (flat side down). A food grater or mandolin can be used, but isn't necessary.

Once vegetable slaw is in your mixing bowl, add starter and 1 tablespoon of salt and massage or burse the vegetables with your hands while mixing thoroughly; this allows the salt and ferment starter to start working. Were gloves if your hands are sensitive.

If using dill relish and wanting a more traditional sauerkraut – add 1 teaspoon Fennel or Carraway seeds.

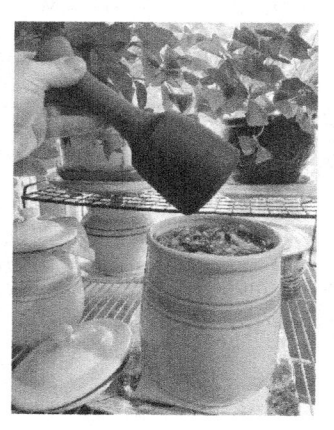

Now that everything is mixed, begin filling the fermenting vessel, or jar. Pack the vegetables in tightly, pressing out all the air. Fill to within 2-3 inches of the top and cover with brine water made with 1 tablespoon coarse salt and 1 cup filtered water. Make sure the vegetables are covered with water, and place a loose-fitting lid on the top.

You will want your jars or containers in a plastic tray or on a plate to prevent any escaping liquid from making a mess. Place in a cool area out of direct sunlight.

1- 2 times daily uncover vegetables and press slaw/kraut matt down (they begin to float right away) under the liquid. By day three a froth of bubbles should come to the surface when you compress the kraut or slaw. If not, move to a slightly warmer area with good air circulation. When it is cold fermentation may take up to 6 days. Take a small sample of your kraut for a taste, when it reaches the tangy taste pleasing to your pallet, pack into glass jars (if using a large fermenting jar) seal plastic lids down tight and place in the back of the fridge. Will keep in the refrigerator up to 6 months.

## Fermented Foods to Brine Ratio

|      | 250 ml | 500 ml | 750 ml | 1000 ml | 2000 ml | 3000 ml | 4000 ml |
|------|--------|--------|--------|---------|---------|---------|---------|
| 2%   | 5 g    | 10 g   | 15 g   | 20 g    | 40 g    | 60 g    | 80 g    |
| 3.5% | 9 g    | 18 g   | 26 g   | 35 g    | 70 g    | 105 g   | 140 g   |
| 5%   | 13 g   | 25 g   | 38 g   | 50 g    | 100 g   | 150 g   | 200 g   |
| 10%  | 25 g   | 50 g   | 75 g   | 100 g   | 200 g   | 300 g   | 400 g   |

|      | 1 cup | 2 cups | 3 cups | 1 qt | 2 qts | 3 qts | 4 qts |
|------|-------|--------|--------|------|-------|-------|-------|
| 2%   | 5 g   | 9 g    | 14 g   | 19 g | 38 g  | 57 g  | 76 g  |
| 3.5% | 8 g   | 17 g   | 25 g   | 33 g | 66 g  | 99 g  | 132 g |
| 5%   | 12 g  | 24 g   | 35 g   | 47 g | 95 g  | 142 g | 189 g |
| 10%  | 24 g  | 47 g   | 71 g   | 95 g | 189 g | 284 g | 379 g |

### *Self-Brining Vegetables* (Beets & Cabbage)

Mix 5-6 grams of Celtic Sea salt for every pound of cleaned, prepared vegetables. Top off with 2% brine solution if needed.

Onions, garlic, broccoli, cauliflower, carrots, beet kvass, horseradish, potatoes, and green beans require a 2% brine solution.

Cucumbers and Peppers (mold easily) require a 3.5%-5% brine solution.

Pepper mash (molds very easily) requires a 10% brine solution.

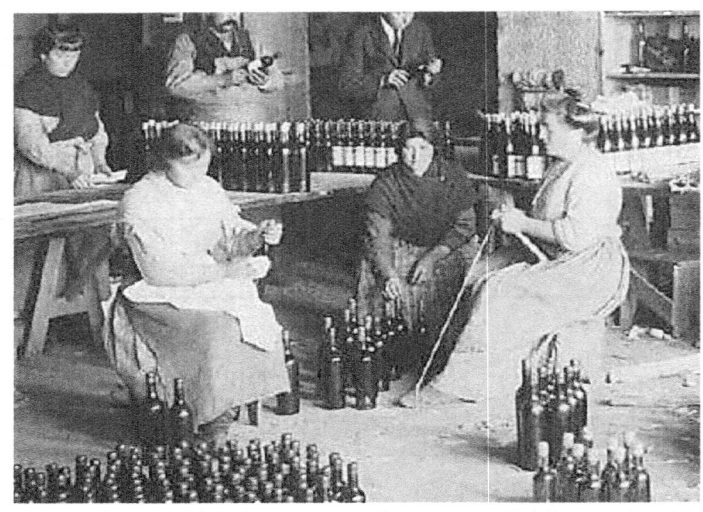

Women bottling and labeling regional wine in Italy during the 1800s.

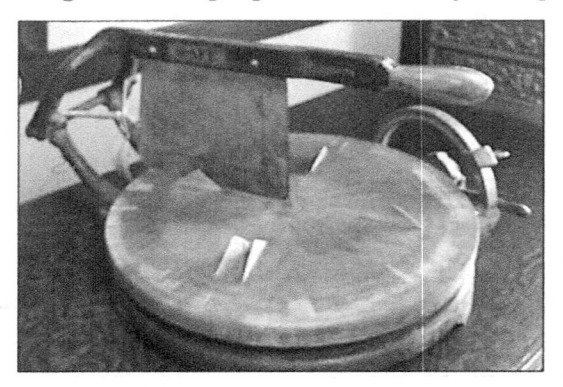

Mercantile cheese wedge slicer, Bowman Museum, Prineville, Oregon

---

177 www.kingarthurflour.com

178 Archaeobotanical evidence reveals the origins of bread 14,400 years ago in northeastern Jordan, 2018, Retrieved October 24, 2022: https://www.pnas.org/doi/full/10.1073/pnas.1801071115

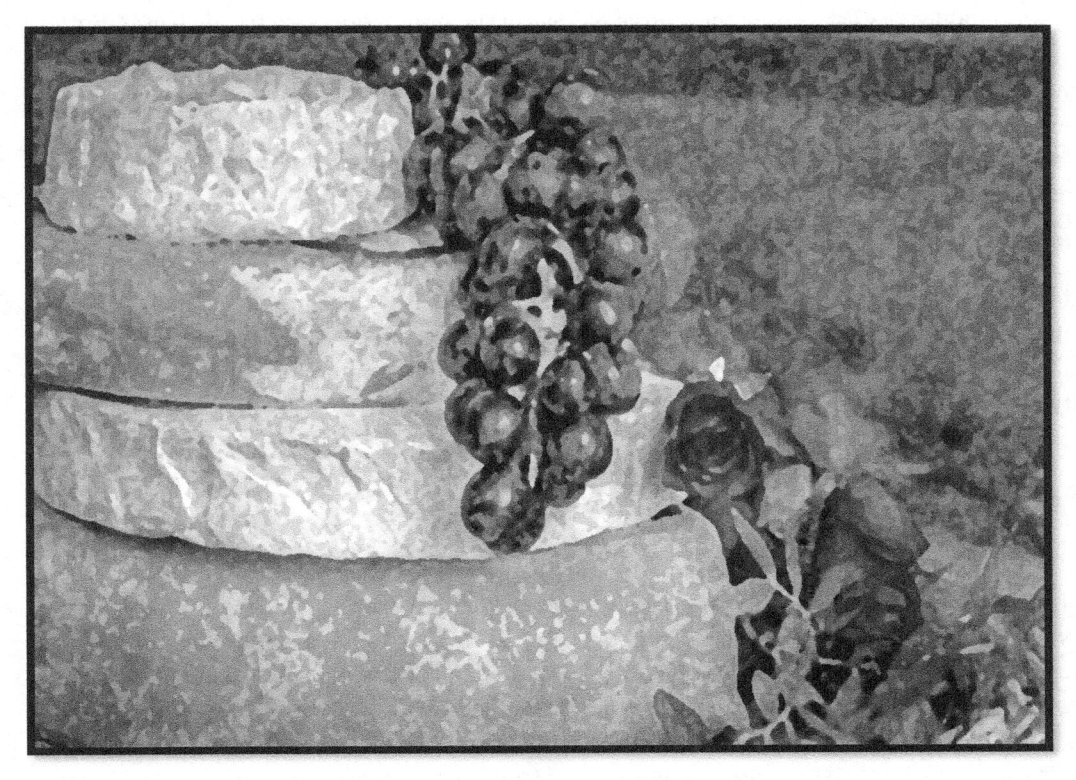

## *Where's the Cheese?*

As you have traveled the pages of this cookery book, you may have noticed a missing member of *our journey with food*; cheese. While many recipes contain butter and ghee, very few contain any form of cheese or milk. Initially, this came about due to the challenges with digesting dairy, next the effects on blood sugars and increased inflammation, and last but not least quality and authenticity. The vast majority of cheeses made commercially are a far cry from traditionally made cultural cheeses.

Tammera believes history supports the use of dairy and the fermentation which led to cheese in its many forms as a major player in dietary cultures from archaic ages to present. Anthropologists believe that around 6,000 BC, herders in Iraq discovered how to make cheese from wild and domesticated goats and sheep followed by bovines later. Egyptian tombs depict the cheese making process and required skill needed, dating to around 2,000 BC.[179]

Newer research has uncovered evidence of cheese and dairy fermentation and use in northern Europe to around 9,000 BC. By piecing together Neolithic pottery shards and ancient human genomes, scientists found a rapid evolution of lactose intolerance among Europeans well after they first started consuming the beverage. How is it that a food in the daily diet of northern

Europeans 9,000 years ago is now the source of 95% of the population's gastric distress? Pottery fragments investigated by archaeologists have confirmed the drinking and use of milk was presumably fresh and fermented.[180] However, dairy didn't enter our diets without some dangers. Dairy is susceptible to *salmonella*, *E. coli*, *listeria*, and *campylobacter*, all of which would have been present in the ancient kitchen and contribute to food preservation and storage advances. Early attempts at storing milk and soft cheeses would have played a part in the development of fired pottery and cheese fermentation.

An additional piece of the puzzle on dairy digestibility is vitamin A. Research has found the vitamin A content of dairy aids in reducing allergies and intolerance.[181] Ancient man's levels of vitamin A would have been significantly higher than that of modern humans due to the feed quality consumed by the animals. Lactose intolerance came about through multiple factors.

*Enter Famine*

In 2015 and again in 2022, hunger stones emerged from the Elbe River in Bohemia and Saxony.[182] The earliest one dating from 1616 is carved with a warning in German; "*Wenn du mich seehst, dann weine*" – "If you see me, then weep." During times of drought followed by famine, humans learned how to store nutrient-dense foods; in this case, cheese. These hunger stones provide additional clues to the conditions that aided the progression of food preservation in the form of cheese.[183] The regions of France and Germany where these hunger stones reside are today world renowned for cheese making. The stressors of famines and pathogens following drought, may have exacerbated milk's typically mild gastrointestinal effects on the lactose intolerant. It follows that during times of famine, vitamin stores in animal fodder and human levels of vitamin A would be depleted, hence opening the door to increased intolerances and leading to deadly bouts of diarrhea and dehydration.[184]

Richard Evershed and colleagues mapped human milk use during the past 9,000 years, creating an enormous database from 6,899 animal fat residues derived from 13,181 fragments of pottery from 554 archaeological sites around Europe.[185] The UK scientists' analysis found virtually no difference between the milk consumption of tolerant and intolerant adults. So how could people have been dairy farmers when lactose intolerant? In nutrition science, the healthier an individual and the state of the microbiome correspond to improved digestion of all foods. When eating a staple food such as dairy and cheese, fermented or fresh, the body develops intrinsic factors early that allow for digestion, but when these foods are absent in the diet the intrinsic factors decline. An example of this would be malnourishment during a famine, following a long period of drought.[186]

> **Principle 26**: *Traditionally prepared dairy, that is naturally fermented and cared for, can provide valuable nutrition for those not allergic.*

## Is Ancestral Cheese and Fermenting the Answer?

Some cultures depend heavily on cheese as a protein and calcium source. Switzerland, per capita, makes and consumes more cheese daily than chocolate.[187] Every day begins with cheese. The challenge is that few individuals outside of Switzerland eat these traditionally made cheeses from sustainable dairy production. Raw milk from local dairy cows (female bovine) feeding on diverse, high alpine meadows is delivered each morning to the cheese makers.[188] While possibly the largest producer and consumer of cheese, Switzerland is a very small land mass compared to Canada, Mexico, and the United States, individually and combined. Local and traditional takes on a whole different challenge within these technology driven countries.

Other countries, of course, are larger than Switzerland and have equally impressive cheese cultures. The Scandinavian nations utilize goat, sheep, bovine, and reindeer milk in their cheese making. Yogurt is a Scandinavian food, and is consumed most every day. Once again, we return to the quality of the food being made with attention to tradition over mass production. There are scores of cheeses from England, France, and Germany additionally. What about Spain, Italy, and Greece, all of which have centuries of dairy cultivation? And cheese milk is not solely from bovines, sheep, and goats. There is camel, a relatively new soft cheese. Yak and horse milk are also used in cheese making.

Traditionally made water buffalo cheese has a home in a small area of the Philippines and Peynir in India. Contrary to the popular conversation, countries in the African continent make cheese: Egypt makes three kinds, Ethiopia, Benin, and Mauritania also have regional cheeses. While these foods may result from European immigrants or local traditions, the authors have not fully explored the topic. But when looking at who produces and consumes dairy and cheese, we also begin to see biases in nutrition information on humans' inability to digest lactose and dairy after infancy. Globally, Tammera found many cultures with centuries of traditional, fermented cheese production. Once again, we look to the *how* food is prepared and made for clues on digestibility on what otherwise would be detrimental to human health.[189]

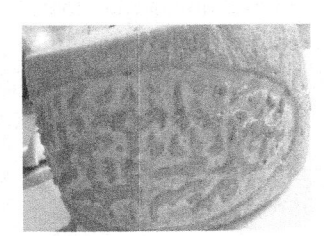

**Rumi** is a hard Egyptian cheese made from cow's milk or a combination of cow and water buffalo milk, often enhanced with peppercorns. When served, the cheese wheels are typically cut into long and thin slices, which easily fit into pita bread. This cheese is aged eight to twelve years. [190]

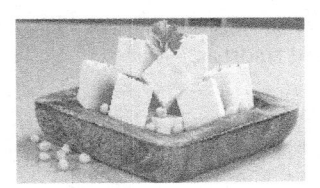

**Paneer** is a moist, fresh cheese with a soft and crumbly texture made from pasteurized cow's milk or water buffalo's milk. Unlike most cheeses, paneer does not involve rennet making it completely vegetarian. India and Bangladesh have been mentioned in the Vedas dating back to 6000 BC. Its name comes from the Persian and Turkish word for cheese, *peynir*.[191]

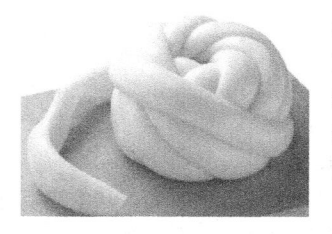

**Oaxacan** cheese is a semi-soft white cheese made from cow's milk. It is named after the Oaxaca state in southern Mexico where it was first produced. The pasta filata cheesemaking process, originally from Italy, was brought to Mexico by Dominican friars who settled in the state of Oaxaca.[192]

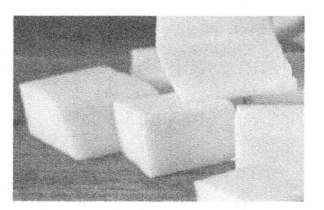

**Queso Chihuahua** is a traditional Mexican cheese made from bovine milk. The cheese is also called Menonita, referring to the Mennonite communities in Chihuahua that first produced it. [193]

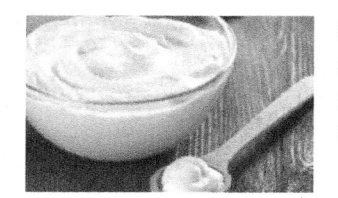

**Skyr** is an Icelandic cultured dairy product made from cheese characterized by its thick and creamy texture. It is said that skyr dates back to the 9th century when Norwegian settlers first arrived in Iceland.[194]

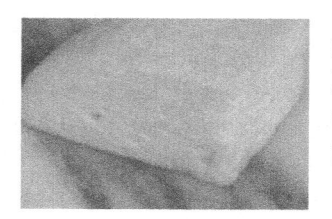

**Byaslag** is a mild Mongolian cheese made with yak or cow milk. Kefir is typically used in place of rennet to separate the curds from the milk. After draining, the curds are wrapped in a cloth, then pressed between wooden boards with weights.[195]

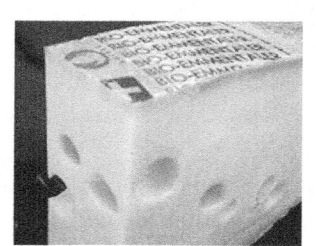

**Emmental** is a hard cheese made in Bern, Switzerland. It is a traditional, unpasteurized, hard cheese made from cow's milk with a mild taste, fruitier aroma, and thin rind. The maturation period ranges from two to eighteen months depending on the variety. Emmental has walnut-sized holes and is considered one of the most difficult cheeses to produce because of the complicated hole-forming fermentation process.

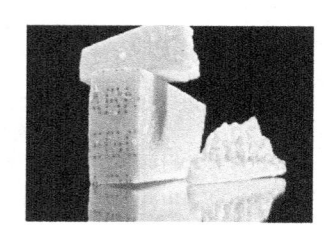

**Parmesan** cheese is considered among the top cheeses by cheese connoisseurs. True Parmesan cheese has a hard, gritty texture and is fruity and nutty in taste. Cheeses mocking Parmesan or inferior Parmesan may have a bitter taste. Parmigiano Reggiano cheese is mostly grated over pastas, used in soups and risottos. It is also eaten on its own as a snack.

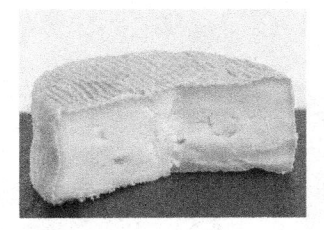

**Munster Géromé** cheese is a soft-washed rind cheese made from milk produced by cows living in the regions between Alsace, Lorraine, and Franche-Comté in France. The cheese is made from unpasteurized cow's milk called crude milk. The soft and creamy cheese also comes flavored with cumin and tastes best when accompanied with a good beer.

*The authors suggest the use of cultural dairy and cheese in moderation and as a condiment providing it is an easily digestible food for the individual.*

## *An American Classic ~ adapting recipes and preserving family legacy*

When it comes to family recipes, we honor the past and future by adapting them. Family recipes go through revisions for ingredients about every three generations. Part of this comes about through technology (kitchen appliances have changed the way we cook from past generations), location, and availability of ingredients. The quintessential American Mac and Cheese is a perfect example of a dish developed for Thomas Jefferson in the 1780s through to Kraft Mac and Cheese in the 21st century. During Chef James Hemings's time at Monticello, the concept of locally produced, organic, clean, artisanal, naturally aged, chemical-free, and fermented cheese would have never been an issue. All foods were locally produced, artisanal, organic, and so forth; an entirely different world from that of the modern cook. With that in mind, how do we adapt and preserve classic family recipes without compromising on health?

### Who Invented the Iconic Mac & Cheese?

James Hemings (1765-1801) was a chef, trained in Paris, born into slavery, and lived much of his life enslaved. At thirty years of age, he negotiated for legal manumission and began his life as a free man. James Hemings was a younger half-brother to Jefferson's wife, Martha Wayles Jefferson. He was a personal attendant to Thomas Jefferson following his election as wartime governor of Virginia in 1779. It was Jefferson's idea that Hemings travel with him to France for the primary purpose of his training in "the art of cookery."

James Hemings - along with many other highly trained enslaved individuals who succeeded him in Washington and at Monticello - serves as inspiration to modern-day chefs and culinary historians alike. These early African American chefs were instrumental in creating and defining American cuisine.

### Macaroni Pie (1784 style)

*For Sauce*
2 tbsp butter
2 tbsp flour
½ cup heavy cream
1 cup chicken stock

*For Macaroni*
3½ cups whole milk
1 tbsp onion, finely minced
½ tsp mustard, ground
1 tsp pepper, ground
16oz elbow macaroni, dried and organic

*For Pie*
2 cups sharp Cheddar cheese, grated
2 cups Gruyere
2 cups Swiss
2 cups Emmentaler
1 cup Parmesan, grated
4-8 tbsp butter
Salt if needed at the table

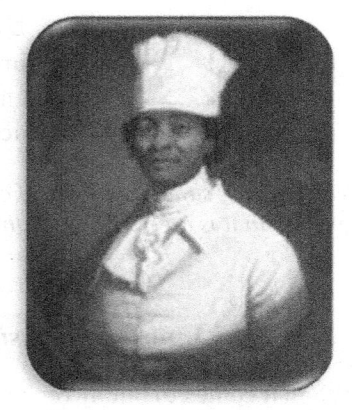

Chef Hemings (1765-1801)

Add milk to a pot, cook on medium-low heat, and add seasonings. Add macaroni, bringing the mixture back up and letting it heat to slightly boil for two minutes. Once the two minutes are done, you then cover, turn off the heat, and set a timer according to the manufacturer's instruction, about 15 minutes. Remove the lid, and check if macaroni has absorbed most, if not all, the seasoned milk mixture.

In a sauce pan, melt the butter over low heat and stir in the flour with a wooden spoon. Cook while stirring for two minutes. Add chicken stock, ⅛ cup at a time, whisking the mixture to a smooth consistency after each addition. When you've added about half the liquid, add heavy cream and the remaining broth whisking the mixture to a smooth consistency. Continue warming on low to medium heat until the sauce thickens. Whisk as needed to prevent it from scorching or getting lumpy. Remove from heat, and add cooked macaroni to the cream sauce. Salt and pepper to taste.

Using a slotted spoon, place enough macaroni into a baking dish to cover the bottom. Place a few dollops/pats of butter onto the macaroni, and then top with some of each type of cheese, enough just to cover the macaroni. Repeat forming layers. Save some of the cheese for topping.

Top with leftover cheese. Place into a 350°F preheated oven for 15-20 minutes for a golden brown on top. Allow macaroni and cheese to rest for 10 minutes, then serve.

~~~~~~~~~~~~~~~~~~

When we asked contributor Sharena Graves about her family's Mac and Cheese recipe, it was interesting to see how the generations following James had modernized his recipe. First, the inclusion of canned milk would have happened in the late 1800s and the use of locally made cheddar cheese versus imported. Onion and mustard may have been dropped due to availability. Then the inclusion of Munster cheese, which came to the Midwest with German and French immigrants, added a smooth creaminess. This ingredient list remained much the same until the 1970s, when the family recipe was adapted to include Campbell's® Cream of Chicken Soup, CheeseWiz® and Velveeta® cheese. These processed foods signified the modern age of convenience and ease of storage. It would be three decades before consumers learned the health challenges resulting from ultra-refined processed ingredients.

The precision of layering macaroni, butter and cheese in the baking dish does not seem to have changed with the generations.

### Mac & Cheese (Sharena Graves)

*My mother had drawn her inspiration for her Mac and Cheese from her grandmother, my great-grandmother, Cassels. My mother changed out a few ingredients over the years and decided to make a cheese sauce instead of layering the noodles with just shredded cheese like her grandmother's original recipe. Mac and Cheese seem to have been a part of my family for generations. My family tree dates to the 1760s when my 6th great grandmother Sally Hemings' brother, Chef James Hemings, classically trained in French cuisine, became the "developer of mac and cheese." The current recipe has once again been adapted.*

*Autor's note:* Sharena further adapted her mother's recipe to lower sodium and processed cheese content after speaking with Tammera.

Serves 10

3-4 cups whole milk (substituted by Sharena for canned milk)
½ cup chicken broth (substituted by Sharena for the Cream of Chicken Soup)
2 large eggs, beaten
1 tsp pepper
16 oz elbow macaroni
8 cups sharp Cheddar cheese, grated
8 cups mild Cheddar cheese, grated
1 8 oz package Munster cheese, sliced
4 cups Colby cheese, grated
4-6 tbsp butter plus for topping
2 cups Mozzarella cheese (DO NOT mix into the sauce)

Cook macaroni according to the directions on the package. Drain and set aside.

1. Add milk to a pot, cook on low heat, and add salt and pepper. Next, slowly add in eggs, stirring well. Gradually add mixed cheese, stirring, so it doesn't stick.

2. Once the cheese is melted into the milk, add it to the macaroni.

3. Using a slotted spoon, layer macaroni and cheese sauce with grated mozzarella cheese and butter into a baking dish.

4. Top with mozzarella cheese.

5. Place into a 350°F preheated oven for 15-20 minutes. It should be golden brown on top when finished. Allow macaroni and cheese to rest for 10 minutes, then serve.

## Easy Cream Cheese Made at Home (Tammera Karr)

8 cups full-fat milk (whole milk), best raw or pasteurized.
5 tbsp lemon juice or 1 large lemon
½ tsp salt or more to taste

*Options*
Pinch dried herbs if desired. Dill, parsley, chive, and garlic powder.
Vanilla

*Equipment*
Cheese cloth for draining, mesh strainer

Pouring the milk in a sauce pan. Heat the milk and bring it to boil over medium-high heat. As soon as it boils, add the lemon juice, and then turn off the heat.

Take off heat while the milk curdles. You'll notice curds forming and a yellow-ish liquid whey forming. Within a few minutes, all your curds should have formed. Line strainer with cheese cloth. Pour the curdled milk through cheesecloth and a sieve to strain all the liquid whey.

Rinse the curds with cold water. This will help to get rid of any extra whey, clinging to the curds. Squeeze the curdled milk as much as possible to drain any last drop of the liquid whey.

Put cheese curds into a food processor or blender and add salt. Blend for 1-2 minutes for a light and fluffy cream cheese.

Be warned though as certain additional ingredients will affect the shelf-life of the cheese. Dried herbs and garlic powder do not affect shelf life. Store the cream cheese in an air-tight container in the fridge for up to 7 days. You can freeze cream cheese, but the texture upon thawing is crumblier and is best used for cooking.

**Cheese Pudding** (*Daily Wants, A Book for Every Home* 1873, pg. 76)

Put into a sauce pan half a pound of good grated cheese, with a pint of milk, six ounces of grated bread crumbs, and two eggs well beaten; stir well, till the cheese is dissolved; then put it into a buttered dish, and brown it in a Dutch oven, or with a salamander. Serve quite hot.

**What is a Salamander?**
One of the earliest accounts by Pliny the Elder states that salamanders had the ability to extinguish fires with their bodies and this gave rise to the notion that salamanders were immune to fire. Somewhat understandable, as the main job a salamander is to put out heat. A salamander in the case of the previous recipe from the 17th and 18th century was a browning element. These were flat and rounded or squared pieces of heavy wrought-iron melted welded to a handle. The metal disc would be heated in coals to a red-hot temperature and then held on the top of the food to brown it or broil it. Alternatively, a flat "kitchen shovel" would be heated in a similar way and used to brown or finish a dish. Today salamanders look like small open ovens mounted above the grill or in a pass through in commercial kitchens. Salamanders produce much higher heat, which can be used to cook everything from vegetables to proteins; cheese melters are made to finish food that's already cooked. Professional chefs use a salamander broiler for several purposes, such as broiling fish, melting cheese or caramelizing sugar.

179 Encyclopedia of Kitchen History, by Mary Ellen Snodgrass: 2004,: 1-57958-380-6, pg. 117-121

180 University of York. (2019, September 10). Earliest evidence of milk consumption found in teeth of prehistoric British farmers. ScienceDaily. Retrieved August 16, 2022 from www.sciencedaily.com/releases/2019/09/190910105353.htm

181 University of Veterinary Medicine -- Vienna. (2018, February 6). Vitamin A in cattle fodder is potentially protecting against cow's milk allergy. ScienceDaily. Retrieved August 15, 2022 from www.sciencedaily.com/releases/2018/02/180206100333.htm

182 Clim. Past, 16, 1821–1846, 2020. https://doi.org/10.5194/cp-16-1821-2020 Low water stage marks on hunger stones: verification for the Elbe from 1616 to 2015.

183 Food, A Culinary History from Antiquity to the Present by Jean-Louis Flandrin and Massimo Montanari, 1996: ISBN 0-231-11154-1, pgs. 41, 171, 232

184 Evershed, R.P., Davey Smith, G., Roffet-Salque, M. et al. Dairying, diseases and the evolution of lactase persistence in Europe. Nature (2022). https://doi.org/10.1038/s41586-022-05010-7

185 Sabeti, P. C, Schaffner, S. F., Fry, B., Lohmueller, J., Varilly, P., Shamovsky, O., Palma, A., Mikkelsen, T. S., Altshuler, D., & Lander, E. S. (2006). Positive natural selection in the human lineage. Science (New York, N.Y.), 312(5780), 1614–1620. https://doi.org/10.1126/science.1124309

186 The Great European Famine of 1315, 1316, and 1317 by Henry S. Lucas, 1930 pgs. 343-377; University of Chicago Press: https://www.jstor.org/stable/2848143 retrieved August 2022

188 Cheese a Love Story by Afrim Pristine, 2021, information retrieved July 2022: https://www.foodnetwork.ca/tag/cheese-a-love-story/

189 National Research Council (US) Panel on the Applications of Biotechnology to Traditional Fermented Foods. Applications of Biotechnology to Fermented Foods: Report of an Ad Hoc Panel of the Board on Science and Technology for International Development. Washington (DC): National Academies Press (US); 1992. 7, Fermented Milks—Past, Present, and Future. Available from: https://www.ncbi.nlm.nih.gov/books/NBK234682/

190 Rumi Cheese information retrieved July 2022: https://www.tasteatlas.com/rumicheese

191 Paneer Cheese information retrieved July 2022: https://www.thehindu.com/news/cities/mumbai/Paneer-and-the-origin-of-cheese-in-India/article14516958.ece

192 Oaxaca Cheese information retrieved July 2022: https://www.cheese.com/oaxaca/

193 Queso Blanco Cheese information retrieved July 2022: https://www.cheese.com/queso-blanco/

194 Skyr Cheese information retrieved July 2022: https://www.tasteatlas.com/skyr

195 Byaslag Cheese information retrieved July 2022: https://www.mongolfood.info/en/recipes/byaslag.html

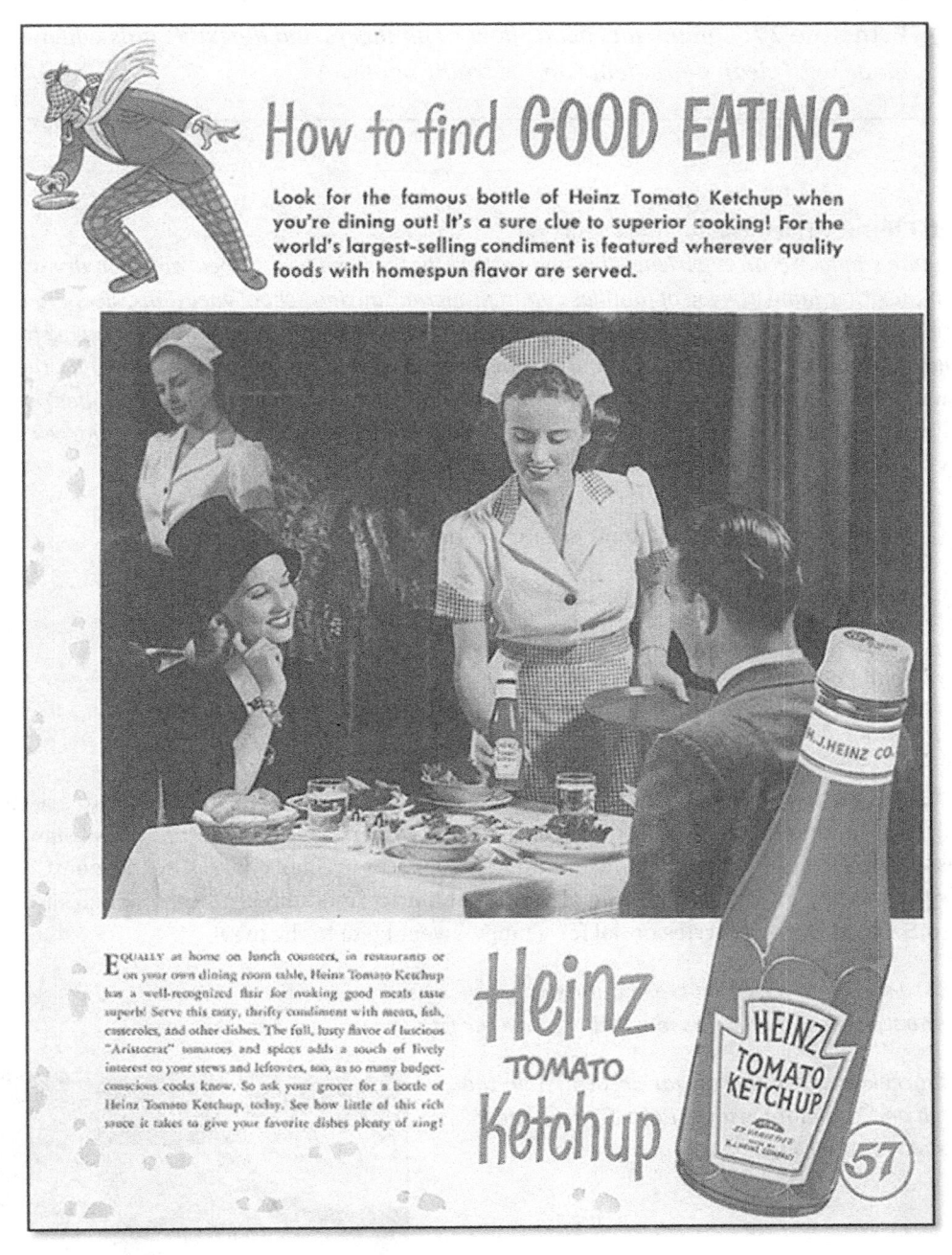

Heinz Tomato Ketchup was first introduced as "catsup" in 1876 in Pittsburgh, PA. In 1907, 13 million bottles of Heinz ketchup were produced. By 2020, over 1.8 billion bottles were sold worldwide.

# Dressings & Sauces

> **Principle 27:** *Condiments act as flavor enhancers and digestive aids when made with clean ingredients and in traditional ways.*

**Mango Chutney** (Medha Mujumdar Murtyy)

*The Indian summer is an experience like none other! On the one hand, unbearably hot, dry weather, and on the other hand, the joy of families coming together during school vacations, sleeping under the stars at night, and the highlight of it all - the world-famous Alphonso mango is a recipe for sheer joy. During summer, Indians use raw and ripe mangoes in dishes ranging from pickles, chutneys, dal, sweets, and the love of every Indian-Aamras, mango pulp eaten with ghee and pepper powder. This sweet and sour mango chutney recipe is made by cooking raw mangoes with fenugreek seeds and is a specialty of western India.*

2 lbs firm mango pieces cut into about 1½ inch square pieces
¼ cup oil
1½ tsp mustard seeds*
1 tsp fenugreek seeds**
½ cup jaggery (see Pantry pg 66)
1 tsp red chile powder
Salt to taste
1 cup of water

Heat oil and add fenugreek seeds, followed by mustard seeds. Allow mustard seeds to splatter (ensure that fenugreek seeds do not burn, or they will impart a bitter taste). Add raw mango pieces and water. Cook on medium heat until mango pieces are half cooked. At this point, add jaggery, red chile powder, and salt and continue cooking on medium heat until mango slices are cooked. Serve alongside curries or dal for a tangy-sweet taste to the meal.

*\* Mustard seeds are a rich source of antioxidants such as kaempferol, carotenoids, and isorhamnetin; these flavonoids may help reduce the risk of coronary heart diseases.*

*\*\* Fenugreek seems to slow sugar absorption in the stomach and stimulate insulin. Both of these effects lowers blood sugar in people with diabetes.*

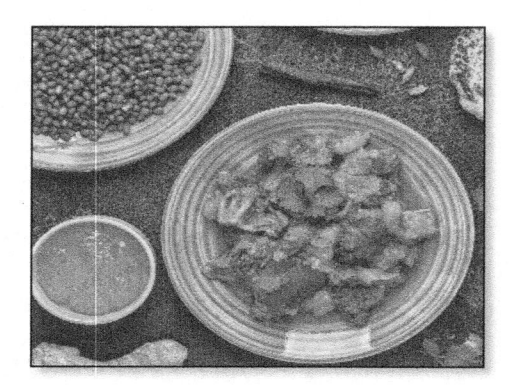

## Homemade Ketchup

4 whole cloves
1 bay leaf
1 cinnamon stick
¼ tsp celery seeds
¼ tsp chile flakes
¼ tsp whole allspice
2 lbs Roma (or Plum) tomatoes roughly chopped
1½ tsp kosher salt
½ cup apple cider vinegar
5 tbsp light brown sugar
1 yellow onion peeled and chopped
1 Anaheim chile deseeded and chopped
1 garlic clove diced
Cheesecloth
Kitchen twine

Prepare a single square layer of cheesecloth that will fit all the spices with room to fold and secure the contents.

Place the cloves, bay leaf, cinnamon stick, celery seeds, chile flakes, and allspice in the middle of the cheesecloth. Fold closed and secure with a length of kitchen twine.

Place tomatoes, salt, vinegar, sugar, onion, chile, garlic, and spice packet in a medium stock pot, 4 quarts or larger (enough to house the tomatoes with some extra room). Cook over medium heat until tomatoes and chiles are soft and onions are translucent and limp (about 30 minutes).

Remove and discard the spice packet. Purée the sauce using a traditional blender or food mill.

Strain the ketchup through a fine-mesh strainer back into the cooking pot. *NOTE:* This step removes any seeds.

Cook over medium-low heat for 20-30 minutes until thickened to your preference.

Store in sealed ½ pint glass jars in the refrigerator for up to 3 weeks.

### Cucumber Catsup (1890 *Buffalo Morning Express*)
Yields 2 pints

6 large cucumbers
1 onion, medium sized, peeled and grated
¾ tsp freshly ground pepper
1 tsp salt
1 cup cider vinegar (about)
1 tbsp whole mustard seed, soaked and drained

Wash cucumbers, drain, cover with cold water and a handful of salt, let stand 1-2 hours. Drain, pare, grate, or grind fine into bowl or glass jar. Add remaining ingredients with just enough vinegar to make a smooth consistency. Mash, mix well, and press through sieve. Put in a jar and cover with remaining vinegar, cork tight; keep in a dry place.


### Ben's Barbecue Sauce (BQ's BBQ Sauce -Chef Ben Qualls)
*I came up with this basic barbecue sauce at work. Didn't have barbecue sauce on hand but had all the ingredients. Voila! BQ's BBQ sauce. As stated, this is a very basic sauce. Feel free to add or remove ingredients to your taste. This recipe will yield about a gallon of barbecue sauce.*

1 (#10) can tomato ketchup (I use Heinz, use whatever you like)
1 lb brown sugar
½ to 1 cup cider vinegar depending on how much tang you want
¼ cup Worcestershire sauce
¼ cup olive oil
1 tbsp ground black pepper
1 tbsp liquid smoke (optional)

In a large mixing bowl, combine all ingredients. Mix until brown sugar is dissolved.

Store in jars in the refrigerator for several weeks. It can be processed in a hot water bath canner. Search under canning basic tomato sauce.


### Avocado Dip (for salmon Miriam G. Zacharias)
Serves 4 or 1 cup

1 ripe avocado, peeled and pitted
¼ cup Libby's mayonnaise
2 tbsp fresh lemon juice
1 serrano chile, seeded and chopped

¼ onion, chopped (for a mild flavor use Walla Walla or vidalia sweet onion)
Salt to taste

Place all ingredients in a blender or food processor and pulse until smooth. Chill.

## Basil Pesto (Tammera Karr)
*Serve pesto on fresh pasta, spread on a halved baguette, and broil, or as a pizza topping. Experiment with other herbs like parsley, thyme, tarragon, and cilantro.*

3 or more cloves garlic
2 cups fresh basil leaves
¼ cup pine nuts
1½ tsp salt
¼ tsp pepper
½ cup good-quality olive oil
3 oz Parmesan cheese, grated

In a blender, combine garlic, basil, nuts, salt, pepper, and half of the oil. Purée, then slowly add the remaining oil. If using immediately, stir in Parmesan. Pesto turns brown when exposed to air. Add Parmesan before serving.

## Strawberry Mango Salsa (Tammera Karr)
*I am one of those people that cilantro tastes like soap for - so I use basil, Italian flat leaf parsley and lovage instead.*
Makes 4-6 cups

½ red onion, cut into thin slivers
½ cup lemon juice, or as needed
¼ cup lime juice
1 jalapeno pepper, seeded
1 lb fresh strawberries, cut into ¼ inch pieces
1 mango, cut into ¼ inch pieces
½ red bell pepper, finely diced
¼ cup chopped fresh basil
Salt, to taste

Place onions in a small bowl of cool water for 5 minutes. Drain water and put onions directly into a serving bowl. Cover onions with lemon and lime juice.

Slice jalapeño in half lengthwise. Remove seeds and wash thoroughly

Finely chop and add to bowl. Add strawberries, mango, bell peppers, and basil. Stir and season with salt.

Let salsa rest for at least 30 minutes for flavors to blend.

### **Traditional Salsa** (Tammera Karr)

*We make up a 16 quart bowl of this and can in ½ pint jars.*
Makes 2 quarts

4 cups peeled, finely chopped tomatoes
2 cups finely chopped mixed chiles; jalapeno, ancho, Anaheim, poblano
2 cups finely chopped sweet onion
3-4 garlic cloves, minced
1 lemon juiced
1 lime juiced
1 tbsp chopped fresh basil
1 tsp sea salt, or more to taste
1-2 crushed avocado leaves

In a bowl, combine all the ingredients. Taste, add extra chiles and salt if desired, and serve.

### **Berry Vinaigrette Salad Dressing or Glaze** (Tammera Karr)

1 cup mixed berries
1 cup balsamic vinegar
¼ cup raw honey, real maple syrup, or stevia to taste
½ cup filtered water
½ cup organic extra virgin olive oil
¼ tsp turmeric, a pinch of black pepper

Place all ingredients in a blender and mix until smooth. Place dressing in a glass jar and refrigerate. This mixture is good for two to three weeks. Use it as a salad dressing or a glaze for salmon, cauliflower, broccoli, or chicken.

### **Cucumber Sauce** *(for salmon or halibut)*
Makes 1 cup

1 cup plain yogurt (substitute coconut yogurt)
2 pickling cucumbers, peeled and finely diced

¼ cup fresh Italian parsley or chives, chopped
2 tbsp fresh lemon juice
Celtic Sea salt and pepper to taste

Combine in a blender and mix.

## Italian Salad Dressing
Serves 8

¼ cup extra virgin olive oil
½ cup water
4 tbsp balsamic or rice vinegar
2 tbsp maple syrup
1 tsp dried basil
½ tsp dried oregano
3 cloves garlic, minced
¼ tsp ground black pepper
½ tsp Celtic Sea salt

Blend well in the blender.
Prep time is about 5 minutes.

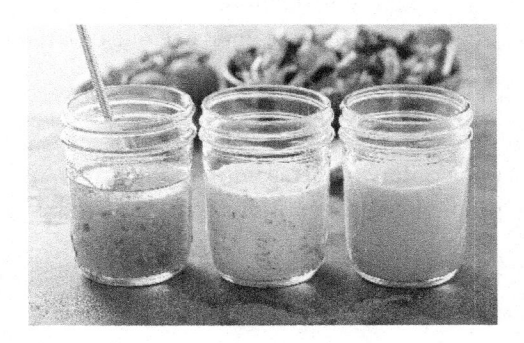

## Poppy Seed Dressing (Chef Christine Wokowsky)

½ cup almond milk
½ cup cashews, soaked for a few hours
2 Medjool dates, pits removed
1 tbsp apple cider vinegar
1 tbsp poppy seeds
Sea salt and pepper to taste

## Libby's Mayonnaise

2 hard boiled egg yolks
1 egg yolk, uncooked
½ tsp Celtic Sea salt
Dash organic sugar (pinch)
½ tsp dry mustard

½ cup extra virgin olive oil
2½ tbsp fresh lemon juice
2 tbsp apple cider vinegar

Combine in a Vitamix® blender or bowl the egg yolks, salt, sugar, and mustard, and blend until smooth. Slowly stir in olive oil, a tablespoon full at a time. Beat after each addition. Add the remaining ingredients with the last two reserves of oil. Beat well. Refrigerate.

## Old-Fashioned Tomato Sauce

2 tbsp organic or Kerrygold butter
1 slice yellow onion
2½ tbsp gluten-free flour or white spelt flour
1 cup stewed and strained organic tomatoes
¼ tsp Celtic Sea salt
Pinch paprika

Cook onion in butter until lightly brown. Add flour, and when well browned, pour in tomatoes gradually while continually stirring tomatoes.

Bring to a boiling point, add seasonings, then run through a strainer or Foley Food Mill for a smooth texture.

## Avocado Cream Sauce (Chef Christine Wokowsky)

½ avocado, chopped
¼ small cucumber, chopped
A handful of fresh herbs like green onions, cilantro, basil, oregano
Juice of half a lemon
1 clove garlic
Dash of cayenne
Salt to taste
1 tbsp almond or coconut milk

Finely chop the herbs and mix in the avocado sauce with salt and cayenne.
Feel free to add a bit of fresh garlic, onion, and leek, as these are all excellent sources of prebiotics.

## French Dressing (*Virden's Camp Fire Brand*, 1920)

1 cup Camp Fire Salad Oil *(substitute your preferred oil)*
⅓ cup vinegar
¼ tsp paprika
Salt, white pepper

Beat thoroughly with an egg beater.


## New Mexico Green Chile* Sauce (Tammera Karr)
*(*Regional Spelling)*

15 lbs fire-roasted Hatch Chile
1 yellow onion
1 purple onion
1½ bulbs garlic
1 tbsp Celtic Sea salt
4 tbsp apple cider vinegar, lime, or tequila
4 cups water

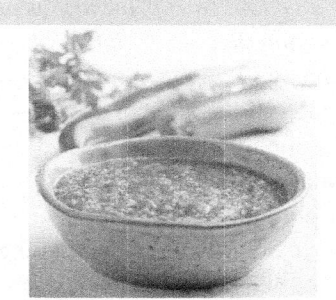

Peel and remove the stem on chiles and the skin removes easily once roasted. SAVE the juice in the container and add chopped chiles, garlic, and onions.
You can use or remove seeds.

Blend all in a Vitamix, blender or food processor. Place sauce in 4-8 oz jars, wipe, and close with Ball canning lids and rings.

Water bath jars for 20 minutes.
Makes 46, 4 oz jars.


## Tahini Sauce (Chef Christine Wokowsky)

1 clove garlic
1 tsp salt
½ cup tahini
½ cup water
½ cup lemon juice

Mash the garlic and salt together. Add the tahini, mixing well. The sauce will thicken. Gradually add the water, blending thoroughly. Then add the lemon juice. Blend well.

Note: This can be a thin or thick sauce, depending upon the use and preference. Simply adjust with lemon juice and water.

## Sauces and Stuffing (*Daily Wants: A Book for Every Home*, by Alexander V. Hamilton, 1873, pg 95)

*The use of sauces has become more general of late, and several forms of these condiments are popular. Taken in moderation, they may be considered healthy, but used in excess they are decidedly injurious. The base of all the meat sauces is the Indian Pickle chutney, soy, garlic, sugar, pepper, and catsup, in various proportions. The Worcester and Harvey's sauces, have so much in common that a description of the latter will be sufficient.*

**Harvey's Sauce** — The following are the ingredients for a gallon; though of course less may be made: — Five pints of best pickling vinegar; ¼ of a pound of good pickled cucumber, cut small; ¼ of a pound of white mustard seed, bruised; ¼ of an ounce of fresh celery-seed, bruised; and one ounce of garlic, peeled, and cut small. Boil until reduced to four pints, in a stone jar. In another jar put four pints of water, one oz of bruised ginger, ¼ of an ounce of bruised mace; ¼ of an ounce of cayenne pepper; one pint of *India chutney* or soy; boil slowly in a stone jar reduced to four pints; then mix the contents of the two jars together, stirring well; boil them together for half an hour, then let the mixture stand till cold. Take the peel of three lemons, cut into strips, dry in an oven, till quite brown and dry. Add hot to the cold mixture. Cover close; let it stand ten days, and strain for use.


## Fruit French Dressing (*Virden's Camp Fire Brand*, 1920)

½ tsp salt
¼ cup orange juice
¼ tsp paprika
½ cup salad oil
½ tbsp powdered sugar
1 tbsp lemon juice

Mix all together and serve with fruit salad.

### Championak Salsa Berden: Mushrooms with Parsley Sauce (Kelsi Sitz)

*The Basque language is unprecedented, matching no other spoken language in history. The Basque tongue does not derive from the Indo-European or Finno-Ugric language strains from which all other European languages stem. Food from the Basque country of Euskadi Herria is as unique as the ancient language, filled with color, flavor nuances, and family.*

Serves 8

24 large fresh mushrooms
1 medium onion, chopped
¼ cup Spanish olive oil
¼ cup butter
½ cup white wine
4 tbsp parsley, minced
3 cloves garlic

Heat oil and butter in a large sauce pan; add chopped onion and cook until soft. Add mushrooms and cover. When they begin to reduce in size, add the wine. Continue cooking for about 5 minutes. Add parsley and garlic and let simmer until the raw flavor of garlic has subsided. Drain and pierce each one with a toothpick.

### Creamy Basque Dressing (*Basque Heritage Cookbook* by Kelsi Sitz)

¾ cup apple cider vinegar
1 tsp salt
2 cloves garlic
1½ cups olive oil
Sugar to taste

Combine the vinegar, salt, garlic, and sugar in a blender. While blending at high speed, slowly add the oil and blend until white. Remove from the blender and pour over any salad for a delicious taste.

### Mint Sauce (adapted by Chef Ben Qualls from 1917 recipe)
Serves 4

¼ cup mint leaves
½ cup boiling water
2 tbsp organic sugar
4 tsp apple cider vinegar or kefir water
⅛ tsp paprika
¼ tsp salt

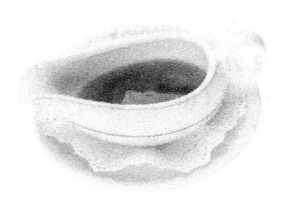

Chop the mint leaves very fine in a food processor. Add boiling water, sugar, and mint leaves in a heat-resistant bowl. Cover and let stand ½ hour. Add the vinegar, paprika, and salt.

### Lamb Gravy (adapted by Chef Ben Qualls from 1917 recipe)
Serves 4

4 tbsp dripping off the roast leg of lamb
2/3 cup water
2 tbsp arrowroot powder or potato starch
½ tsp salt
Fresh ground black pepper to taste

Place ½ of the drippings in a sauce pan. Add arrowroot powder, whisk together, and allow to brown on medium heat. Add water, salt, and 2 tablespoons of meat drippings slowly. Boil 1 minute. Add pepper to taste.

### Nona's Salmon Spread (Miriam G. Zacharias)
*GREAT on bagels, too!*

10 oz salmon, skinned, boned, and drained (if using canned)
1 8 oz package of cream cheese, softened
1 tbsp lemon juice
3 tsp grated onion
¼ tsp salt
Dash of Worcestershire sauce
Dash of Tabasco sauce
½ cup pecans or parsley

Mix all ingredients except pecans and parsley, sprinkle with pecans or parsley (or both), and chill.
Serve with your favorite crackers, along with some sliced pears.

## Dressings & Sauces

### Raisin Sauce (Sun Maid Raisins 1921)

*This comes from a Sun Maid Raisin advertising booklet with 97 recipes. The inside cover contains an endorsement from J.H. Kellogg.*

2 cups seeded raisins
½ cup sugar
1 tbsp lemon juice
1 tsp grated lemon rind
½ tsp salt
1 tbsp flour

Wash the raisins, put in with 2 cups of water, and boil slowly 10 minutes. Add salt, sugar and flour which has been mixed smooth with a little cold water; boil 3 minutes; add lemon juice and rind.

This makes a good breakfast fruit.

### Lemonade Syrup (*Healthward- Cooking and Eating for Health-Happiness and Success*, 1935, pg 59)

2 cups sugar
Water
Lemon rinds
Orange rinds

After juice has been extracted from the lemons and oranges, place the fresh rinds in a 2 quart Cookware Sauce Pan, cover with water, add 2 cups of sugar and simmer 10 minutes.
Remove the rind. Keep the flavorful syrup in cans near the ice. It is ready for the addition of lemon juice when a cool drink is desired.

This cook book was a marketing tool from Dr. Burnettes Cookware Company, Hartford, Michigan.

**Introduction for Cookware buyers**:
Uncertainty has interfered with success in cooking, but our latest Cockware, with the patented ventilator and heat control, has eliminated the guess work. Now you can cook without water and preserve the precious mineral salts and vitamins which ensure genuine results in maintaining your health and vigor.

This 100-page cook book promoted the "state of the art aluminum cookware."

**Now Some Practical Cooking Advice From 1864.**

*"The secret of good cooking is: first, be a critical judge –
know excellent cooking from poor cooking;
second, find a fascination in the science, and become thoroughly familiar with
what and what not to do;
third, find genuine pleasure in the practice – mastering the basic recipes and the
operation and control of your range –
and above all, THINK".*

"Home Comfort" Cook Book,
Wrought Iron Range Company 1909

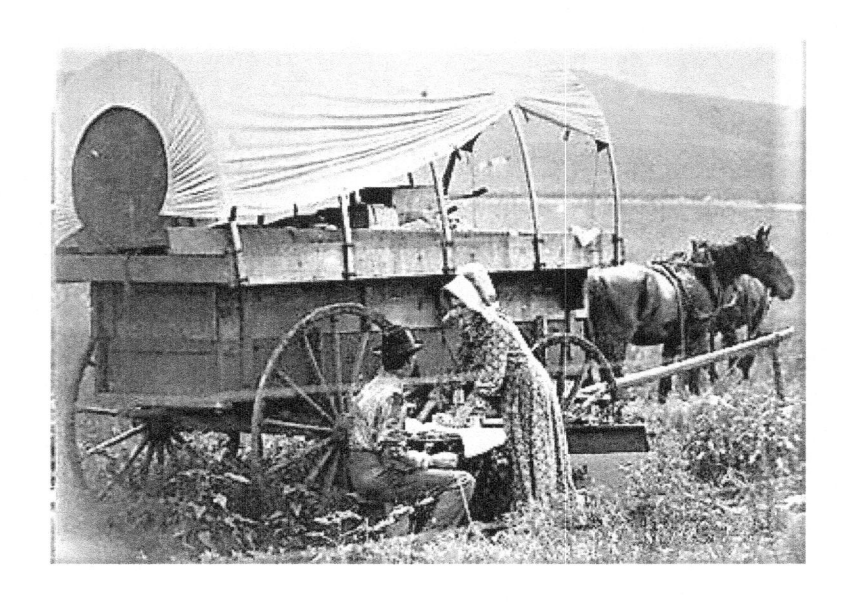

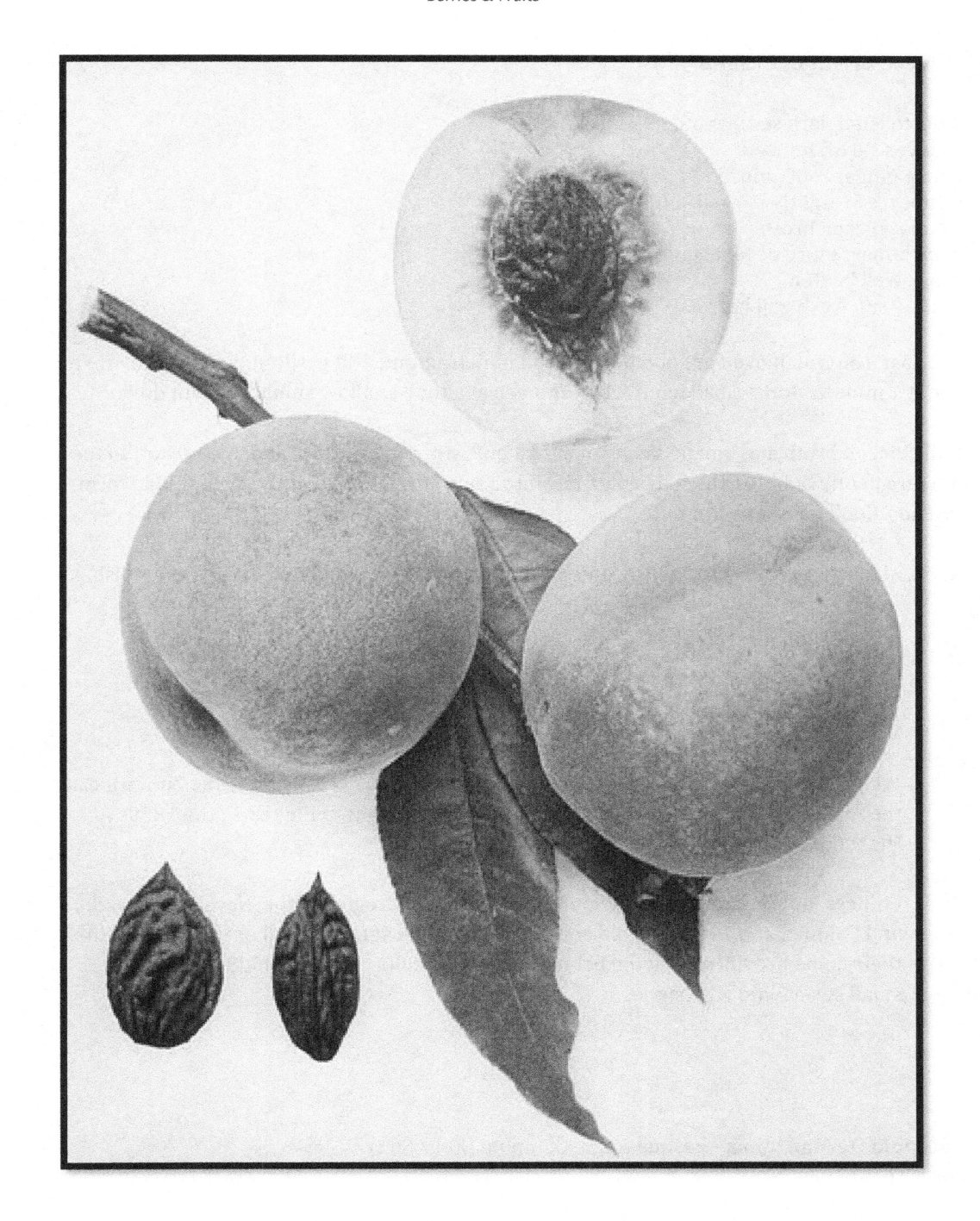

# Berries & Fruits

**Chinese Bright Eyes Soup**

2 tsp toasted dark sesame oil
3 cloves garlic, minced
1 tbsp ginger root, minced
8 cups fresh, tightly packed spinach leaves
3 cups chicken broth
1 tsp tamari sauce or to taste
1 egg, well beaten
½ to ¾ cup fresh goji berries

In a cast iron Dutch oven or soup pot, heat oil until fragrant. Add garlic and ginger. Stir fry for about 1 minute. Add a small hand full of spinach at a time to allow spinach to wilt down.

Add chicken broth and tamari sauce. Heat to a boil, stir several times and lower heat, so the mixture gently bubbles. Drizzle beaten egg into soup, stirring constantly. Eggs should form threads. Cook for about 1 minute.

Add goji berries, remove from heat, and let stand while you ready bowls. Serve and relish.

### *Goji Berries or Wolfberry Fruits*

*Wolfberry*, *matrimony vines*, or *goji berries* were a staple in the diet of the Zuni tribe of the American Southwest. Matrimony vines were brought to the U.S. in the 1880s in Utah, Colorado, and New Mexico.

Chinese laborers came to the mountains of eastern Oregon, Idaho, Nevada, Colorado, and California to work the gold and silver mines. Most Chinese laborers returned to their home provinces, leaving behind a rich food culture and the hidden delight of small sweet wild goji berries.

**Compota De Manzanas** - Basque Apple Compote (Kelsi Sitz)
Serves 6

6 medium tart or winter apples
¾ cup organic sugar
Spanish red wine
1 stick cinnamon

Peel and quarter apples. Place apples in a pot, cover with red wine and add the sugar and cinnamon stick. Boil until the apples are tender, and serve hot.

### **Baked Apples with Blackberries** (Tammera Karr)

2-4 tart apples, cored
¼ cup blackberries
4 tbsp organic butter
5 tbsp organic coconut sugar
¼ cup water

Place apples so they do not touch the sides of the pan. Fill centers with coconut sugar and blackberries. Top each apple with a pat of butter. Cover pan with a tight-fitting lid.

Bake in the oven at 350°F for 45-60 minutes, depending on the size of the apples.

### **Blackberry Sorbet** -Traditional Irish Dessert
Serves 4

1 lb fresh blackberries
4 oz organic sugar
½ cup water
2 egg whites

Blend fruit and strain seeds (this can be done with a food mill). Dissolve sugar in water and boil for 5 minutes to make syrup. Add blackberries and boil for a few more minutes. When the liquid has cooled, fold it into stiff-beaten egg whites.

Freeze in an ice cream machine or in ice cube trays, stirring once an hour to prevent large ice crystals from forming.

### **Blackberries & Peaches** (Tammera Karr)

6-8 peaches, sliced (more if you like)
4 cups blackberries (more if berries are small)
Place fruit in the bottom of a 9x13 inch glass baking dish.

*Crumb Topping*
1 cup almond flour
1 cup coconut sugar

½ cup organic butter
1 cup gluten-free rolled oats

In a stand mixer, combine ingredients and mix well until butter is well incorporated. Spread topping over fruit. Bake for 35-45 minutes at 350°F.

Times will vary based on the thickness of fruit, oven variances, and elevation.

### Moms Peach Cobbler (Mira Dessy)

*This particular recipe is one of our summertime favorites and it comes from my mom. It's simple and so easy to put together. It makes a perfect dessert after just about any meal.*

*Topping*
5 tbsp cold unsalted organic butter
1 cup Pamela's baking mix
2 tbsp organic yellow cornmeal
2 tbsp sugar
1½ tsp baking powder
½ tsp salt
½ cup organic whole milk
½ tsp vanilla

*Filling*
3-4 peaches, peel, pit, and slice thick
2 cups blackberries, rinsed
2 tsp organic cornstarch
⅓ cup sugar
1 tsp vanilla extract
1 tbsp brandy
Toss with fruit to coat

Preheat oven to 375°F
1. Cut butter into pieces.
2. In a bowl with a pastry blender or in a food processor blend or pulse together baking mix, cornmeal, sugar, baking powder, salt, and butter until the mixture resembles coarse meal.
3. If using a food processor, transfer to a bowl.
4. Add milk and vanilla and stir until the mixture forms a dough.
5. Drop topping by rounded spoonsful onto the filling (do not completely cover it) and bake in the middle of the oven 40 minutes or until the topping is golden and cooked through.
6. Serve with ice cream or lightly whipped cream.

### Apple Crumble (Betty Sitz)

*This recipe works for rhubarb, apples, peaches, blackberries, or pears.*

*Crumble Mix*
1 cup Bob's Red Mill Gluten-Free Rolled Oats
1 cup Bob's Red Mill Gluten-Free flour
1 cup Kerrygold butter, soft
½ cup maple or coconut sugar

Combine with a pastry cutter.

Place sliced fruit in a 9x13 inch baking pan, and add ½ cup water for dry fruit like apples and rhubarb. Place 5-6 knobs of butter around the top, and sprinkle with cinnamon.

Cover the fruit with the crumble mix, and bake at 350-375°F for 35-40 minutes. Juice should look thick where visible.

You can combine cranberries with apples and add a pinch of clove with the cinnamon for a holiday crumble.

> "Flummery" - This delight came west with pioneers from New England. It became popular in areas along the west coast, where berries grew with profusion. Flummery could be found at logging camps' tables, where my grandmother Kate cooked. Logging camps were judged by their cook – a poor cook meant the logging boss had a hard time getting workers; a great cook could name their price and would be found at the biggest and most prosperous camps. Berries most commonly used were blackberries, wild blackcaps, and raspberries.

### Wild Berry Flummery (Kate Morgan, 1920)

2 cups fresh berries, stems removed
2 cups water
3½ tbsp arrowroot
3-4 tbsp water (for arrowroot)
½ cup organic honey or sugar

In a sauce pan, simmer berries in 2 cups of water 10-12 minutes. In a cup, blend arrowroot and 4 tablespoons water, and stir gently into simmering berries. Then stir in honey and a dash of salt. Let cool. Serve in small bowls with thick clotted cream.

### Fried Sweeting (Kate Morgan, 1930)

*Tammera's paternal grandmother was a marvel in the kitchen, she could peel potatoes and fruit with almost translucent trimmings. This skill came from years of being a logging camp cook, feeding as many as 100 hungry lumberjacks at a time in the 1920s and 1930s.*
Serves 6

6 sweet apples
6 tbsp molasses
Organic butter or lard

Wash and core apples and cut each into three or four rings. Heat a little fat in a frying pan, lay the apples in, cover, and cook slowly, turning at the end of 15 minutes. When both sides are brown, pour 1 tablespoonful of molasses over each slice, cook 5 more minutes, and serve very hot.


### Triple Berry Bars (Tammera Karr)

*Berry Filling*
½ cup water
¼ cup arrowroot powder
3 cups fresh or frozen berries (raspberries, strawberries, blueberries, and blackberries; altogether or individually)
1 tsp fresh lemon juice
⅓ cup raw honey
4 tbsp chopped nuts

*Gluten-free oatmeal crumble*
1½ cups gluten-free rolled oats
2 cups plus 2 tbsp almond or coconut flour, divided
1 tbsp arrowroot powder
¼ tsp Celtic Sea salt
½ cup raw honey
¼ cup organic almond butter
¼ cup coconut or almond milk
1 tsp vanilla

In a shaker or blender, combine water and arrowroot powder, pulse blend a few times to mix well, then add to a sauce pan on medium heat. Frequently stir to keep the mixture smooth. Add chopped or blended berries to the pan, bring to a low boil over medium heat, then turn off the heat. Add lemon juice, honey, and nuts, stir, and set aside.

*Crumble topping*
Heat oven to 350°F. Line a 9x9 inch baking pan with parchment paper. Reserve some crumb mix for topping.

Combine oats, nut flour, arrowroot powder, and salt in a mixing bowl. Mix. Next, add almond butter, honey, nut milk, and vanilla. Spread mixture into the baking pan, careful not to tear parchment paper.

Place in oven and bake for 20 minutes or until golden. Remove from oven, spread berry mixture over the top of crumb mix, sprinkling any saved crumb mix over top of berries. Bake additional 10 minutes. Allow to cool and cut into bars.

### Apricot Silk (Tammera Karr)
*This is a perfect sauce to use with roast pork or poultry; on ice cream, toast, pancakes, and waffles; or incorporated into salad dressing.*
Makes 6-7 pints

2 lbs ripe apricots with peal; washed, halved and pitted
½ cup water
1½ cups organic sugar
2 tbsp lemon juice, fresh squeezed

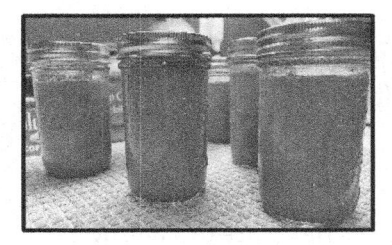

In a large stainless steel sauce pan combine rinsed apricots and water. Bring to a slow boil on medium high heat, stirring occasionally, until apricots are soft; about 20 minutes. Transfer smaller amounts to a food mill and purée – do not liquefy.
Measure 6 cups of apricot purée.

In a stainless steel sauce pan, combine apricot purée and sugar. Stir until sugar dissolves. Bring to a boil over medium high heat, stirring frequently. Reduce heat and boil gently, frequently stirring, until the mixture thickens and holds a soft syrup or jelly shape on the spoon. Stir in lemon juice.

Using a wide mouth jar funnel, ladle apricot silk into clean pint jars (there should be 1 inch of head space). Cover with fresh Ball or Kerr lids that have been heated in hot tap water, screw the retaining ring down finger tight.

Option 1: Once jars are filled and lids are in place, place them in a pressure canner (be sure to follow your canner directions), heat and vent for 10 minutes and place weight on the vent, bring to 5 pounds pressure and hold 8 minutes. Turn off heat and let the canner cool. Once cool, remove the jars and let rest on the counter for 24 hours. Check jars to be sure they have sealed, then place them in the pantry. Shelf stable for 18 months.

Freezer Option 2: Once jars are filled and lids are in place, allow them to cool for 24 hours on the counter. Once cool, place in the freezer.
*Note*: Thawed sauce may be thinner after freezing. Use within 3-6 months.

*One of the delights of childhood for my husband and me was spiced crabapples. These treats were found at the homes of grandparents or individuals living on homestead properties. Pioneers brought foods west they were familiar with, and the crabapple holds importance with Irish immigrants as a flavor of home, who homesteaded in the Pacific Northwest in the 1880s.*

~ Tammera Karr

### Crabapple Jelly

2 cups crabapple juice
1 tsp fresh lemon juice for each cup of crabapple juice
⅔ cup organic sugar for each cup of crabapple juice

Traditional jams and jellies did not use pectin until much later. Apples contain high levels of natural pectin, so adding it is unnecessary. Use a mix of ripe and slightly unripe fruit for the best taste.

Place approximately 5 pounds of fruit in a large sauce pan with 1-2 cups of water. Cover and cook on medium heat until the fruit falls apart and becomes very liquidly.

With a jelly strainer or cheesecloth, strain juice from the pulp.

Measure juice and lemon juice into a stainless steel 8 quart sauce pan. Heat juice to a boil over medium-high heat. Add sugar and stir constantly until sugar dissolves. Increase heat to high and cook, skimming off any foam and frequently stirring, until jelly passes one or more softball tests on wax paper; approximately 10-15 minutes but may take longer at higher elevations.

Pour into glass jelly jars and seal. Process in boiling water bath for 15 minutes at 5,000 feet, or at recommended time for water bath canning at your elevation.

### Ginger Poached Peaches with Goat Cheese & Blueberries (Tammera Karr)

Serves 12; Cook time 20 minutes

6 peaches, organic ripe freestone (Redhavens, Hucrest or 49's work great)
⅛ cup crystallized ginger
¼ cup organic or Kerrygold butter
8 oz goat cheese
1 cup blueberries
2 cups Crater Lake ginger vodka or ginger beer

Cut peaches in half and remove the stone. Place chunks of butter around the bottom of a cast iron Dutch oven, and place peach halves in the bottom with the center stone indentation facing up. Add ginger beer or vodka to the Dutch oven, cover, and poach on medium heat for 10 minutes. Leave the lid on, turn off the heat and let rest while preparing the cheese filling.

Form goat cheese into a small log approximately 2½-3 inches across.

Blueberries are best if they have been slightly stewed in their juice and cooled; however, fresh can also be used. With a slotted spoon, separate the berries from the juice and spread berries on parchment paper in a jelly roll pan (you want the berries as dry as possible).

Roll the cheese over the berries coating the cheese roll entirely with blueberries, and place the roll in the refrigerator to cool and firm back up.

Once the cheese roll has firmed up, using a cheese wire or dental floss, cut 1 inch slices off the cheese log. Place each slice in the center of your peaches, and cover and return to medium heat for 10 more minutes. Cheese and blueberries should still be in the center of the peaches but melted.

Place a peach in a dessert dish, spoon some of the liquid over each, sprinkle small crystalized ginger pieces over each peach, add a minutest leaf to the side for garnish, and serve warm.

### Sherry's Easy Baked Figs (Sherry Holub)

12 medium-sized, ripe Black Mission figs
3 tbsp balsamic vinegar
2 tbsp olive oil
4-5 springs of fresh rosemary
3 cloves of garlic
Goat cheese crumbles

Preparation: Pre-heat oven to 400°F.

Slice figs in half and place cut side up in the baking dish. Slice the garlic cloves and sprinkle over the fig halves. Sprinkle goat cheese crumbles over the fig halves (no specific amount, just to taste).

Mix the balsamic and olive oil and drizzle over the fig halves. Place rosemary springs on top. Place uncovered baking dish into oven for 15-18 minutes or until figs are just starting to brown.

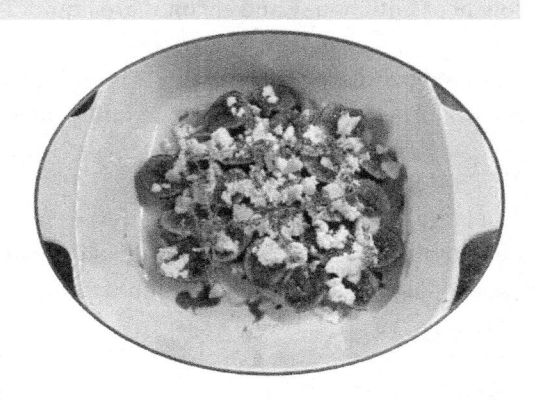

**Karen's Awesome Banana Nut Muffins** (Karen Langston)
Makes 6-12 muffins

6 eggs, pasture-raised
1 cup organic ripe banana, mashed
½ cup organic walnut pieces
¼ cup coconut oil
¼ cup raw honey
⅓ cup Aroy-D coconut milk or homemade almond milk
¾ cup coconut flour, sifted
½ cup almond flour, sifted
1-2 tsp organic cinnamon
1-2 tsp Chinese Five Spice
1 tsp baking soda
2 tsp Celtic Sea salt
1 tsp organic vanilla extract

Preheat oven to 400°F.

Lightly grease a muffin tin or use non-bleach muffin paper cups.
Place eggs in a bowl of hot water and let sit to come to room temperature.
In a medium bowl, peel bananas and break them into small pieces, then mash with a big serving fork. Set to the side and let the flavors marry and release the essential oils making favorable muffins.

In a small pot, add ¼ cup coconut oil, ¼ cup honey, and ⅓ cup coconut milk, and gently heat over low heat until honey and coconut are liquid. Turn it off and let it cool.

In a food processor, pulse walnuts into small pieces. Or place between non bleached parchment or waxed paper and crush with a rolling pin or the bottom of a cup.

*Dry Ingredients*
In a large bowl, place a fine wire strainer (colander) and add coconut flour, almond flour, cinnamon, Chinese Five Spice, and baking soda; sift all ingredients into the bowl by tapping the side and lightly shaking the contents through the strainer; you will have a fine feathery mixture. Add Celtic Sea salt. Set bowl aside.

*Wet ingredients*
Ensure your bowl is big enough to hold wet and dry ingredients.
Take eggs out of the water and pat dry with a clean towel. Crack eggs into the bowl and whisk until well mixed. Add stove mixture, coconut oil, honey, and coconut milk and whisk into eggs; add organic vanilla extract.

Slowly add dry ingredients into wet ingredients and mix using a fork to make a batter. Gently mix into banana mixture just to incorporate; do not over mix; you want to keep the fluffiness as much as possible. Fold in walnuts. Use a spoon to scoop up and drop the batter into each cup. Do not pat down; it will make the muffins too dense.

Pop the pan into the oven and bake for 20-25 minutes. Check muffins with a clean, sharp knife; poke into the middle; if it comes out gunky, continue baking another 6-8 minutes and check again. If the knife comes out clean, they are ready! Take them out of the pan immediately and let them cool on a wire rack. Then enjoy. Keep the rest refrigerated or freeze.

You can easily double the recipe. I make big batches and freeze them for a quick, healthy snack on the go.

## **Lemon Bliss Bars** (Tammera Karr)

*Crust*
1½ cups graham flour
2 tbsp flour
¼ tsp sea salt
3 tbsp butter of ghee
¼ cup maple syrup
1 tsp vanilla extract

*Filling*
1 tbsp fresh lemon zest
¾ cup fresh lemon juice, about 3 or 4 lemons
4 large eggs
½ cup maple syrup
1 tbsp arrowroot starch

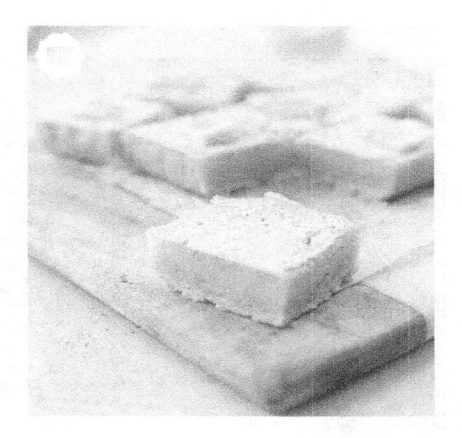

*For the Crust*
1. Preheat the oven to 350°F.
2. Add all dry ingredients into a bowl and mix well.
3. Add the wet ingredients in and mix well. This becomes a sticky mixture.
4. Take the wet mixture out and press it into a lined tin or springform pan until the bottom is completely covered.
5. Bake for another 15 minutes

*For the topping*
1. Add the eggs, lemon juice, zest, and maple syrup in a bowl, and mix well.
2. Add the arrowroot starch and whisk until clump free.
3. Add this mixture straight on top of the crust as soon as this comes out of the oven.
4. Bake an additional 20-25 minutes to cook topping.
5. Take it out of the oven and let it rest 30-40 minutes. Remove from tin and slice into squares. Serve with fresh clotted cream.

406. Common sense in the use of sugar. (*Theory and Practice of Cookery* 1900-1912, Pg 259 New York Public School textbook for grades 6-8)

Because sugar dissolves readily, a small quantity of it are easily digested; but if more than a little is taken at once, some of it is likely to ferment in the stomach, causing distress, and interfering with the digestion of other foods. It may ferment in the mouth and make the teeth decay.

Do not eat sweets just before meals; they will take away your appetite for more substantial food. Use sugar sparingly on oatmeal and in beverages; a little tastes as sweet as more to one who has not blunted his taste by using too much. Do not be tempted by sweets in the bakeshop; they are bad for teeth, complexion, and health.

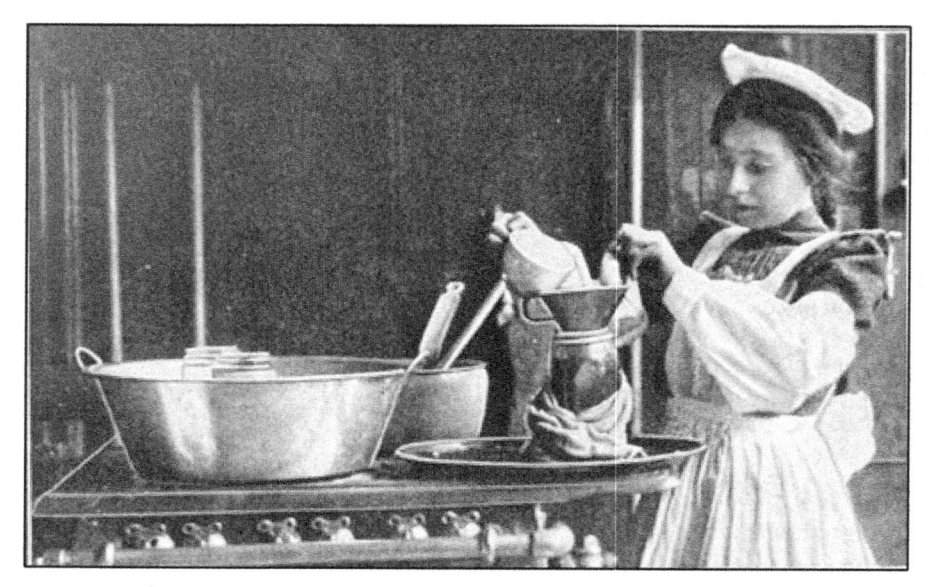

Image of a 6th grade student filling canning jars with fruit, New York public school, pg. 285

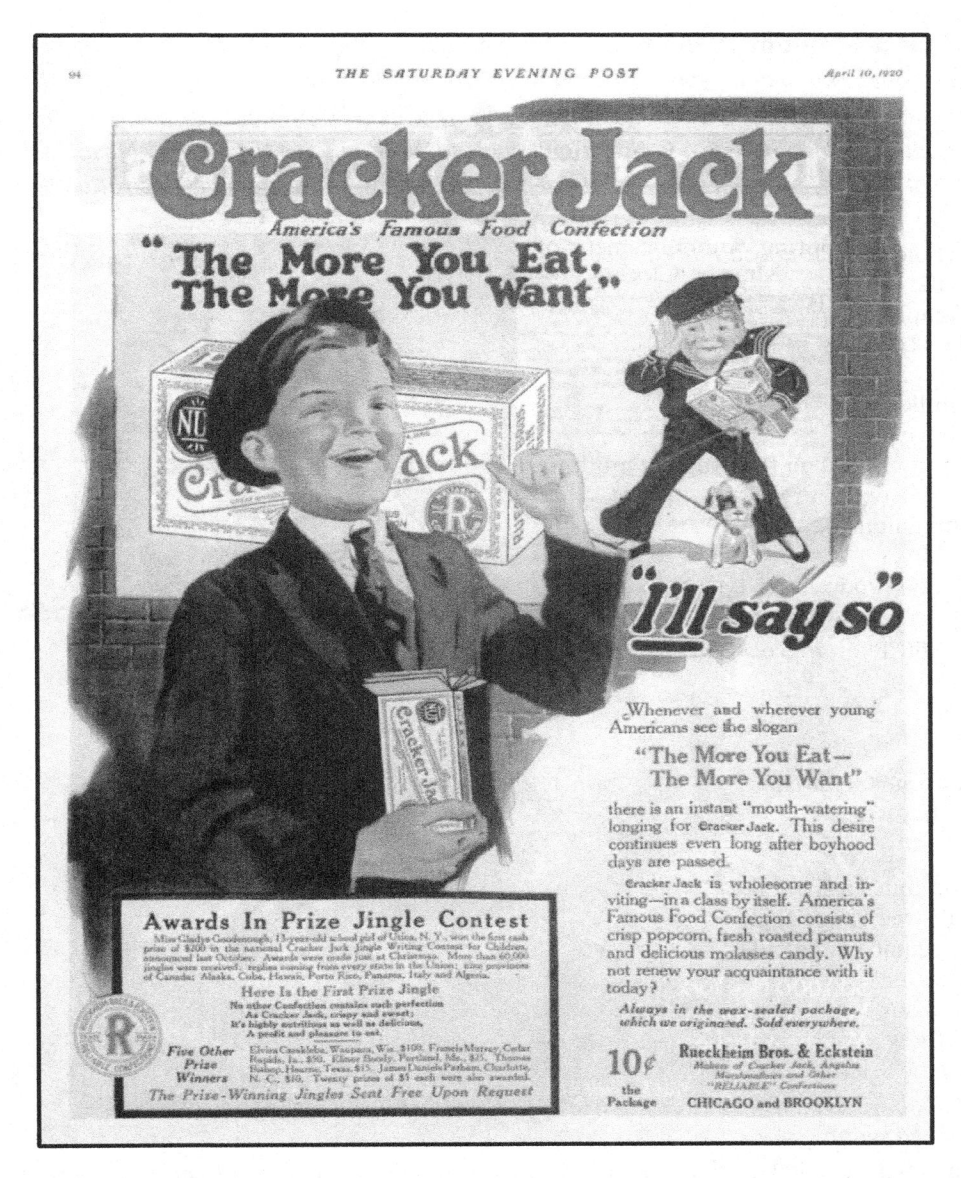

Frederick Rueckheim, in 1893, came up with a new popcorn creation for the Chicago World's Fair. When his brother Louis arrived from Germany, they established the F.W. Rueckheim & Bro. Company. In 1896, the name Cracker Jack was officially registered, and the familiarly sticky and sweet candy we know today was born. In 1912, Rueckheim Bros & Eckstein began adding tiny prizes to each box of Cracker Jack. In 1918, Sailor Jack and his dog Bingo were added to the packaging.

# Desserts for Special Occasions

### Banana Crunch Muffins YUMM (Nicole Hammond)

*It is important to me that my food is delicious, nutritious, and beautiful in presentation. This seriously brings me great joy. I care a lot about my health and my family's health, and I have a background in Health Science and Nutrition Coaching. Now halfway through my Master's degree program at Pacific College of Health and Science, I learn new ideas and gain inspiration daily.*

1 cup whole wheat or coconut flour
1 cup oats
¼ cup maple syrup
3 mashed bananas
2 eggs
½ cup milk of your choice
¼ cup olive oil
½ cup granola and more to top the muffins
2 tsp vanilla extract
1 tsp cinnamon
1 tsp baking powder
½ tsp baking soda

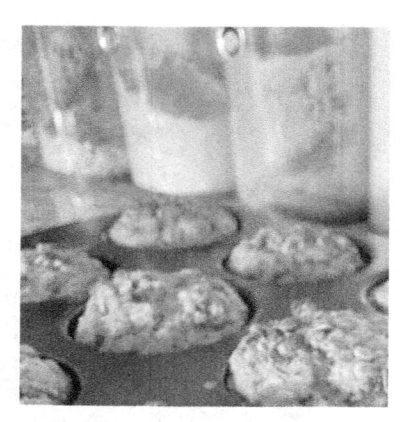

Bake at 350°F for approximately 20 minutes or until golden.


### Flan (Basque Custard)
Serves 10-12

½ cup organic sugar
6 organic free-range eggs
4 cups organic whole milk
1 cup organic sugar
1 tsp vanilla
1 tsp nutmeg
⅛ tsp Celtic Sea salt

*Caramelized sugar*
In a heavy 8 inch skillet, cook the ½ cup sugar over medium high heat (do not stir) until the sugar begins to melt. Shake the skillet occasionally. Reduce heat to low and cook about 5 minutes more or until sugar is golden brown, frequently stirring with a wooden spoon. Remove the skillet from heat and immediately pour the caramelized sugar into a 10 inch quiche or custard dish. Quickly rotate the dish to coat the bottom evenly.

In a large bowl beat eggs.
Add milk, 1 cup sugar, vanilla, nutmeg, and salt. Stir well; do not beat.

Place the custard pan in a large roasting pan, then place on the oven rack. Pour egg mixture into caramel-coated pan. Pour boiling water into the roasting pan to encircle the custard pan at a depth of 1 inch.

Bake in a 325°F oven for 40-45 minutes or until a knife inserted near the center comes out clean. Cool on a wire rack. Cover and chill at least 4 hours or overnight.

To serve: Unmold onto a serving plate with sides.

### **Pizzelles** (Cynthia Edmunds)

*Pizzelles are Italian cookies. They are crisp and very delicious! It does require a special cooking iron to make these, which are readily available online. In my house these are always made around the holidays, especially when guests were coming over.*

3 eggs
¾ cup granulated sugar
½ cup melted unsalted butter OR vegetable oil
1 tbsp vanilla extract*
1¾ cups all-purpose flour
2 tsp baking powder
Extra oil for the pizzelle iron

In a large bowl, beat the eggs until lemon in color, 2-3 minutes. Beat in sugar until well-mixed. Add remaining ingredients, beating until smooth.

Heat the pizzelle iron according to directions. When iron is at appropriate temperature, lightly oil. Place a rounded tablespoonful of batter into center of each design and cook 1-3 minutes (depending on your iron) until lightly browned and steam stops coming from the iron. Remove and cool. If preferred, you can lightly dust with powdered sugar.

Pizzelles should be a bit crisp. If they are soft, they have not cooked long enough.

*You can substitute anise extract and add 1-2 tablespoons anise seed for a licorice-like flavor.

** To make chocolate pizzelles, add ¼ cup cocoa powder and add an extra ¼ cup granulated sugar.

### **Cookies That Bring Joy** (*Saint Hildegard's Kitchen*)

12 tbsp plus 1 tsp organic butter
¾ cup organic sugar
2 tbsp organic blackstrap molasses

⅓ cup raw honey
4 egg yolks
2½ cups spelt flour
1 tsp sea salt
2 rounded tbsp of "Spices of Joy" mixture

*Spices of Joy*
1 tbsp nutmeg
1 tbsp cinnamon
1 tsp clove

With a mixer combine sugar and molasses; set aside. Melt butter under low heat, add sugar blend, honey, and slightly beaten egg yolks. Add flour, Spices of Joy, and salt, and combine gently. Refrigerate after mixing.

Roll out onto a floured surface. Cut into shapes or use a cookie cutter.
Bake on a baking sheet at 400°F for 10-15 minutes until just golden, watching closely.

> *"Take one whole nutmeg, add equal amount of cinnamon and a pinch of cloves, grind this together until it forms a fine powder; add the flour and a little water. Make small cookies and eat these often. They will reduce the bad humors, enrich the blood and fortify the nerves."*
>
> *"Children may eat up to three cookies a day, adults may eat five. These cookies may help strengthen the five senses and may prevent aging. They may remove hate from the heart, assure good intelligence, reduce harmful juices (secretions), and make one have a joyful spirit."*
>
> ~ Hildegard of Bingen
> 12th century Benedictine Abbess

## Welsh Cookies (Cynthia Edmunds)

*This is a story of lost heritage. I was given this recipe when I was a teenager, something my grandmother would make. I never really thought about where it came from and was never told. Turns out, after doing a lot of genealogical research, I have a fair bit of Welsh ancestry on my father's side. I still don't have the answer as to where exactly this recipe came from. Was it handed down through my relatives? And I'll never know at this point after my paternal grandparents are deceased, as is my father, but I like to think this is something that was handed down through a few generations to reach me. Even if it isn't, it's still delicious!*

*As for the cookies themselves, sometimes they are called Welsh Cakes. They are made more like pancakes and vaguely resemble a scone in texture. Traditionally they are made with dried currants, but you could do a more modern twist by adding cranberries, blueberries, etc., if you like.*

Makes 40 cookies

3 cups all-purpose flour
2 tsp baking powder
½ tsp nutmeg
¼ tsp salt
2 sticks (½ lb) unsalted butter, slightly softened and cut into pieces
1¼ cups granulated sugar
7 oz dried currants
2 eggs
¼-½ cup milk
Extra sugar for sprinkling

In a large bowl combine the flour, baking powder, nutmeg, and salt. Add the butter, cutting with a pastry cutter or two butter knives until crumbly. Stir in the sugar and the currants. Make a well in the center and add the eggs and ¼ cup of milk. Combine with a fork until dough forms. If the dough is too dry you can add a little more milk.

On a floured surface roll the dough out until ¼ inch thick. Using a round cookie cutter or clean glass, cut into rounds.

Heat a griddle on low medium heat. Lightly butter the griddle, then place the rounds on the griddle. Cook until lightly browned, about 3-4 minutes. Flip and cook another 3-4 minutes, until lightly browned. The cookies are perfectly done when the edges are dry but not hard. Remove to a wire rack and immediately sprinkle with some sugar.

Serve warm with tea and enjoy!

## Ginger Molasses Cookies

Makes 20 cookies
Bake at 350°F

1½ cup blanched almond flour
1 tsp coconut flour
1 organic egg
¼ cup organic butter
¼ cup blackstrap molasses
1 tbsp ground ginger

½ tsp ground cinnamon
¼ tsp ground allspice
¼ tsp ground clove
¼ tsp salt
¼ tsp baking soda

*Roll in:*
1 tbsp granulated sugar or succinate
1 tbsp ground cinnamon

Line a baking sheet with parchment paper.
Combine almond flour, coconut flour, baking soda, spices, salt. Mix well to combine.

Add and stir to incorporate egg, molasses, softened butter, and dry ingredients in mixing bowl.

Chill dough for 30 minutes.

Remove cookie dough from the refrigerator and roll into 1 inch balls. Roll cookie dough balls in cinnamon and sugar mixture to coat thoroughly and place on cookie sheet. Do not flatten cookies before baking.

Bake for 8-9 minutes.
Remove from oven. Cool on baking sheet before moving to a wire cooling rack or tray.


## No-Bake Cranberry Nut Energy Bites
Makes 12 bites

9 Medjool dates, pitted and cut in quarters
⅓ cup agave
1 tbsp almond butter
1 tbsp chia seeds
1¼ cup whole grain oats
¼ cup pistachios, shelled
⅓ cup sliced almonds
¾ cup dried cranberries
1 tsp vanilla extract
⅓ cup white chocolate chips

Add dates, agave, almond butter, chia seeds, oats, pistachios, almonds, cranberries, and vanilla in a food processor with a metal blade. Pulse until roughly chopped but not pulverized.

Place oat mixture into a medium mixing bowl. Add white chocolate chips and stir together. Place in refrigerator and chill for about 20 minutes.

Once chilled, use your hands to shape into 1 inch balls, pressing your hands firmly together to shape. A touch more almond butter can be added to help shape and hold, if necessary. Repeat with the remaining mixture.

Note: Store in an airtight container in the refrigerator for up to 1 week.

**Arroz con Leche** (Roseanne Romain adapted from *A Taste of Old Cuba*)
*Rice pudding is such a soothing sweet to me. I remember loving it as a kid, and I still love it to this day. Arroz con Leche is one recipe passed down from mom or grandma to their sons and daughters in Cuban culture. I love that Cuban cuisine is very similar to Italian cuisine. Every family has its own unique version of all the classic dishes. Every cook will have their own special recipe that stays within the family. These are the little things that make tradition and bind families together. It's so cool.*
Serves 8

½ cup Valencia rice
1½ cups water
¾ cups sugar
⅛ tsp salt
5½ cups whole milk
2 cinnamon sticks
1 tsp lime zest
⅛ tsp anise seeds
Ground cinnamon for garnish

Rinse the rice.

Bring your 1½ cups of water, salt, and sugar to boil.
Add rice, stir, cover, and simmer for about 20 minutes or until the water has absorbed and the rice has softened.

While the rice is cooking: scald your milk, anise, and cinnamon sticks in a separate pot. Be careful not to allow it to over boil.

Once the rice has absorbed the water, add the scaled milk to the rice. Stir constantly and bring the mixture to a soft rolling boil. Lower heat to a simmer. Keep the lid off the pot and stir often for the next 40-60 minutes.

The mixture should get very thick; you should be able to draw a line with your finger on the back of your spoon. The rice should be open and very soft.

Transfer to a shallow bowl, and cover with some plastic wrap to avoid creating a skin. Poke some holes in the plastic wrap with a paring knife to allow the pudding to breathe and cool.

Once cooled, refrigerate until thoroughly cold. Sprinkle some ground cinnamon over the top before serving.

*Notes:* This recipe is taken form *A Taste of Old Cuba* by María Josefa Luriá de O'Higgins

## Ashure ~Turkish dessert (Nour Danno)

*This recipe takes prep work, so read it fully.*

½ cup barley
2 oz of dried figs (optionally, also have some for garnish)
2 oz of raisins
2 oz of dried apricots
6 cups water
⅓ cup cooked or canned chickpeas
⅓ cup cooked or canned white beans
2 oz peeled almonds
1 apple
1 tsp salt
1 cinnamon stick
½ cup almond milk
1 cup sugar (or honey)
Pomegranate seeds (optional)
Grated coconut (optional)
Blanched almonds (optional)
Roasted hazelnuts (optional)
Pistachio (optional)

Start by soaking the barley overnight. When ready the next day, wash the figs and then boil for three minutes, drain them, and set aside. Repeat with the raisins; wash, boil for three minutes, drain, set aside. Wash the apricots and immerse them in water for 30 minutes. Drain the apricots, save the water you soaked them in, and then dice them.

In a large stock pot, cook the barley in six cups of water (or according to its package instructions).

Add water if necessary. Cut the apple into large pieces (you will be removing them from the final dish). Halfway through cooking the barley, add the apple and the cinnamon stick and continue cooking until the barley is very tender; almost like porridge. Toward the end of cooking the barley, remove the apple and the cinnamon stick. Add the raisins, the apricots, and their soaking water to the barley, then put in the chickpeas, white beans, almonds, salt, sugar (or honey), and almond milk. Mix it all well and simmer for 10 minutes.

While simmering, dice the cooled figs. Mix them into the barley at the end of cooking.

Transfer into pudding cups or ramekins and let it cool down. Top with more figs or any of the other optional garnishes. Serve at room temperature or refrigerate and serve cold.

### **Hungarian Walnut Cookies** (Chef Ben Qualls)

*Called Kifli, meaning crescent, these delicious cookies were usually served at Christmas time. My grandmother, and later, my mother, made them every year (well, almost) when I was growing up. These cookies are great any time of year, though, not just at Christmas. They go well with a good cup of coffee or tea.*

1 cup butter, softened
1 package (8 oz) cream cheese, softened
2½ cups all-purpose flour

Filling:
3 large egg whites
¾ tsp vanilla extract
⅓ cup sugar
3½ cups ground walnuts
Flour and sugar for rolling pastry

In a large bowl, cream butter and cream cheese until blended. Gradually beat flour into creamed mixture. Divide dough into 3 portions. Shape each into a disk. Wrap and refrigerate 1 hour or until firm enough to roll.

Preheat oven to 375°F. For filling, in a small bowl, beat egg whites and vanilla on medium speed until foamy. Gradually add sugar, 1 tablespoon at a time, beating on medium after each addition until well blended. Stir in walnuts.

Generously coat a work surface with equal parts of flour and sugar. Roll 1 portion of dough into a 12 inch round about ⅛ inch thick, sprinkling with additional flour and sugar as necessary to coat well. Cut into 8-10 wedges. (Like cutting a pie.)

Place about 2 teaspoons of filling onto each wedge. Roll up starting at the wider end. Bend slightly to form a crescent shape. Place 2 inches apart on greased baking sheets. Repeat with remaining dough and filling.

Bake until bottoms are golden brown, 9-11 minutes. Remove from pans to wire racks to cool completely. Dust with confectioners sugar.

### Raw Lemon Cheesecake Bars

*For the crust*
1 cup raw pecans
½ cup walnuts
3 large Medjool dates, pitted
1 tbsp coconut oil
¾ tsp ginger root powder
Pinch of salt

*For the lemon cheesecake layer*
1½ cups raw cashews, soaked
¼ cup dairy-free milk or unsweetened coconut milk
¼ cup fresh squeezed lemon juice
2 tbsp coconut butter
2 tbsp coconut oil
2 tbsp raw honey
1 tsp vanilla extract
Zest from one lemon
Pinch of salt

*Make the crust*
Line an 8x8 inch baking pan with parchment paper. Set aside.
Put the pecans and walnuts in a food processor fitted with a steel blade. Pulse several times to break up the nuts. Add the Medjool dates, coconut oil, ground ginger root, and a pinch of salt. Process until the mixture begins to come together as a dough. Press the nut mixture evenly into the bottom of the lined pan. Set aside.

*Make the filling*
Put the cashews, dairy-free milk, lemon juice, coconut butter, coconut oil, honey, vanilla extract, lemon zest, and a pinch of salt into a high powered blender. Start on low, gradually increase to high, and process until completely smooth.

Scrape the mixture on top of the crust and smooth the top. Cover and place in the freezer for 4-6 hours or overnight.

Let sit at room temperature for 15-20 minutes before cutting and serving.

*Notes:* Don't let this dessert sit at room temperature for too long or it will get very soft. It's best when served chilled.

## 5-Minute Guilt Free YUMM-OHH Pudding (Karen Langston)

*If you want to eat this pudding right away but want it cold, refrigerate the ingredients overnight, then make.*

2 ripe avocados, medium sized
1 ripe organic banana
¼ cup fair trade cocoa powder (if you want it chocolatier, add 1-2 tbsp)
¼ cup coconut milk (I use Aroy-D)
1 tbsp honey
¼ tsp organic cinnamon
¼ tsp organic vanilla extract

Peel the avocados, remove the pits, spoon out flesh, and add to food processor. Peel the banana, and break into chunks; add to the food processor. Add remaining ingredients; blend until smooth and no avocado clumps remain. Serve in bowls.

## Rhubarb-Berry Spoon Cake (Mark's Kitchen)

Serves 8

1 cup fresh rhubarb, chopped
¾ cup fresh strawberries, chopped
¾ cup monk fruit sweetener, divided
1 tbsp lemon zest
1 tbsp arrowroot flour
½ cup coconut flour
1 cup fine almond flour
1 tbsp baking powder
8 large pasture-raised eggs, room temperature
½ cup plain unsweetened goat or sheep yogurt (or substitute with dairy-free)
1 tbsp vanilla extract
1 tbsp coconut oil, melted (plus a bit extra for greasing)

*Garnish*
Blueberries
Coconut whipped cream

Preheat the oven to 350°F. Brush 8 individual 6 inch oven safe ramekins with coconut oil. (Alternatively, you can bake one large cake in an 8x8 inch baking dish. Begin checking the cake for readiness around 40 minutes of baking time. It's done when golden brown and a toothpick inserted in the middle comes out clean.)

In a small mixing bowl, add the rhubarb, strawberries, 2 tablespoons of monk fruit (reserve the rest for the next step), lemon zest, and arrowroot flour. Stir to combine and set aside.

In a separate mixing bowl, whisk together the coconut flour, almond flour, salt, baking powder, and the remaining ½ cup plus 2 tablespoon of monk fruit.

In a third mixing bowl, whisk together the eggs, yogurt, vanilla, and melted coconut oil. Once smooth, begin adding the dry ingredients in intervals until fully incorporated and no lumps remain. The batter should have the consistency of pancake batter.

Gently fold the strawberry-rhubarb mix into the cake batter.
Pour the cake batter into the greased ramekins and bake for 35 minutes on a middle rack in the oven until golden brown and a toothpick poked in the center comes out clean.

Serve with optional blueberries and coconut whipped cream.

### Sicilian Olive Oil, Almond Flour Cake (Roseanne Romaine)
*Being a pastry chef and being Sicilian, this recipe is close to my heart. Oddly I had to learn a lot about my cultural traditions. My grandma passed when I was rather young, and my mom, the youngest of nine, seemed to have missed a lot of the traditional cooking methods. She remembers the constant pot on the stove and the daily loaves of bread being baked, but not the recipes. These have passed, unfortunately, with my older aunts. I am told I had uncles who loved to bake, and rumor has it they were pretty good.*
Serves 8

1 lemon, zested
2 tbsp lemon juice
¼ cup local honey
½ tsp vanilla
¼ cup extra virgin olive oil
2 large eggs
¼ tsp salt
1½ cups almond flour
1½ tsp baking powder
8 fresh figs

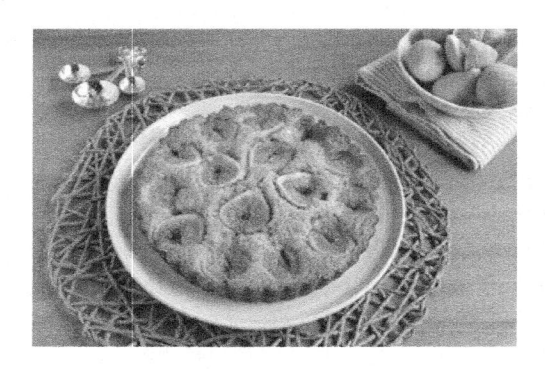

Heat oven to 350°F
Butter a 9 inch glass pie pan well.
In a medium bowl whisk together lemon zest, lemon juice, honey, vanilla, oil, eggs and salt.
In a large bowl whisk together the almond flour and baking powder.

Add the wet ingredients to your dry ingredients and stir until smooth. Pour your batter into the greased cake pan.

Slice your ripe figs in half, and arrange in a circular pattern on the top of your batter with the seeds facing up to create a flower effect.

Place the cake on the middle rack of the oven and bake for 35 minutes or until a knife comes out clean from the center.

Allow the cake to cool before serving. This cake is delicious as is or can be served with some fresh whipped cream, cultured sour cream, mascarpone cheese, and vanilla gelato.

### Coconut Milk Ice Cream (Tammera Karr)

To make this you need an ice cream maker. I like the Rival® 1 quart maker where you freeze the bowl, no messing with ice and salt; it's just the right size for 2-4 servings. Ready in 20-30 minutes.

1 can organic coconut milk
⅛-¼ cup raw honey or real maple syrup
Pinch xanthan gum (optional)
1 tsp real vanilla

Blend in a food processor, blender or by hand until smooth. Add flavorings listed below. Stir in chunk flavorings before placing in an ice cream freezer bowl. Follow mixer recommendations for freeze and set time.

*Additional additions*
¼ cup dark chocolate chunks
¼ cup mixed frozen berries
¼ cup chopped nuts

### 18th Century Apricot Ice Cream (Dr. Juneisy Q. Hawkins)

*While ice cream may sound like a modern-age food, a food from the age of refrigeration and freezers, people have been eating ice cream since well before those things came around in the 19th and 20th centuries. In fact, if we use the term "ice cream" loosely to mean frozen sweets, wealthy ancient Romans were eating it at least since the 1st century CE.*
Yields 1¼ quarts

12 ripe apricots (about 2½ lbs)
2½ cups heavy cream
¾ cups white granulated sugar; if using caster sugar, 6 oz

Blender or food processor
2 quart ice cream machine

1. Set a large pot of water to boil. Take your apricots and score an X at the bottom of each one.

2. Prepare a large bowl with ice cubes and water.

3. When the water in the pot is boiling, carefully drop the apricots in the boiling water. Allow the water to come back up to a boil and leave the apricots in the boiling water for 60 seconds.

4. Remove the apricots from the boiling water and immediately transfer them to the ice bath to stop the cooking. When cool enough to handle, peel the apricots, cut them in half, remove the pit, and cut them into chunks.

5. Add the cream and sugar to a small pot. Set it over medium heat, stirring frequently, until bubbles begin to rise at the edges of the cream. If using a thermometer, at this point the milk should register 180°F.

6. Place the chopped apricots and the milk and sugar mixture in a blender or food processor. Blend until smooth. You may have to do this in batches, depending on the size of your appliance.

7. Set a fine mesh strainer over a large bowl and pour the mixture through it. With the back of a rubber spatula, push the mixture though the strainer, but do not scrape the pulp that accumulates on the outside of the strainer into the bowl.

8. Cover the bowl with plastic wrap. Allow the mixture to cool down on the counter, then put it in the refrigerator for at least 4 hours or until it is no warmer than 40°F. If you are using an ice cream machine with a compressor, you may be able to skip the refrigeration part.

9. Churn the mixture according to your ice cream machine's instructions. Once fully churned, transfer the mixture to a freezer safe container or to silicone molds if you are feeling fancy.

10. Allow the ice cream to fully freeze, which can take several hours. Take it out of the freezer about 10 minutes before eating.

The flavor of this ice cream is truly fruity. The apricot flavor comes through clearly, and it's a little tart. It's perfect for those who don't like their sweets too sweet.
https://www.historicalfoodways.com/apricot-ice-cream-from-the-18th-century/?fbclid=IwAR2rccXKMKTUEor0naIWwBRkH3CUkupsS-Rmk5O3HgAYdHaz1hgXkRuXGuI#recipe


### Mincedmeat (Chris Smith *The Cookery of England, 1977*)
*Chris, who is from England, and Tammera have had long debates on mincemeat. Even the spelling of the word came into the conversation, mince meat, mincemeat or minced meat, mincedmeat. So, in fairness here is his version dating back to the 1760s.*
Makes 24 small pies

1 lb raisins
¼ lb sultanas
½ lb dark chunky marmalade
½ lb suet
½ lemon
½ tsp mixed spice
1 large glass brandy

½ lb currants
¼ lb candied peel
½ lb demerara sugar
1 lb good cooking apples
¼ tsp nutmeg
A good pinch ground ginger

Wash all the dried fruit. Grate the rind of the lemon. Peel, core and slice the apples. Put all the dry ingredients through a mincer. When minced, stir well, add lemon juice and brandy, stir again, fill into jars and tie down so they are airtight. Keep in a dry, cool place.

All mincedmeat should be prepared at least a fortnight before Christmas, and to make it in November is still better.


### Food of the Gods Chocolate Mousse (Tammera Karr)

1 cup organic sugar
¾ cup organic butter
¼ cup organic cocoa powder
1 tsp Mexican vanilla
½ tsp cinnamon
1 oz Mexican tequila
Small pinch cayenne pepper
3 large organic eggs

Soften and cream butter and slowly add sugar, cocoa, and spices, and then tequila and vanilla. Mix on medium high speed until well-blended. One at a time while mixer is running, add raw eggs (with a pause of 60 seconds between each one). Turn the mixer to high and beat for a smooth froth (about 2 minutes).

Place a small amount into small dishes and place in the refrigerator to firm up (about 30 minutes). Serve with a topping of fresh organic whipped cream and a sliver of organic dark chocolate. This is very decadent and rich; it melts like silk in the mouth and will make chocolate lovers sigh.


### Ricotta Pie (Miriam G. Zacharias)

1 lb of part skim ricotta (the 15 oz packages work ok)
3 eggs
¾ cup sugar
1 tsp vanilla
½ tsp orange extract

½ tsp lemon extract
1½ tsp flour

Mix well in a bowl by hand; do not use an electric mixer. Pour into regular depth pie crust. Bake 50-60 minutes at 350°F. Cool to room temperature, then refrigerate.


## Mock Apple Fritter (Michael Karr)

*If you are hungry for something sweet but need to be careful with sugar and gluten, here is our solution.*

2 cups of Libby's Baking Mix
2 cups chopped apple
3 tbsp coconut sugar
1 tsp cinnamon
¼ cup applesauce
¼-½ cup water, approximately

Combine baking mix, sugar, cinnamon, and apples. Mix well.
Add applesauce and mix well. Add water slowly while stirring (you may not use all or might need a little more); you want a thick, muffin-like batter.

Butter a cast iron skillet or a glass baking pan. Add dough.

Bake at 375°F for 15-20 minutes, depending on size and depth of your pan. Check at 15 minutes with a butter knife inserted in the center. If it comes away clean your mock apple fritter is done. Sprinkle a little cinnamon and maple sugar on top. Let cool, then cut into small squares.


## Apricot Tansy (Chris Smith *The Cookery of England, 1977*)

Serves 4

1 lb fresh apricots
Butter
Caster sugar
4 eggs
2 tbsp double cream
A very little nutmeg

Stone the apricots, quarter them, and gently fry in butter until they are quite soft. Sprinkle with about 2 ounces sugar and set aside in the pan.

Beat together the eggs, cream, 1 tablespoon caster sugar, and the nutmeg, and set aside. Just before serving, make the pan with apricots hot so that they are just sizzling. Put in a little more butter if at all dry. Stir the egg mixture and pour it over the apricots; stir it very gently among them. After about 2 minutes, it should have set at the bottom. Turn it on to a plate.

Melt a little more butter in the pan and slide it back, the un-browned side (which has the most egg) downwards. Fry 2 minutes more and serve at once. It should be a little soft but not liquid in the middle. Sift sugar over it and serve thick cream separately.

**Salted Caramel Pecan Pie**

*Crust*
1 cup of cashews, soaked for 3 hours, rinsed, and strained
1 tbsp coconut oil or ghee
1 tbsp honey
1 tsp vanilla
½ cup shredded coconut

*Filling*
One packed cup pitted Medjool dates, soaked for 3 hours in 1 cup of water (save the soaking water)
¼ cup coconut oil or ghee
1 tbsp vanilla
½ tsp pink salt

*Fold-In*
2 cups salted roasted pecans, plus more to garnish

Pre-heat oven to 400°F.

Purée the cashews, oil, honey, and vanilla crust ingredients in a food processor fitted with the S-blade for about 1 minute. Add the shredded coconut and purée to form a ball.
Using wet hands press the crust into a greased 9 inch glass pie dish. Do NOT pre-bake the crust.

Add all of the filling ingredients, including the soaking water, to the blender and puree until smooth. Fold in the pecans, then add the filling to the unbaked crust. Garnish the pie with more pecans.

Bake for 10 minutes, then reduce the heat to 350°F and bake for 10 minutes more. Allow to cool on the counter, then refrigerate to set.

Serve with whipped coconut cream.

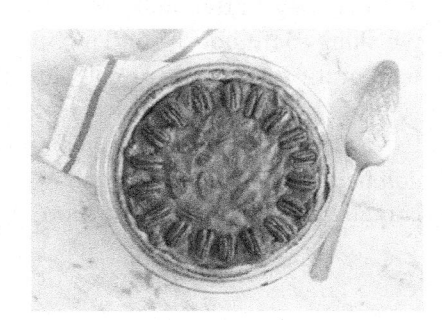

## Spiced Truffles

8 oz 100% dark chocolate
¼ cup clarified butter
⅔ cup maple syrup
½ cup coconut milk
⅛ tsp coarse Celtic Sea salt
3 tbsp cocoa powder
⅛ tsp ground clove
¼ tsp ground cinnamon

Shave chocolate and place in a medium bowl.

Warm honey, butter, milk, and salt in a sauce pan. Once warm, pour the mixture over chocolate, whisking continuously until mixture becomes smooth. Let the mixture come to room temperature, then cover tightly and refrigerate until chocolate is firm, about 2-3 hours.

Use a tablespoon or melon baller and scoop out truffles. Roll into balls, slightly smaller than a golf ball, and gently roll around in cocoa powder. Refrigerate until serving. Store in an airtight container in the refrigerator for up to a week.

## Natillas – Custard Cream (Kelsi Sitz)
Serves 6

8 egg yolks
4 cups whole milk
1 cup organic sugar
1 cinnamon stick
Powdered cinnamon
1 tbsp corn starch or arrowroot

Put 2 cups of milk in a sauce pan with the cinnamon stick and bring to a boil. Beat the egg yolks with the sugar in a large bowl. Dissolve the corn starch or arrowroot in the rest of the milk, stir well and add to the egg and sugar. Once the milk is boiled, remove the cinnamon stick and add the egg, sugar and thickener mixture. Cook until the custard thickens, do not boil. Serve in individual bowls with a sprinkle of cinnamon on the top.

### Dad's No-Bake Cheese Cake  (Sharena Graves)

*My father started making this cheesecake when he was a young adult. He loved to bake and create new dishes and one day become a baker. He started off making this cheesecake for his mother and family gatherings. When my father married, my mother and her girlfriends tasted the cheesecake. After that, more requests for his cheesecake started pouring in from her workplace, church events, friends, and so on.  As I got older, his cheesecake quickly became popular among my friends, cousins, and godchildren.  And I plan to use this recipe for generations to come.*

8 oz cream cheese, full fat (soften)
1 can of condense sweetened milk
¼ cup lemon juice
1 tsp real vanilla
Graham cracker crust

Set cream cheese out at room temperature until it's soft.
Blend softened cream cheese with condensed milk on low until mixed (about 2 minutes.)
Add lemon and vanilla.

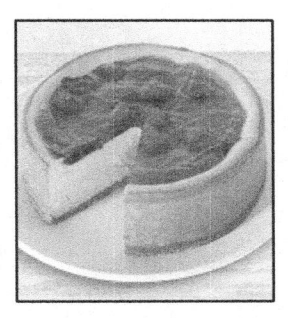

Stop blender, mix with a spatula, and then blend on high for 3 minutes.
Batter should be thick, no lumps. If it's thin, let it sit in the refrigerator for about 10-15 minutes to thicken up.

Pour batter onto crust and place in refrigerator for 24 hours.
Add topping the following day.

*Cherry topping*
2½ cups of cherries
Water
½ tsp vanilla
1 tsp maple syrup
1 tsp or more of roux for thickening (butter and flour mix)

Add cherries and about ¼ cup of water or more to a pan.
Smash some of the cherries to release juices.
Add vanilla and maple syrup.
Let the mixture come to a simmer and add the roux.

Simmer until thick.  Let it cool before adding to the cheesecake.
Enjoy!

> **Principle 28**: *Special foods are always a part of Cultural events, so be kind to yourself and those around you and savor the flavor and connection of traditions.*

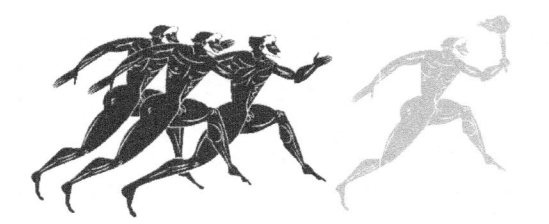

Cheesecake dates back over 4,000 years to the Greek island of Samos. Anthropologists excavated cheese molds there, which date to circa 2000 BC. Cheesecake was considered a good energy source. There is evidence it was served to the athletes at the first Olympic Games in 776 BC. Cheesecake history also includes a simple wedding cake made from flour, wheat, honey, and cheese. Food historians have recovered what may be the earliest know written recipe for cheesecake, dating to 230 AD.[196]

---

[196] The Rich History of a Favorite Dessert, retrieved September 2022: https://www.cheesecake.com/History-Of-Cheesecake.asp

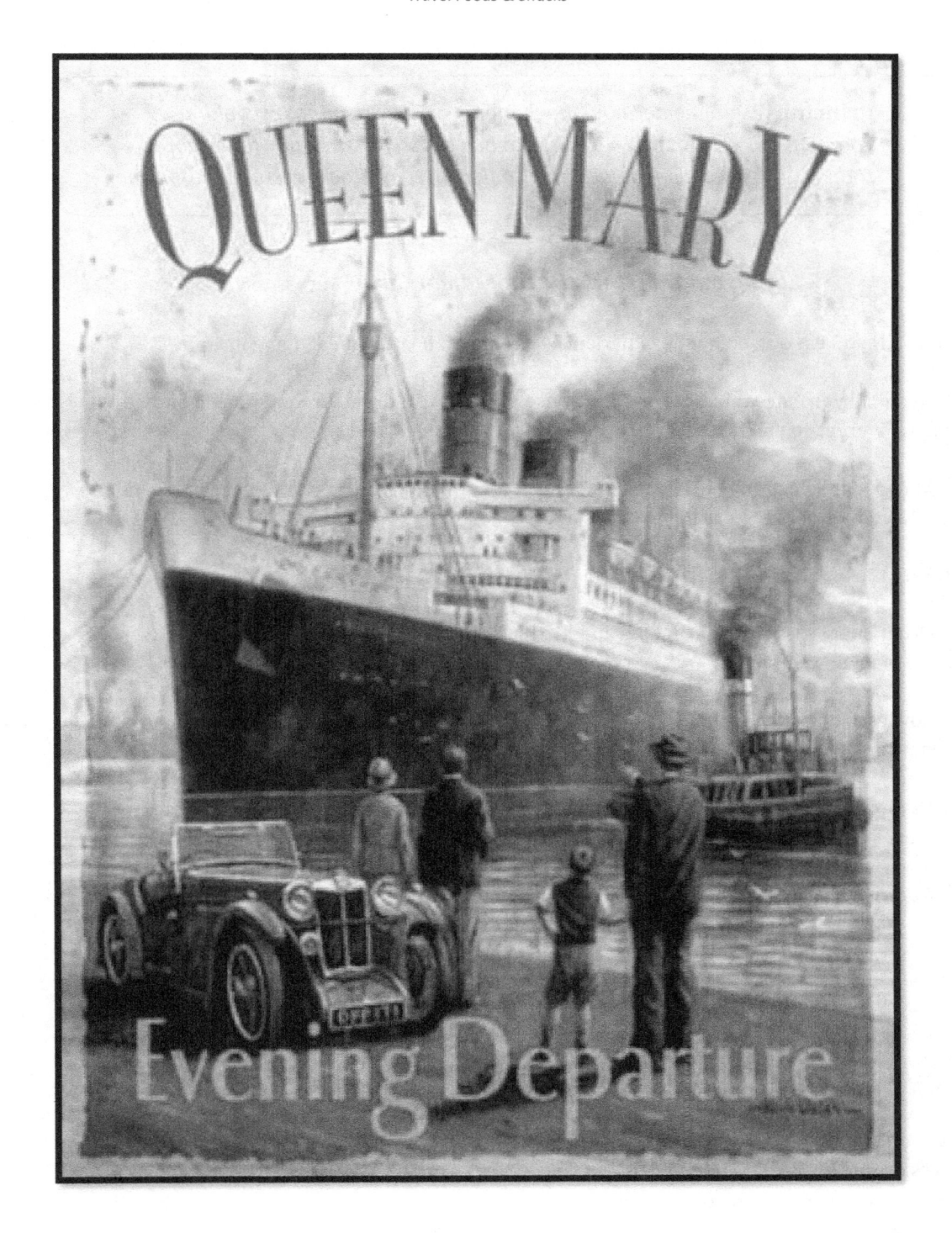

## Travel Food & Snacks

> **Principle 29:** *Consider how much money you are saving by cooking yourself! For example, it costs less to buy grass-fed steak for four people than it does to buy a feedlot steak cooked in a mediocre restaurant for one.*

### *7 Eating out tips from the Ingredient Guru* (Mira Dessy, NE)

You CAN still eat out, enjoy the experience, and have a healthy meal doing it.

1. Avoid all you can eat buffets or steakhouses. These restaurants frequently encourage you to overeat so you feel like you are "getting your money's worth."

2. Make your selection before you get to the restaurant and are possibly overwhelmed or sidelined by smells, the setting, or specials.

3. Skip the bread or chips basket.

4. Order soup, a small salad, and an appetizer, or two appetizers and a small salad in place of an entree.

5. Low carb does not mean low calorie. Restaurants may choose to add fat or sugars to enhance the flavor, but it boosting the calorie count.

6. Ask for your salad dressing on the side. This allows you to manage how much dressing you use.

7. Ask for salsa instead of sour cream or butter for your baked potato.

For more information, go to: https://theingredientguru.com/

### *Travel Tips; for plane, train, boat, bus, or car*

**Seasonings:** Bring salt, pepper, and spices from home with you. Plan and pack small glass or safe plastic jars with herbs and spices. Spices at the grocery store are insanely expensive, compounding the cost when you only use a little during your vacation. Even if the kitchens are well stocked the spices are probably years old.

**Travel kit:** When traveling by car, carry a small camp stove, cutting board, wooden spoon, spork, cup, and a sharp knife for impromptu or planned picnics.

**Dehydrated individual servings**: Bone broth, coffee, tea, oatmeal cups, and creamers are lightweight and easy to pack in a carry-on.

**Veggie sticks**: Sliced fennel bulbs (helps prevent gas), snap peas, carrots, celery, red bell peppers, and raw yam.

**Fruit:** Sliced apples, pears, and pineapple, whole strawberries and cherries, and peeled citrus. When combined in a container pineapple helps keep apples and pears from browning.

**Finger steaks:** Make marinated meat finger strips of well-done elk, venison, pork, beef or chicken. Ensure the meat is chilled thoroughly or frozen before tucking it into your carry on.

**Water:** Keeping yourself well-hydrated can help prevent you from catching a prevalent virus on planes and in airports. Packets of Airborne® to load one or more water bottles helps support your immune system. These types of products also contain vitamin C and B vitamins for energy.

**Meal replacement bars and nut bars** are handy for breakfast or snacks while sightseeing and require no refrigeration. Watch the sugar content and nuts. These may add to water retention and inflammation.

**Hand sanitizer** made with peppermint or clove oil and ethanol are safer than those using synthetic chemicals. Your skin will fare better steering clear of antibacterial products.


### Trail Mix in Minutes (Tammera Karr)
*Use one bag each of the following from Costco® or a bulk food store; it costs a fraction of the prepackaged store brands, and there are no processed fats or added sugars. Substitute more low oxalate seeds and nuts for almonds if chronic inflammation is a challenge.*
Approximately 8 quarts

Raw almonds (or oxalate free seeds)
Raw pecans
Coconut flakes
Dried cherries
Dried blueberries
½ bag of dried cranberries
1 small bag of organic dark chocolate chips

Combine all ingredients in a large 16 quart mixing bowl or container. Blend thoroughly with a spoon or your hands. Fill quart freezer bags or glass pint jars, place in the freezer for easy grab and go.

## Dining Out Tips for Gluten Sensitivity

- ✓ Avoid the busiest time of day to eat out.

- ✓ Always use gluten and dairy sensitivity enzymes 20 minutes before eating. This helps reduce the severity of the reaction if one occurs.

- ✓ Check menus and offerings beforehand. Even while waiting, you can look at the offering on the Internet.

- ✓ Talk to the food service management staff about what they offer that is gluten-free. Be thorough in your questioning and polite.

- ✓ Sandwich, omelet, and salad bars can be options if they have gluten-free meats and sauces.

- ✓ Bring your own condiments or do without.

- ✓ Select individually wrapped gluten-free foods.

- ✓ Politely request the server making your salad or food change their gloves to reduce cross contact.

- ✓ When possible, take a portion of food you have pre-prepared.

### Granola (Tammera Karr)

2 lb bag gluten-free Old Fashioned oats
1 cup dried cranberries or blueberries
1 cup chopped raw pecans
1 cup slivered raw almonds (or seeds)
1 cup Bob's Red Mill® Coconut Flakes
1 cup melted organic butter
½ cup warm local honey

1 tsp ground cinnamon
¼ tsp ground clove
1 tsp real vanilla

Mix dry ingredients with spices, breaking up any clumps of dried fruits. Add melted butter and warm honey, mixing well to distribute honey and butter evenly through the mix. Heat oven to 300°F.

Place raw granola on a jelly roll pan(s); spread out evenly and not too thick. Place in oven for 15 minutes. Stir to prevent burning or over-toasting on bottom and edges, and cook for additional 15 minutes. Stir once more. If edges are brown and the mixture has a beautiful golden-brown color, set out to cool.

Cooking times vary on local ingredients and elevation. Approximate cook time: 30 minutes. When cool, place in glass mason jars with lids and store in refrigerator or freezer to preserve oil freshness.

### Beef Heart Jerky (Tammera Karr)
*This tastes the same as jerky made from the loin or large cuts of beef. Nutrient-dense. Easy to make in a food dehydrator.*

1 beef heart trimmed (usually 3-4 lbs)
¼ cup tamari sauce
⅛ cup cider vinegar or sweet rice vinegar
1 tsp of smoked paprika
1-2 tsp of garlic powder
1 tsp of chili flakes
1-2 tsp of Celtic Sea salt
½ tsp of pepper
2 tsp turmeric powder
¼ cup raw honey
4 tbsp liquid hickory, pecan, apple smoke (Colgin®)
1 quart water

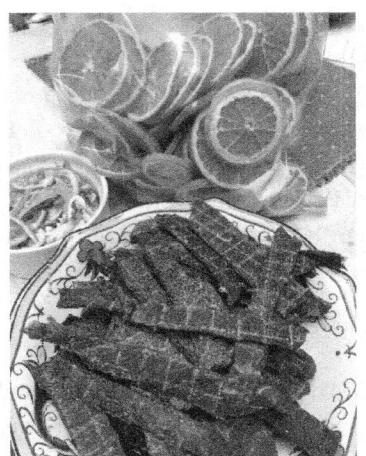

Begin by trimming the beef heart of excess connective tissue, fat, and valves. Once the beef heart has been cleaned, slice the meat into thin strips or pieces. The thinner the slices the better they dry in a dehydrator.

Place the beef heart slices into a glass bowl and add tamari sauce, vinegar, honey, water, liquid smoke, and spices. Cover, refrigerate, and marinate for 24 hours. Turning over the contents three times during marinating ensures equal coverage of the meat.

The next day, preheat dehydrator to 150-170°F (meat setting in owner's manual). Place the slices onto the dehydrator racks. Make sure there is space between the slices. Allow to dry for 5-8 hours.

The jerky is ready when it is dry, chewy and crispy.

Store in an airtight **NON Metal** container (meat will spoil in stainless steel or other metal containers) in the pantry, freezer or refrigerator to preserve freshness.

## *Ice Cold*

Summer travel, camping, rolling blackouts, forest fire evacuations, power outages, and the pandemic have affected millions of people worldwide. The pandemic launched the second golden age for RV travel and family camping trips. With each of these, keeping food fresh and reducing waste is paramount. Ice chests and crushed or block ice are the standard go-to, but the pool of water and soggy food are a common result. Even when using contained blue ice products, they fail to keep food cool enough for more than a few hours.

*Consider:* Dry ice will keep your food or drinks colder and will evaporate instead of melt.

**Method:** [197, 198]

1. Dry ice can be used with most coolers if there's a way to ventilate them. To ventilate evaporating gas from the cooler, use a lid that doesn't seal shut entirely or a drainage cap (usually located near the bottom of the cooler). If you need a small cooler or just want to use the dry ice for a day, choose a foam free biodegradable or urethane-insulated box (3 inches thick). For longer dry ice use or for a larger cooler, choose a rotomolded or plastic cooler.

2. Cut pieces of cardboard to protect the plastic from cold and lay them on the bottom and the sides of the cooler.

3. To prevent damage to the cooler, leave the lid slightly cracked or unscrew the drainage cap a little. **Wear gloves to protect your hands when you handle the dry ice.**

4. Buy 10-20 pounds (4.5 to 9 kilograms) of dry ice for every 24 hours. A 40-60 quarter cooler (37-56 liters) usually requires 10 pounds (4.5 kg) of dry ice for one day. Most dry ice is available in large blocks or chunks. Blocks will last longer than small pieces or pellets of dry ice. Wrap blocks of dry ice in newspaper. The newspaper will insulate and slow down the evaporation. Newspaper can also prevent touching the dry ice with bare hands. Pack the gaps with newspaper and cover the dry ice with a piece of cardboard, providing an even surface for food and added insulation.

5. To quickly freeze fish, meat, or game, place food on the bottom of the cooler with the dry ice on top. Put the dry ice in the bottom of the cooler to keep food and drinks cold.

6. Dry ice will evaporate (releasing $CO_2$) on its own over several hours or days, depending on how it's stored. If you need to dispose of dry ice, do not put it in a sink. Take the cooler outside, place cooler with the lid off or askew in a safe location away from children or animals.

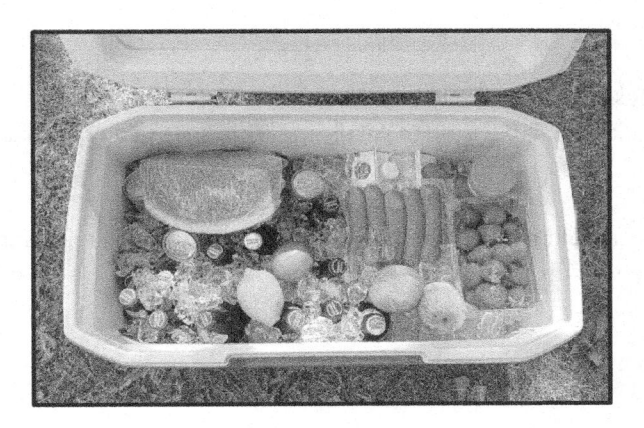

## *After Arriving at Your Destination - Guidelines*

- Eat a breakfast that contains protein and complex carbohydrates; naturally fermented vegetables, oatmeal, nuts, and fruit.

- Have at least one glass of warm water with fresh lemon pulp and rind. This will activate the liver and bowels reducing constipation.

- Minimize dairy as it can be mucus-forming and lead to chest, nasal and constipation.

- Make lunch your biggest meal.

- Begin each meal with a salad and use vinegar as the dressing or on steamed vegetables. Adding as little as a tablespoon of vinegar to a meal can lower the overall glycemic load, reduce blood sugar, blood pressure, and stimulate healthy digestion, reducing the likelihood of GERD or heartburn.

- Make dinner your smallest meal and load up on vegetables. You will rest better and have more energy for the next day of sightseeing.

- Take your time eating. Meals generally last up to 5 hours in many countries, this allows for conversation, savoring and digesting the foods before you.

- Go easy on the coffee as it can increase muscle cramps and lower back pain if kidneys are overworked.

- Keep alcohol, fried foods, and desserts to a minimum. All these can elevate blood sugars, making you feel fatigued the next day.

- Get out and move every day.

- Drink water: 4 glasses a day of 6-8 ounces will prevent water retention, light-headedness, headaches, and low back pain. Tip: Drink in small sips. This keeps you from running to every bathroom in town.

- Eating healthy while traveling can prevent unwanted weight gain, jet lag, and water retention while keeping energy levels up.

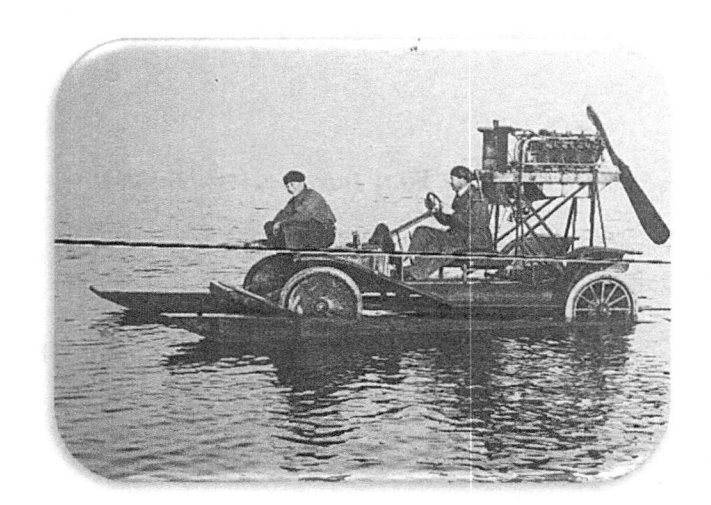

---

[197] How to Use Dry Ice in a Cooler PDF: retrieved August 2022. https://www.wikihow.com/Use-Dry-Ice-in-a-Cooler

[198] Dry Ice Safety Tips: https://penguindryice.com/

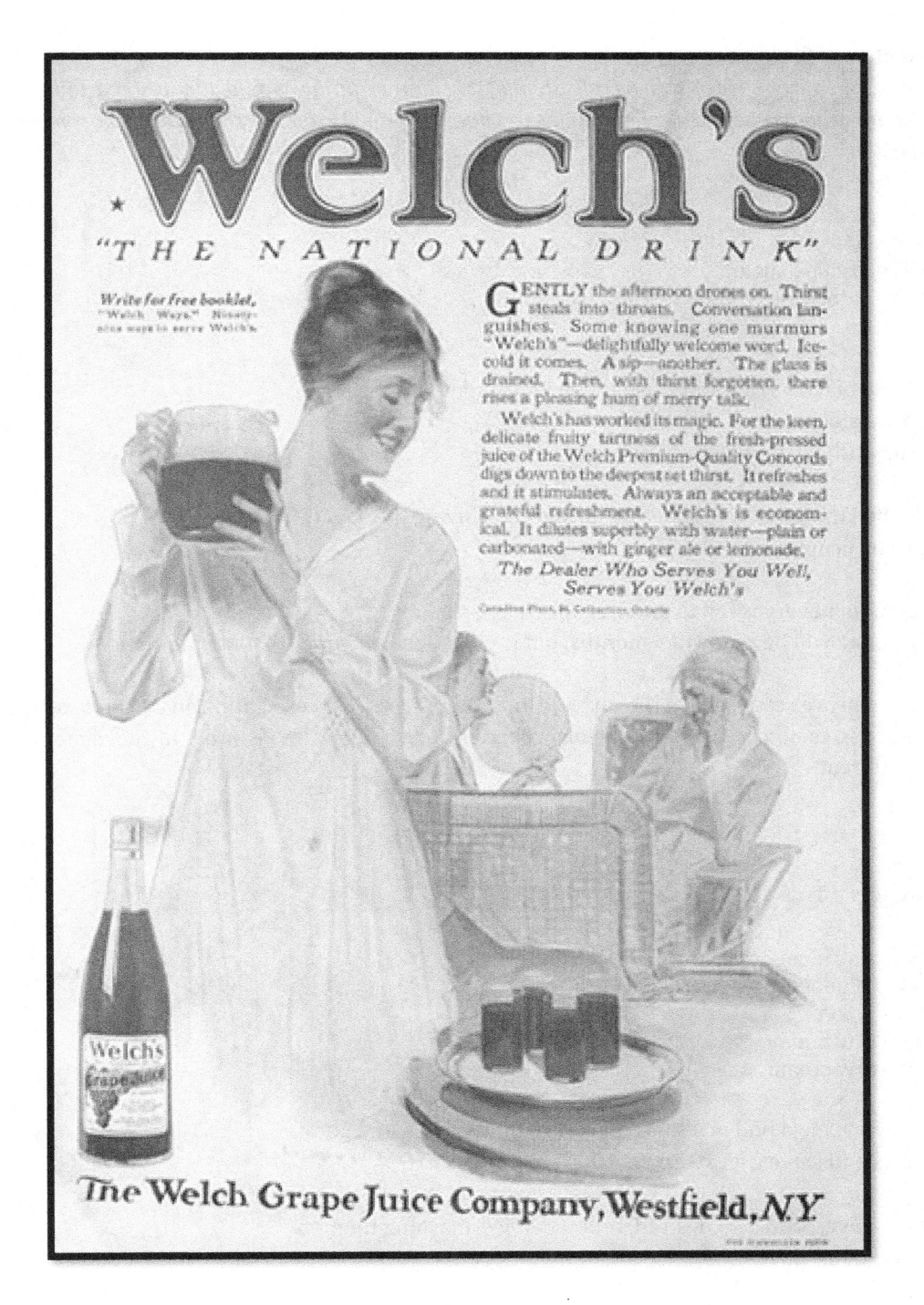

# Beverages

## Blackberry Liqueur

*This has medicinal use as well as refreshment. My mother-in-law would administer 1 tablespoon blackberry liqueur with 1 tablespoon Certo® liquid pectin to stop diarrhea whenever someone got the flu.*

1½ pint canning jar
2½ lbs of fruit
7 oz of organic sugar
24 oz Crater Lake vodka

*Method*
Pick the blackberries and wash them. Pour them into the jar.
Add the sugar.
Fill up with Crater Lake vodka.

Seal the jar, upend, and shake jar to start dissolving the sugar.
Place in a cupboard.

Return to it every week to admire, upend and shake.
The vodka will be ready in 3 months, but it will infuse and mature if kept for longer.

When you are ready, strain the mixture and filter through cheesecloth. You can add sugar or honey to sweeten to taste. Use the blackberries in an adult crumble or dip in chocolate for a special treat.


## Blueberry Tea

12 organic blueberries (fresh or frozen)
2-3 tsp blueberry leaves (dried)
2 cups water
1 tbsp raw honey
1 tbsp raw cream

Bring water to a boil in a sauce pan, turn off the heat, and add berries and leaves; let steep for 10-15 minutes.

Strain leaves, and if so desired, retain berries, mashing them to release more flavor.

Add honey and cream.
Serve over ice or hot.

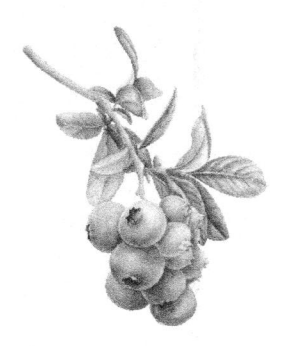

### *Fire Cider*

Since the early 1980s, Rosemary Gladstar, an herbalist who many consider to be the godmother of American herbalism, has been teaching one such recipe to her many students and has been sharing it freely throughout the herbal community and beyond. From its inception, she called it Fire Cider and describes it as a "spicy, hot, deliciously sweet, vinegar tonic."

This creation was copyrighted in her herbal course materials and featured in several of the books she authored. Since then, it has been shared, enjoyed, modified, and even sold ~ with Rosemary Gladstar's blessing,

**Fire Cider** (Chef Christina Wokowsky)

*Fire cider is a traditional folk drink made with herbs stewed in apple cider vinegar. It's a potent tonic that's been used for generations as a remedy to ward off sickness and boost health. This tonic uses grated fresh horseradish, ginger, garlic, onions, and hot peppers in apple cider vinegar for 3 to 4 weeks, then finishing with honey to balance the acidity.*

1 qt (4 cups) of raw unfiltered apple cider vinegar (at least 5% acidity)
⅓ cup grated horseradish and ginger roots
¼ cup peeled and diced turmeric
6 cloves garlic, minced
½ cup peeled and diced onion
1 or 2 habanero chilies split in half
1 large lemon, sliced with rind
2 tbsp chopped rosemary
2 tbsp chopped thyme
½ cup chopped parsley
1 cinnamon stick
1 tsp allspice berries
½ tsp whole cloves
1 tsp black peppercorns
¼ cup raw honey, or more to taste

Place herbs in a half gallon canning jar and cover with enough raw, unpasteurized apple cider vinegar to cover the herbs by at least three to four inches. Cover tightly with a tight-fitting lid.

Place jar in a warm location and let it infuse for three to four weeks. It is best to shake every day to help with the maceration process. After three to four weeks, strain out the herbs and reserve the liquid.

Add honey to taste. Your Fire Cider should taste hot, spicy, and sweet. "A little bit of honey helps the medicine go down."

Rebottle and enjoy! Fire Cider will keep for several months unrefrigerated if stored in a cool pantry. But it's better to store in the refrigerator if you have room.

*How to take*: A small shot glass daily serves as an excellent preventative tonic. Or take several teaspoons throughout the day if you feel a cold coming on.


**Cranberry Spritzer** (Nicole Hammond)

1 tbsp apple cider vinegar
2 tbsp lemon juice
¼ cup pure cranberry juice
¼ cup mixed berries of choice
2 basil leaves
1 cup ice
4 oz sparkling water

Combine ingredients. Serve over crushed ice and garnish with berries or basil.

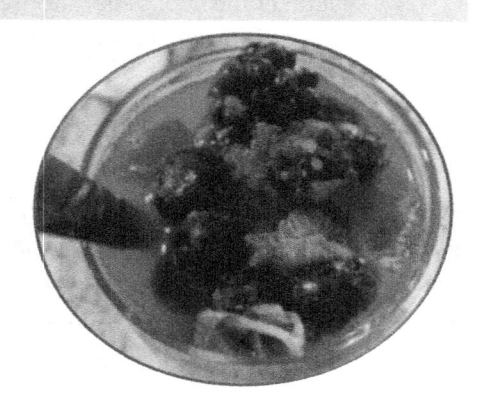

**Berry Lemonade** (Tammera Karr)
Servings 6

2 lemons, juiced
1 lime, juiced
1 pint raspberries
1 pint strawberries
½ cup unrefined cane sugar, or to taste
5 cups filtered cold water

Put lemon and lime juice into a large pitcher.
Mash berries and press through strainer. Add berry juice to pitcher. Stir in sugar until dissolved. Add water and stir again. Just before serving, add ice.

## Ginger Beer

Servings 10-12

1 lb fresh ginger, grated
½ cup fresh lime juice
1 cup unrefined can sugar, or to taste

In a sauce pan, bring 3 quarts of water to a boil, then remove from heat. Add ginger and steep overnight. Strain mixture through a fine-mesh sieve, pressing ginger to release flavor.

Pour into a pitcher or bottle using a funnel. Add lime juice and 1 cup sugar; stir vigorously. Cover and store at room temperature letting mixture steep (and dregs settle) 24 hours. Decant to a second bottle with a tight-fitting screw top and refrigerate for 3-5 days.

## Sorrel for the Holidays

*This drink has its history in the Caribbean and enslaved Africans. This drink and eventually the idea for Kool-Aid can be credited to the ingenuity and wild food knowledge of the individuals who crafted the red beverage.*
Serves 8

½ lb ginger, peeled and mashed
½ tsp ground cinnamon
5 whole allspice berries
2 lbs fresh sorrel flowers and buds
1½ to 2 lbs unrefined cane sugar
1½ cups sweet red wine
1½ cups dark rum

Mix 2 quarts water with the ginger, allspice berries and ground cinnamon in a large sauce pan.

Bring to a boil, then add sorrel buds, and turn off the heat.

Place the cover on the sauce pan, refrigerate and let it steep for two to three days. Once the sorrel has steeped, strain the mixture, and discard any solid pieces.

Sweeten the mixture to taste with sugar. Be sure to mix until the sugar has dissolved.

Lastly, add rum and wine.

Mariposa Farms https://mariposafarms.com/where-to-buy/

## Hot Toddy

1 tsp wild honey
2 oz boiling water
1 wee dram (1½ oz) good Irish Whiskey or Scotch
3 whole cloves
1 stick cinnamon
1 thick slice organic lemon

Pour honey, boiling water, and whiskey into a mug. Add cloves, cinnamon, and a lemon slice. Let the mixture stand for 5 minutes so the flavors can mingle. Drink while warm.

## Crabapplejack

*Traditional applejack is a brandy that has been distilled from apple juice. This is an easy way to make a special holiday treat or gift.*

2 cups small crabapples
1 fifth of good brandy
½ cup organic sugar, or to taste
1 40 oz wide month glass jar

Wash and remove stems from crabapples. Place in glass jar, and add brandy. Cap bottle, and place in a cupboard or dark location that is room temperature or slightly cooler. Let steep for 8-10 weeks, and gently shake the bottle once or twice a week.

After 8-10 weeks, strain out and discard apples. Filter brandy through a funnel lined with a paper coffee filter into a brown or blue glass bottle or jar. Add sugar.

Return to the shelf and let mellow for 2-4 weeks before serving.

## Teas, Coffees, and Cacao

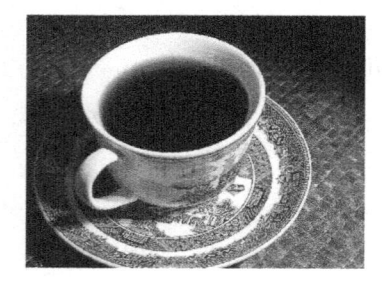

The world is just a happier place with coffee, tea, and cacao! The flavonoids contained in them contribute many health benefits, including reducing the growth of harmful bacteria. They are rich in antioxidants and plant compounds that support the heart and brain, fighting cancer and they taste delicious. As always, opt for organic whenever possible; non-organic free-trade sources are often sprayed with high levels of pesticides.

## Camp Coffee also known as Church Coffee (1900s–1950s)
*Calcium and trace minerals from egg shells gives coffee a smooth, mellow taste and reduces acid. This tradition would also add supplemental essential minerals into the daily diet.*

1 cup boiling water
2 tbsp cold water
2½ level tbsp ground coffee
3 egg shells per cup, washed

Measure coffee, and crush egg shells based on the number cups. Place both into a percolator filter with 4-9 cups water. Place over flame or fire, let boil 5-10 minutes, counting from the time the water begins to perk. Or add cold water, coffee, and eggshells to a French press, cover with boiling water, and steep for 5-10 minutes.

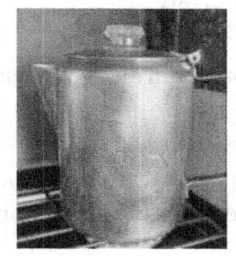

## Flaxseed Tea (1891)

1 tbsp flaxseed
1 tsp licorice root, ground
1 pint boiling water

Wash the flaxseed thoroughly, put in boiling water and set it aside in a warm area for 4 hours. Strain before serving.

An excellent drink when fever is accompanied by a cough.

## Flaxseed Lemonade (1902)

2 heaping tablespoons of whole organic flaxseed to 1 quart of boiling water. Let stand until it thickens, then strain over the juice of 1 lemon and sweeten to taste.

Very good for colds. A little-powdered gum Arabic may be added while it is still hot.

## Instant Turmeric Golden Milk - Dry Mix
Makes about 16 (12 oz) servings

1½ cups coconut milk powder
4 tbsp turmeric powder
2 tsp ground cinnamon
1 tsp ground ginger
½ tsp ground black pepper
½ tsp vanilla bean powder (optional but delicious)

¼ tsp Himalayan salt or sea salt

Add all ingredients to a blender and purée for about 5-10 seconds. This will get rid of any lumps in the mix.

Store in an airtight glass jar in a cool, dark cupboard. Makes about 20-24 servings.

*How to use*
When ready to use, scoop out 3 tablespoons of the mix into a mug.
Add 12 oz (1½ cup) hot water.

Add natural sweetener of choice (raw honey, sweetener, sugar, etc.).
1-2 teaspoon per 8 oz mug is just about the right sweetness.


## Grandmother's Family Spring Bitters (1891)

1 oz mandrake root
1 oz dandelion root
1 oz burdock root
1 oz yellow dock root
2 oz prickly ash berries
1 oz marshmallow
½ oz turkey rhubarb
1 oz gentian
1 oz English chamomile flowers
2 oz red clover tops

Wash the herbs and roots and place in an earthen vessel, pour over 2 quarts of water that has been boiled and cooled. Let soak overnight. In the morning, bring back to the stove and simmer on low for 5 hours. DO NOT boil.

Strain and add ½ pint of good gin.
Keep in a cool place.
One half of a wine glass taken as a dose twice a day.


## Orangeade (*The New Century Home Book* by Frank A DePay, 1900, pg 221)

Beat one egg light and put it into a tumbler. Fill the glass nearly full of cold water, add the juice of one orange, sweeten, and shake well.

> *July*
> The market is full of delights in July:
> Fresh vegetables, berries, red cherries for pie!
> Good housewives and telephones seldom agree, so market yourself!
> You can buy as you see!
>
> *A Thousand Ways to Please a Husband*
> ~ Louise Bennett Weaver, 1917

**Raspberry Drink** (*The New Century Home Book* by Frank A DePay, 1900, pg 220)

Put into a preserving kettle a pint of red raspberries and a quart of currents, and mash them thoroughly. Set the kettle over a moderate fire and let it heat gradually. After the mixture begins to boil pour it into a jelly bag and let it drain into a large bowl. When it is clear and cold, ice it, sweeten to suit, and serve in small glasses.

**Green Tea Ginger Moscow Mule**

*A refreshing and spicy herbal cocktail for summer afternoons.*
2 drinks

2 oz Crater Lake vodka, optional*
1 oz fresh lime juice
4 oz sparkling water
4 oz boiling water
1 tsp maple syrup
2 green tea bags
2 ginger tea bags
Lime wedge for garnish

Pour 4 ounces freshly boiled water over the tea bags, cover and let steep until cool. Squeeze the bags of any excess tea.

Fill two copper mugs or small glasses with ice. Add vodka or sparkling water, syrup and lime juice. Fill about ¾ of the way with the cooled tea and top off with sparkling water. Gently swirl it with a spoon once to mix.

Garnish with a lime wedge and enjoy.

*\*If alcohol is a concern, replace vodka with extra sparkling water and lime juice to your taste preference.*

### Slippery-Elm Tea (1891)

Put a teaspoonful of powdered slippery-elm into a tumbler, pour cold water upon it, and season with lemon and sugar.

Soothing to the dry or sore throat, aids in moving the bowels.

### Corn Silk Tea (Tammera Karr)

*Corn silk has a long history of medicinal use for supporting healthy kidneys in American Indian and Asian herbology. The soft silky threads found on ears of corn can be saved for making tea or a broth by freezing or drying. A gentle corn on the cob flavor.*

1½ cups water
¾ oz corn silk

Boil water, add silk and steep for 10 minutes.

### Horchata made from Chufa (tiger nuts) [199, 200, 201, 202, 203]

*Horchata from chufa is a very popular and refreshing summer drink in the region of Valencia, Spain, where many acres are grown for that purpose. Chufa and Horchata were brought to Spain by the Moors in the 8th century. The Spanish brought them to the New World.*
*Cyperus esculentus (also called chufa, tigernut, atadwe, yellow nutsedge, and earth almond) is a species of plant in the sedge family widespread across much of the world. It is found in most of the Eastern Hemisphere, including Southern Europe, Africa, Middle East, Madagascar and the Indian subcontinent.*

1 lb chufa
1 lb sugar
2½ qts of water
1 cinnamon stick

Clean the chufa well by rubbing them between your hands while rinsing them in clean water. Repeat until chufas are clean (rinse water until it remains clean when chufa are rubbed between your hands). Cover with 4 inches of water and soak for 12-14 hours.

After soaking, rinse the chufas again in clean water, change the water until it is completely clear, then drain off all the water. Mash the chufas or put them in a blender, to make a soft paste. Add a little water if needed.

Add the 2½ quarts of water to the paste that you have made and put in the cinnamon stick. Let it sit in a cool place (like a refrigerator) for 2 hours.

Add the sugar and stir until the sugar is completely dissolved. Strain the mix through a mesh filter to remove the larger particles and then through a damp fine-cloth filter. If the cloth filter did not strain the liquid enough, there are two options here: Repeat until the strained liquid does not have any large particles left or fold or double fold your damp cloth filter and pass the liquid through the filter slowly.

The smooth milky liquid can be served as is, placed in the refrigerator to be served chilled later or, placed in the freezer, occasionally stirring to prevent it from freezing solid and served in a slushy form.

## Mexican Coffee

*Brew up your preferred organic coffee and add the following to suit your taste.*

¼ tsp vanilla
Sprinkle of cinnamon
Sprinkle of clove
Sprinkle of cayenne pepper
1 tsp heaped organic cocoa powder

Place in the bottom of the cup, add a little coffee to blend ingredients, then finish filling your cup. Add organic sugar if you must.

## Paleo Eggnog Recipe

Serves: 4
Prep: 10 minutes

Egg yolks
1 tsp vanilla extract
3 tbsp maple syrup
Pinch of nutmeg
½ tsp cinnamon
4 cups full fat coconut milk, heated

1. Place the egg yolks, vanilla, maple syrup, nutmeg and cinnamon in a blender and blend for one minute.
2. Pour in the hot coconut milk, then blend 2 minutes longer.
3. Pour into drinking glasses and serve. Alternatively, cool and serve over ice.

## Spiced Cider

1 qt apple or pear juice
½ tsp organic ground cinnamon
⅛ tsp organic ground cloves or allspice

Add juice and spices to the sauce pan. Bring the mixture to boil then turn off and let cool. Serve warm or cold. You can also add cranberry juice or sliced orange without the peel to cup. Note: If you use whole spices be sure to remove them after juice cools or it will taste bitter over time.

*Wassail* appears in English literature as a salute as early as the 8th century epic *Beowulf,* in references such as "warriors' wassail" and "words of power." [204]

## Wassail Recipe [205]
Makes about 4 quarts

4 cups freshly pressed apple cider
1 cup orange juice
1 cup cranberry juice
2 pints heavy winter ale*
3 cups port*
4 small tart and sweet apples, peeled and cored
1 lemon
1 lime
1 orange
1 tsp ground cardamom
3 small or 1½ large cinnamon sticks
15 whole cloves
6 whole allspice
1 tsp grated fresh ginger
4 tbsp coconut sugar
1 tbsp cold butter

*Two pints sherry or Madeira wine and 1 cup rum are often substituted for ale and port, resulting in a sweeter flavor and lighter body.

Preheat oven to 350°F. Pack 1 tablespoon of sugar and ¼ tablespoon of butter into the core of each apple. Place apples in a small baking dish and fill the dish with ½ inch of water (to keep apples from burning or sticking to the bottom).

When the oven is preheated, bake apples uncovered for 45 minutes-1 hour or until tender and soft, but not mushy. Drain the water. Quarter each baked apple.

Combine cardamom, cloves, allspice, and ginger in a small piece of cheesecloth, and tie closed with twine to form a spice packet.

In a large stock pot or slow cooker, combine apple cider, cranberry juice, orange juice, (plus ale, port or rum, and wine as desired), and the juice of one lemon and one lime.

Place cinnamon directly into liquid and stir to infuse. Submerge spice packet in a stock pot. Stir apples into stock pot. They'll ultimately float on top and begin to soften, fall apart, and add a creamy quality to the liquid.

Simmer on medium high (never boiling) for two hours until hot spices are thoroughly infused and apples have begun to dissolve. Remove spice packet and pour into "wassail bowl" if not using a stock pot or slow cooker. Be prepared to reheat until the wassail bowl is empty.

Garnish the wassail bowl with floating thin slices of the remaining lemon, limes, and oranges on top. Serve in small mugs with a sizable piece of apple in each mug.

*Wassailing is a Twelfth Night tradition that has been practiced in Britain for centuries. It has its roots in a pagan custom of visiting orchards to sing to the trees and spirits in the hope of ensuring a good harvest the following season. During the visit a communal wassail bowl – filled with a warm spiced cider, perry or ale – would be shared amongst revelers.* [206]

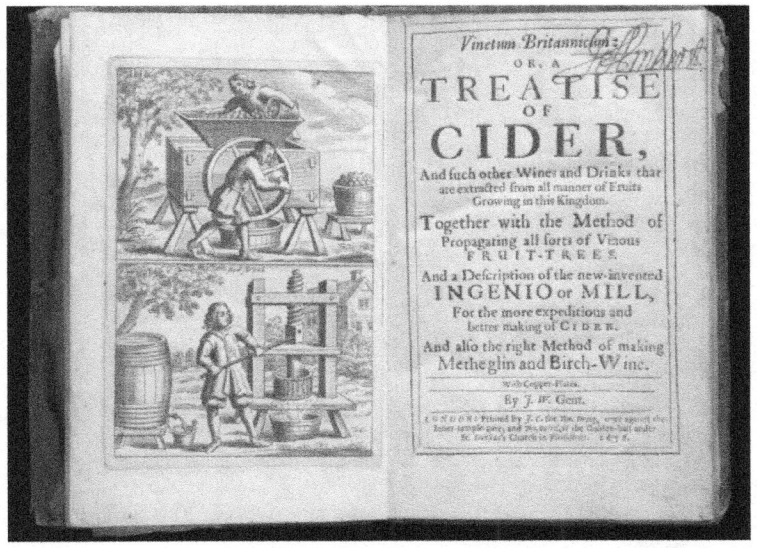

Treatise of Cider published in 1676, Scotney Castle, Kent, England

199 Darby, W: Food gift of Osiris

200 Manniche, L: An Ancient Egyptian Herbal

201 Wilson, H: Egyptian Food and Drink

202 Chafa.com-Glendale Enterprises; Bu Joanna Linsley-Poe  2012

203 https://ancientfoods.wordpress.com/2012/03/23/tigernuts/

204 http://www.history.org/Almanack/life/Christmas/hist_wassail.cfm

205 http://www.history.uk.com/recipes/traditional-wassail-recipes/

206 Ritual and revelry, the story of wassailing by Sally-Anne Huxtable Head Curator, National Trust, Heelis, Kemble Drive, Swindon. England:  https://www.nationaltrust.org.uk/features/ritual-and-revelry-the-story-of-wassailing

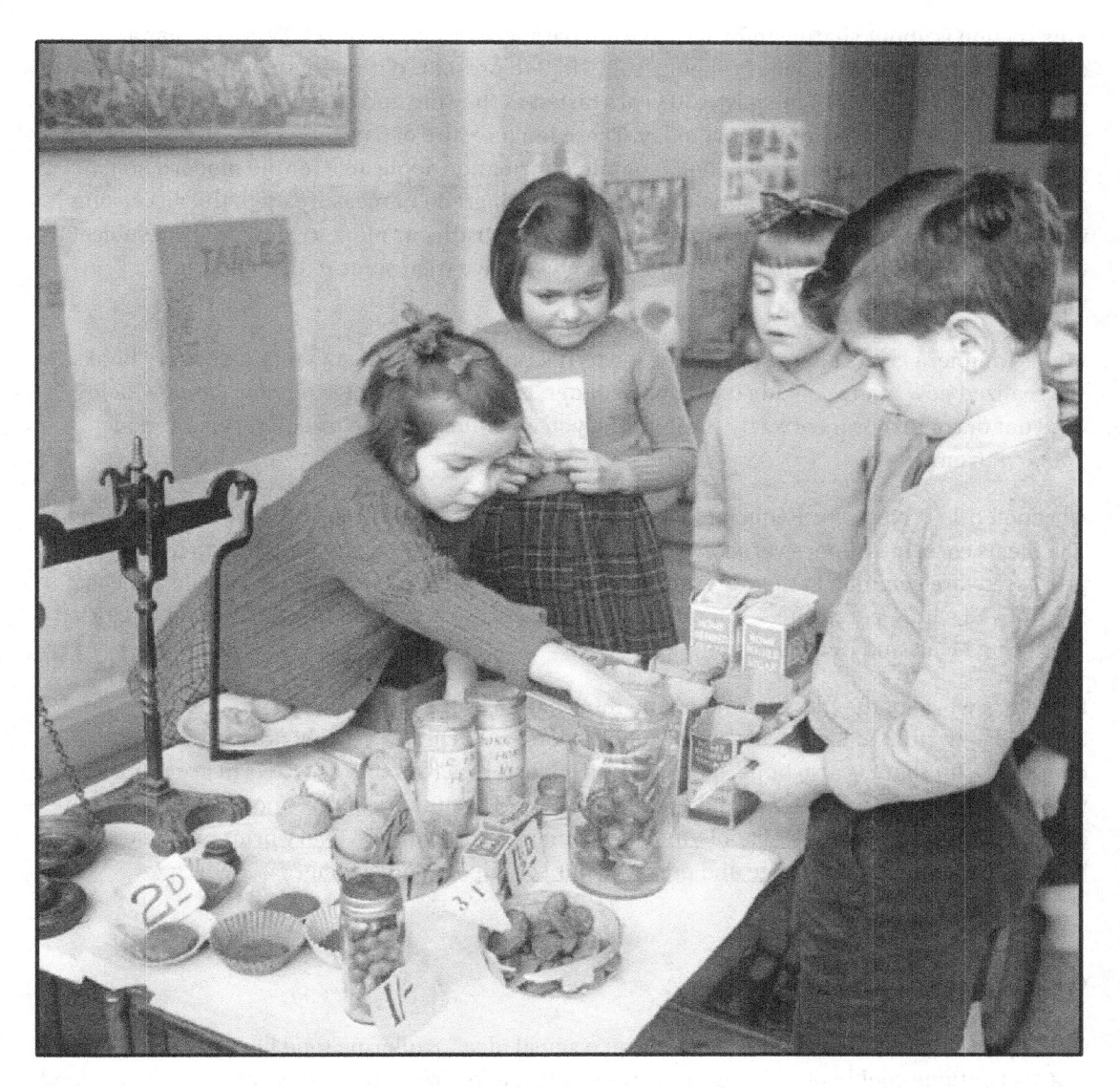

Children were learning math by adding up the cost of a shopping list in a classroom grocery shop at Fen Ditton Junior School, Cambridgeshire, England, in December 1944.

# *Wisdom from the Past*

This section is about sharing information from past generations of cooks. Tammera has a collection of antique cookbooks ranging from 1872 to present. Within these books there are insights into why foods of the past 150 years tasted as they did and sustained individuals who burned far more calories than most today. There is a measure of frugality; ingredients, time, and portion size. All these venerable books contain information applicable for the modern holistic nutritionist, good wife, and personal chef. Does every ingredient measure up to the discerning views of the modern nutrition professional? No, and in truth our modern views will be subject to the same disdain and rejection 150 years from now; as we treat some of the foods and ingredients shared here.

While Tammera cooks almost every day, it was not until researching in vintage cookery books she realized how many cooking terms, once understood by the average person, are now being used out of context or incorrectly. That is why you will find a section titled "Terms Used in Cooking" from 1942.

A section titled "Meals for Reducing" was found in a 1932 cookbook called *Meat Tops the Menu*. The meals contain far more variety, vegetables, fiber, and lower sugar content than the processed fare common in the 21st century North American manufactured weight-loss meals. For fun and a little perspective, Tammera has included a section from this 1932 cookbook titled "Reducing Meals and Recommendations."

In today's world of the Internet and digital information, some of the once commonsense knowledge written in historical cookery books along with cultural food history is in danger of being lost. But there is also hope. Libraries and collectors across the cyber world are utilizing technology to preserve culinary and literature works. <u>The authors of this book freely share digital copies with students, schools, and disadvantaged individuals. Every print book purchased helps share cookery knowledge and preserve our combined food heritage.</u>

**What comes around goes around**

Once upon a time someone said, "There is no original idea." Exploring food history through the pages of antique cookbooks has certainly proved this to be true. It also illustrates how much food memory we have when we allow the senses to flow. Great cooks rarely follow recipes and constantly use all their senses from selecting the ingredients to judging the perfect temperature or serving surface to compose the master piece of food art.

Words like new, healthy, trendy or fad are often used when describing a dietary model or ingredient. Example, wheat free, dairy free, and egg free menus are not unique to modern times. Tammera has historic nursing textbooks and cookbooks that have chapters on this very topic, and they are far more useful than many modern adaptations. "Infant Feeding and Invalid Cookery" took up 24 pages in *The Settlement Cook Book* from 1942. Older works called cyclopedias contain volumes of information on everything imaginable pertaining to food and maintaining a household before convenience stores and Internet shopping.

The 1892 edition of the *New Cyclopedia of Domestic Economy and Practical Housekeeper* contains 603 pages. Within the pages are detailed illustrations of every kind of cooking implement, directions on butchery and harvest, preservation, maintenance of the wood stove, and construction of buildings. A veritable treasure trove of information for the DIY crowd.

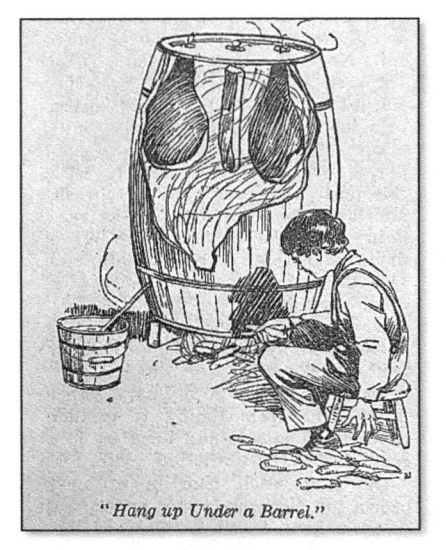

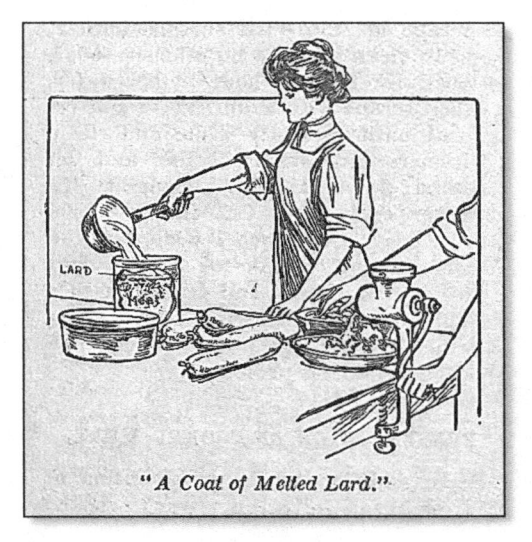

Preserving of Meat and Vegetables (pgs 595 and 597) *Household Discoveries and Mrs. Curtis's Cook Book*, 1906.

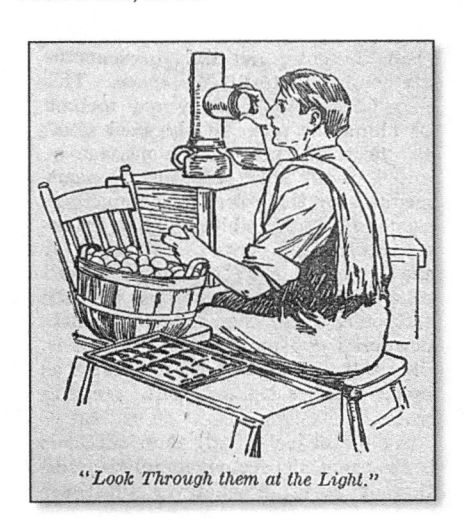

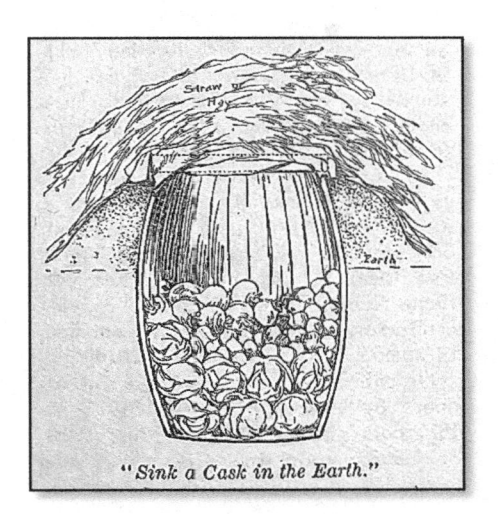

Candling eggs and preserving meat and vegetables (pgs 601 and 605) *Household Discoveries and Mrs. Curtis's Cook Book*, 1906.

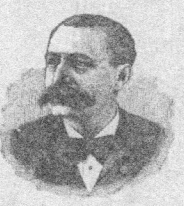

Booklets that contained helpful hints were effective advertising that drove customer loyalty in the 1880s through the 1970s.

We even found recipes for "building a campfire" and "camp cookery."

> **Just a reminder:** The historic recipes are as written. No modern editing of directions or wording has been done; these are how we found them. That means do not use a bare hand to turn the potatoes simply because it does not tell you to use tongs!
>
> Some recipes may contain * to direct you to a note from the modern authors. More than one version of a recipe may be present for technique and comparison.

In a previous section on utensils, we shared information about the knife, fork, and spoon. Here is a view from 1904 that gave us quite a chuckle.

**Knife and Fork** (1904) *Consolidated Library of Modern Cooking and Household Recipes* Volume 1 pg. 49, 50–64, 65

So much has been written about the man who conveys food to his mouth with his knife that it is hardly necessary to point out that it is not proper. The knife is however used exclusively for cutting the food, and should always be held in the right hand....Likewise the fork is found in the right hand when the knife is not in use, and should not be made to take the place of a spoon, except for such dishes as peas, beans, etc.

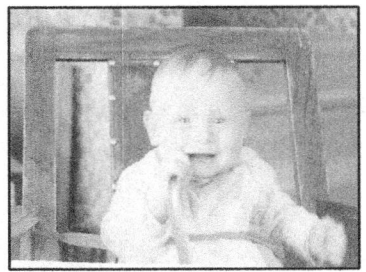

Michael Karr 1956, Idaho

It is equally bad manners to turn the fork into a shovel by loading it with a combination of various foods and then transporting the whole to the mouth. **The Spoon**: You should never drink your coffee, tea or bouillon from a spoon, or allow the spoon, which is furnished simply for the purpose of stirring or testing the temperature of the contents of your cup, to remain in it. This is as bad as to lift a spoon full of soup and attempt to cool it by blowing upon l, which is, as we all know, a habit taught in the nursery.... Numerous foods must, of course, be eaten with a spoon, such as fruit salads, oranges and grapefruit, cereals, hot puddings with sauces.

**Breakfast:** The formal breakfast – or perhaps it would be more accurate to say the company breakfast, for this meal is not as a rule very formal – is much in favor with people of the leisure class, and also with artists and *litterateur*, who frequently have considerable time to kill. It is an exceedingly pleasant mode of entertainment when successfully conducted and also possesses the advantage, for people of limited income, of being as inexpensive an affair as one wishes to make it....The menu for the affair may be more or less elaborate, but should begin with fruit, include some fish, an omelet or other forms of eggs, meat, dainty biscuits, and tea, coffee and chocolate.

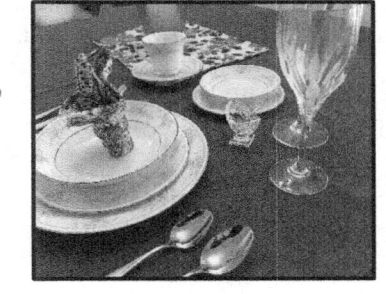

### Terms Used in Cooking (1942) [207]

Cooking is the art of preparing food by the aid of heat and for the nourishment of the human body. The principal methods of cooking are broiling, boiling, stewing, roasting, baking, frying, sautéing, braising, fricasseeing, and steaming.

**Baking:** Cooking in an oven.

**Basting:** Moistening with gravy or liquid at frequent intervals.

**Blanching:** Pouring boiling water over food, sometimes cooking a few minutes, and plunging into cold water immediately.

**Boiling:** Cooking in boiling water. Boiling point 212°F.

**Broiling**: Cooking by direct exposure to heat or over a glowing fire.

**Fricasseeing**: Stewing pieces of meat or fowl and serving with thickened gravy or sauce.

**Frying:** Cooking in hot fat deep enough to cover food to be cooked.

**Grilling:** Broiling.

**Marinating:** Allowing food to stand in French dressing or mixture of oil and vinegar or lemon juice.

**Masking:** To completely cover food with sauce or mayonnaise.

**Roasting:** Cooking uncovered, without water, in an oven.

**Sautéing:** Cooking in a small quantity of fat.

**Scoring:** Making light cuts in lines on the outer surface.

**Searing:** Browning rapidly at high temperature in a skillet or broiler.

**Simmering:** Cooking at just below the boiling point.

**Steaming:** Cooking over boiling water or in a steamer.

**Stewing:** Cooking slowly in liquid, covered, at low temperature for a long time.

**Trying Out Fat:** Heating fatty meat, usually pork or bacon, until fat becomes liquid and can be poured off.

## How to Try Out or Render Fat (*verbatim*, 1947) [208]

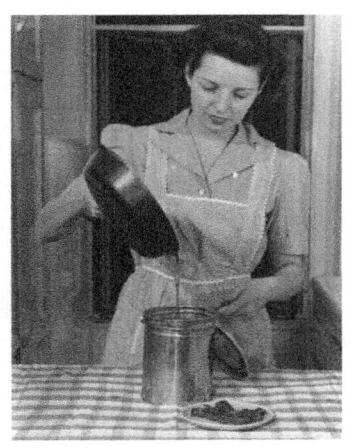

Every bit of fat from scraps of meat, bacon drippings, roasts, soups, and poultry may be made into a mixture for general cooking purposes. The scraps should be "tried out" together, provided there are no special flavors. A mixture of soft fats and hard fats usually makes of whole a good medium fat. Drippings in which onions or other strong flavors are present should be tried out and kept separate for meat and vegetable cookery.

Chop the fat into fine pieces. For each pound of fat allow ½ cup of water. Heat to boiling and as water boils away any extraneous odors are carried off. When the last sputtering begins, remove from heat, then strain through several thicknesses of cheesecloth into clean jars. Label clearly for any differences. If the crisp cracklings left after straining are of good flavor and color, they may be salted and used as an appetizer, for crackling bread, meat and vegetable dishes or muffins.

## Shortening (1947) [209]

The term shortening includes clean, sweet fat of any kind used in pastry, doughs, and batters. The most commonly used are butter, and solid vegetable fats, margarine, salad and cooking oil, lard and bacon or poultry drippings. They may be used interchangeably for "shortening" in a recipe, allowing for the difference in flavor. Since some contain more water than others a larger amount is needed to give the same shortening quality.

## How to Clarify Fat (1947) [210]

If fat that has been tried out from scraps and drippings needs to be clarified, let it harden, remove from container, scrape away and discard any sediment that has settled in the bottom of the cake. If fat has acquired, through use, a slightly burned or disagreeable flavor, * for each pound or pint of melted fat add a medium-sized potato cut in ¼ inch slices. Heat gradually.

When the fat ceases to bubble and the potatoes browned, strain the fat through several thicknesses of cheesecloth placed over a strainer, ** and set away to cool. When ready to use, again scrape away and discard sediment from the bottom of cake. Since the potato is porous, it helps to clarify the fat as well as purify it by gathering into its pores much of the sediment in the used fat.***

*If your fat tastes, looks, and smells bad – DUMP IT.
**Do not use a nylon strainer, it will melt.
*** This has been disproved.

### How to Care for Fats (1947) [211]

Since the four factors that are instrumental in making fat rancid are light, moisture, air and warmth, all fats should be kept in a dark, dry, cool place and as far as possible away from air.

Oils, particularly, are affected by air. If oil is bought in quantity and used a little at a time, it should be transferred from the large container to small ones. Each container should be filled completely full to exclude air, and should be sealed or stoppered. The containers should be kept in a dry, cool place, but not so cold that the contents will congeal. The middle shelf of a refrigerator is usually satisfactory. *

*Modern refrigerators may be too efficient (cold)

### Trying Out and Storing Lard (1906) [212]

Lard – The leaf fat which adheres to the ribs and belly of the hog makes the so-called "leaf Lard," which is of the best quality. Hence it is a good plan to try out the leaves separately. But any part of the hog fat not used for other purposes may be tried out to make an ordinary quality of lard. A set kettle, or other large kettle, held over a campfire by means of a tripod out of doors on a clear, calm day, is the best utensil for this purpose. Cut the fat into small pieces 1 or 2 inches square, and add 1 ounce of soda for each 25 pounds of meat. Stir frequently as soon as the fat melts and the scraps begin to brown. Melt with very gentle heat, taking care not to burn. Toward the last, the lard must be stirred constantly to prevent burning. The lard will be done when the steam ceases to rise. When the scraps are brown and shriveled, throw in a salt to settle the sediment, and strain through a cheese-cloth strainer into tubs or jars. Tie over the tops a layer of cotton batting to exclude the air. Lard will keep better in small jars than in large ones. Good lard should be white and solid without any offensive odor. Store in a cool, dry place. The lard from the intestines will not keep as well as leaf lard, hence should be rendered separately. It will keep better if soaked for 3 or 4 days in strong brine, changed each day.

### Lard (*European and American Cuisine* 1906, pg 348)

Most of the lard now is adulterated with potato flour, salts, carbonate of soda, and caustic lime. We seldom get it pure; unless able to pay a high price to reliable party or dealer.

### 845- To Melt Lard (1872)[213]

Take the inner fat of a newly killed pig and strip off the skin completely and carefully, slice it and put it into a jar, a sprig of rosemary may be placed with it, and set the jar in a pan of boiling water; let it melt, and when perfectly fluid pour it into dry clean jars, and cover them closely; it may be kept some time in a dry place, and when used may be mixed with butter for pastry, for frying fish, and many other purposes in cooking.

**Bleaching Lard** – The addition of about 1 pint of boiled white lye from hickory ashes, strained through cheesecloth into the fat before boiling, tends to bleach it.

**To Preserve** (*Home Comfort Range Cook Book*, 1929 pg 146) – Lard may be kept sweet and fresh, even in warmest weather by adding to the rendering or remelting kettle, a handful of slippery elm bark. No salt or further preparation is necessary for this purpose. Tins, crocks or jars in which lard is placed should always be thoroughly sterilized before filling.

**Meat Tops the Menu** –1936 (published by the National Livestock and Meat Board)

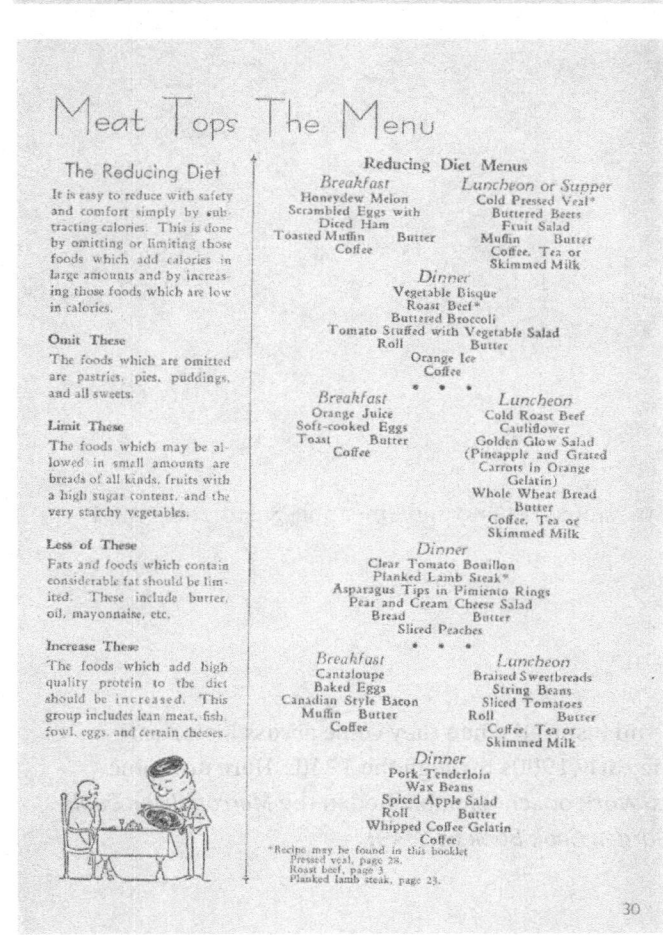

**Meat for Reducing**: Taking off extra pounds is popular in theory, but in practice it is another story. Many a person makes a sober promise to "go on a diet, tomorrow," and tomorrow never comes. Why? Because so many roads to slenderness are too hard to follow! Perhaps this is just as well. Some reducing diets are actually dangerous, for they do not provide the food elements essential to health. Others fail because they do not satisfy the appetite and are given up, for being hungry and uncomfortable just does not seem worth the effort....You should consult your doctor before going on a diet to ensure that the excess weight is not due to physical conditions that require medical treatment....In order to obtain the desired high protein diet, it should include liberal quantities of lean meat.

**No Extra Cooking**: The meat dish provided for the family will fit into the reducing diet menu. You may have to leave off the sauce or cut off the fat, but you won't need to cook something different.

**Amount of Meat**: The meat should be weighed or measured after cooking. An ounce of cooked meat is about 3 inches long, 1 inch thick, and 1 inch wide.

**Your Correct Weight**: Average weight is based on height and age, but it is impossible to make up a table of the most desirable weights which will fit everybody.

**Your Age**: If you are under thirty your health will be better if you weigh a little more than the average: after thirty, the reverse is true.

**For 135 pounds**: You may have a serving of meat weighing 5 ounces for luncheon and one weighing 7 ounces for dinner, if you have 135 pounds as your goal in reducing.

**For 175 Pounds**: If your weight should be 175 pounds, your reducing diet meals may contain 7 ounces of meat at lunch and 10 ounces at dinner.

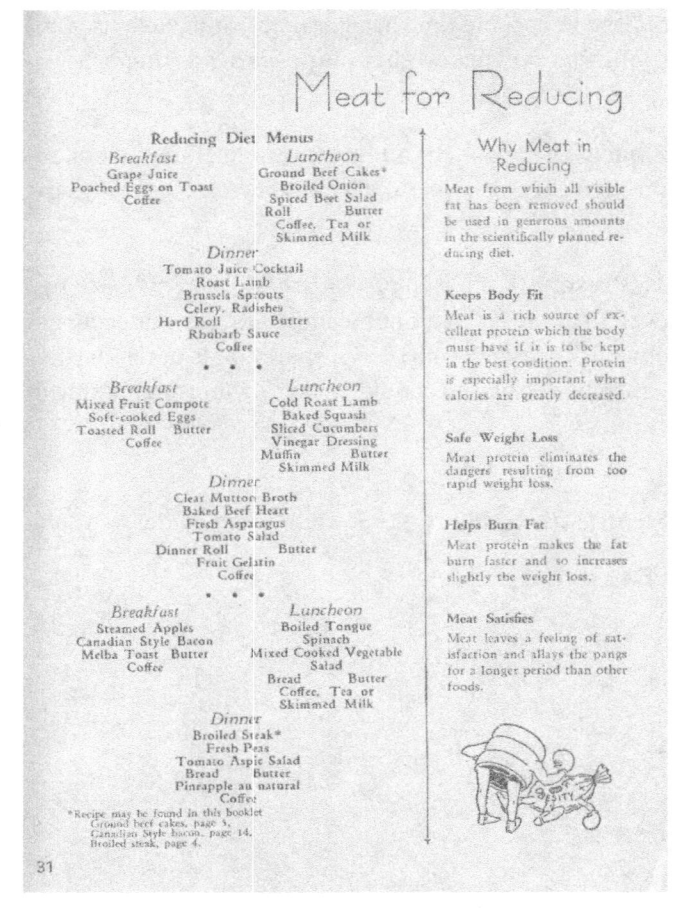

**Dinner:**

Beef broth, Lamb en Brochette, browned parsnips, Tomato and Pineapple Salad, roll, butter, sliced peaches and coffee.

## What is in that Lunch Box?

Tammera and Ben are always fascinated and inspired when they come across historical information on what folks ate between the early 1900s through the 1940s. Here are some examples of lunches carried from home to work or school published in the *Metropolitan Cook Book* in 1922 and the *Better Homes and Garden Cook Book* in 1949.

### Sandwich Fillings *(Metropolitan Cook Book, 1922)*

*Meat*
Minced ham with cream or salad dressing.
Left-over meat, minced, with cream or salad dressing.
Dried beef, plain or frizzled. (Sounds like my hair some days.)
Slices of beef, ham, chicken, or lamb, sprinkled with salt or spread with a little salad dressing.
Broiled slices of bacon.

#### 7 Complete Lunch Boxes

| Filling Dish or Sandwich | Drink or Soup Accompaniment | Raw Salad or Vegetable | Dessert or Fruit |
|---|---|---|---|
| Nut Bread Sandwich / Carton of Cottage Cheese | Tomato Juice / Salted Crackers | Carrot Sticks / Green Pepper Rings | Stewed Apricots / Lemon Cookies |
| Corn Bread / Ham Roll-ups | Hot Cocoa or Milk | Deviled Egg in Leaf Lettuce | Orange / Graham Cracker and Chocolate Bar Stack-ups |
| Potato Chips / Chicken Salad | Orangeade or Chocolate Milk | Chinese Cabbage Rings and Olives | Banana / Oatmeal Cookies |
| Baked Beans / Brown Bread | Hot Spiced Apple Cider | Chopped Cabbage and Green Pepper | Cracked California Walnuts / Potato Doughnut |
| Macaroni Salad / Veal Bird | Cream of Tomato Soup | Lettuce / Cheese-Stuffed Celery | Baked Cup Custard / Honey Nut Brownies |
| Hot Chili | Milk / Crackers and Cheese | Sliced Pickles / Celery Curls | Bunch of Grapes / Sponge Cake Bars |
| Chicken Drumstick / Bran Muffin Sandwich | Split Pea Soup | Cauliflower Salad / Cheese Dressing | Individual Apple Pie or Red Apple |

*Better Homes and Garden 1949, pg 17*

*Fish*
Tuna or salmon, plain or mixed with dressing.
Sardines, minced with lemon juice added.

*Egg*
Hard-cooked, chopped and mixed with dressing.
Scrambled, plain or in milk, or with bits of chopped bacon.

*Cheese*
Creamed cheese with chopped nuts, olives or peppers, or a combination of these.
Sliced cheese with onions and mustard on rye bread.
Cottage cheese with onions and cream or salad dressing used with brown bread. Pimento may also be added.
Add India relish to well-seasoned fresh cottage cheese.

*Fruit*
Chopped dates, butter, orange, or lemon juice.
Chopped dates with peanut butter or cream cheese.

*Vegetable*
Plain lettuce with salad dressing.
Sliced tomato with dressing.
Diced pickled cucumber with cottage cheese.
Pickled beets, chopped and mixed with cottage cheese.
Chopped celery, apple, nuts or olives with salad dressing. Mashed leftover beans mixed with tomato sauce or salad dressing and chopped sour pickle or green pepper relish.


**Additional Lunch Box Suggestions** *(Metropolitan Cook Book, 1922)*

Vegetable soups made with meat stock in a thermos bottle.
Whole vegetables and fruits.
Potato salad, Boston baked beans.

Desserts – nuts and raisins, dates and figs. Plain cookies, sponge cake or griddle cakes.

Custards, cereal puddings, and gelatin. Rich cakes or cookies should not be included in school lunch boxes. **(Hmm…interesting. Good advice for us to return to.)**


*From the ornate Turkish lunch boxes to ones depicting classic American TV in 1963; lunch has been a meal on the go.*

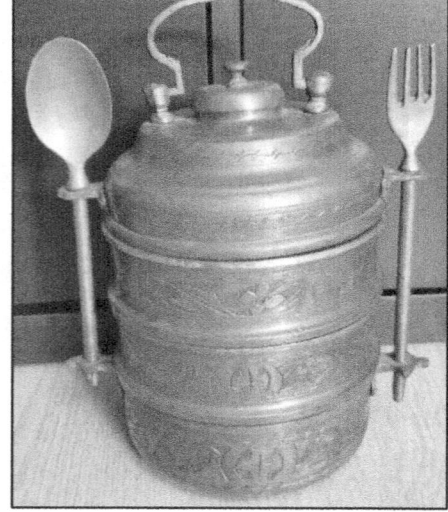

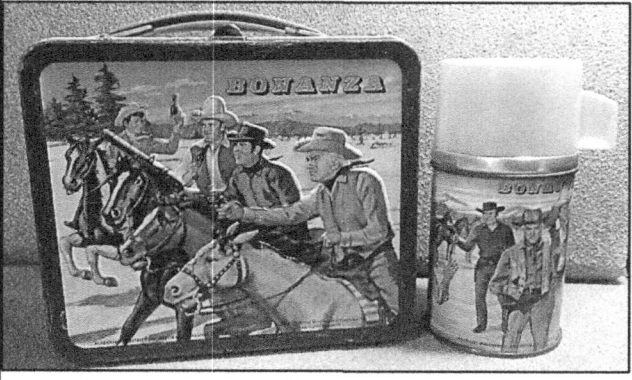

The *Better Homes and Garden Cook Book* from 1949 devotes the first four chapters to nutrition, meal planning, economical food selections, and preparation information. There are pages on foods vitamin content, calories, substitution charts and lists.[214]

## Meal-Planning and Meal-Making

MEAL-PLANNING IS A GAME that's fun if you play it with imagination and zest. If you play it well, you win satisfaction for yourself and cheers of enthusiasm from your family. It's important to plan well-balanced meals, but it's equally important to make those meals appetizing and attractive, with plenty of variety.

1. Plan meals for several days at one time. You will avoid monotony and duplication as well as saving time and money.
2. Keep seasons in mind and make the best use of food when it is at its best.
3. Remember, the eye eats first. As you plan meals think how they will look.
4. Be sure there is contrast in color, in texture, and in flavors. Do not repeat the same food or same flavor in one meal.
5. Avoid serving potatoes at the same meal with other starchy foods: macaroni, spaghetti, rice, and noodles.
6. Season foods carefully and wisely to bring out the best flavors; a good cook tastes food to see that it is well seasoned.
7. Serve hot foods hot and cold foods cold.
8. Introduce new food occasionally and take a family vote; vary the method of preparing those dishes that are served often.
9. Plan desserts that are really a part of the meal. Serve a filling dessert with a light meal, a light one if the meal has been heavy.
10. Arrange all food attractively at serving time. Keep a few simple garnishes on hand. The family will appreciate these touches.

*Better Homes and Garden 1949, pg 13*

**Food Placement in Refrigerator** (1942) [215]

In a mechanical refrigerator, green and salad vegetables should be kept in covered hydrators; berries and ripe fruit in a shallow pan. Eggs should be kept on lowest shelf in a basket, uncovered. Meats should be unwrapped and kept uncovered or covered lightly with oiled paper in the defrosting tray under freezer unit. Wrap fish in wax paper to prevent odors. Milk, cream, and butter should be placed next to the freezing compartment. Store ice cream and other frozen items in freezing compartment. Variety meats and fish, unless frozen, should be used within 24 hours after purchase. Do not use space for pickles and jellies.

In an **Ice-Box** place milk, butter, fresh meats, and soup stock at the bottom where the temperature is lowest; place strongly flavored foods near the top.

**To Build a Camp Fire** (1942) [216]

Build a campfire, if possible, in a hollow spot on the ground or pile up stones along three sides to form a low wall to protect the fire from the wind. Gather a number of light, dry chips and twigs. Make a little criss cross pile of the driest ones and light fire with paper. Add bark and twigs a little at a time and gradually increase the size of the wood until the fire burns briskly. Set grill firmly over the fire before it gets too hot and start coffee or any food to be boiled. When flames die down and a good mass of coal has accumulated, the fire is ready for boiling, roasting, or baking. If needed, add additional wood beneath the hot embers. See that the fire is completely out when leaving the camp. Charcoal or coke may be used.

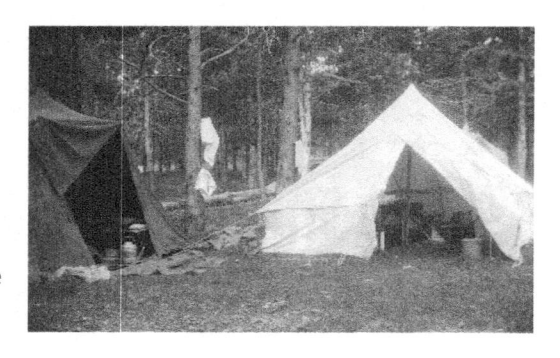

**Camp Cookery** (1942) [217]

*To Broil Steak* – Broil individual cubed steaks 5 to 10 minutes or place steak 1½ inches thick on grill, and broil 20 to 30 minutes.

*To Bake Fish when Camping* – Clean fish and remove entrails. Cover fish well with heavy wrapping paper. Place in hot embers and let bake ½ hour, more or less depending on size. Rake out the fish, take off paper, season with salt and pepper. Scales and skin will stick to paper.

*To Bake Potatoes* – Take medium sized potatoes. Place in ashes close to bright coals. Turn occasionally. Let bake from ¾ to 1 hour.

*To Roast Corn* – Remove silk. Twist husks tightly around ears. Soak in water ½ hour. If roasting in glowing embers, wrap in wet newspapers. If roasting on a grill, place ears above flame. Turn to roast evenly.

*To Grill Chicken* – Clean and season. Broil slowly over glowing coals, turning every 5 minutes, and rubbing with melted butter to which lemon juice has been added.

*To Bake Birds, Fish and Small Game with Clay* – Cut open, draw, and wash them well. Cover with a thick layer of clay, place in the midst of a hot fire. Let bake about 1 hour. Take out and break open. The skin or feathers will stick to the clay.

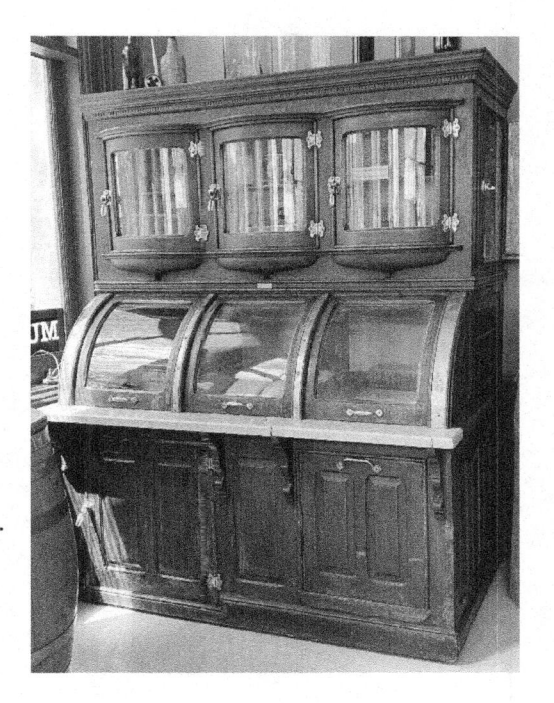

~~~~~~~~

After years of presenting seasonal nutrition classes to area high schools and community centers; Tammera believes it is clear we have done a huge disservice to our youth by removing this very basic of self-sufficiency and survival education from schools. We are now facing three generations of individuals subsisting off commercial, industrial foods, devoid of the seasoning of past generations; care, intention, and love.

> *"BAD cooking is a waste –*
> *waste of money and loss of comfort. Whom God has joined in matrimony,*
> *ill-cooked joints and ill-*
> *boiled potatoes have very often put asunder."*
>
> - Smiles

## *Buy a Beer and Get a Sandwich for Free*!

Signs on outer doors, walls or flyers from beer parlors or taverns announced to potential customers that a free sandwich came with every beer purchased.

This rare sandwich cupboard is approximately 10 feet wide and 12 feet tall. This *icebox* or cold case for sliced bread, meats, cheese, condiments, lettuce, and so forth could be found in taverns in North Eastern Oregon, parts of Idaho and Washington from the late 1800s through the 1950s. Block ice was placed in galvanized tin compartments accessed from a door on the upper rear side section. The cold then settled and permeated the glass-fronted areas keeping food fresh and accessible to customers.

Wallowa County Museum, Joseph, OR.

MENUS.

## Sunday.

### Breakfast.
Oranges.
Oatmeal, with Cream 243.
Broiled Mutton Chops 122.    Tomato Sauce 140.
Favorite Warmed Potatoes 173.
Eggs on Toast 248.    Graham Gems 230.
Wheat Bread 213.    Coffee 408.

### Supper.
Potted Ham 134.
Cheese Cream Toast 198.    Celery Salad 154.
Cold Raised Biscuit 223.
Gooseberry Jam 387.    Citron Cake 260.
Tea 410.

### Dinner.
Oysters on Half Shell.
Mock Turtle Soup 32.
Boiled Halibut 48, Sauce Maitre d'Hotel 142.
Roast Haunch of Venison 91, Currant Jelly 383.
Potato Croquettes No. 1 174.
Creamed Parsnips 180.    Celery.
Pickled White Cabbage 162.
Chicken Patties 77.
Baked Lemon Pudding 353.    Jelly Kisses 330.
Raisins.    Nuts.    Fruit.
Coffee 408.

## Monday.

### Breakfast.
Baked Apples 425.
Boiled Rice 244.    Pork Cutlets 130.
Waffles 231, with Maple Syrup.
Potato Fillets 173.
Toast 246.    Coffee 408.

### Luncheon.
Cold Roast Venison 91.
Broiled Oysters 63.    Potato Salad 155
Rye Drop Cakes 232.
Canned Peaches 390.    Tea 410.

### Dinner.
Macaroni Soup 33.
Boiled Leg of Mutton 121, Caper Sauce 140.
Potatoes a la Delmonico 174.
Steamed Cabbage 178.    Cheese Fondu 197.
Cucumber Pickles 159.
Boston Cream Pie 294.    Sliced Oranges.
Crackers.    Cheese.
Coffee 408.

## Tuesday.

### Breakfast.
Raspberry Jam 387.
Hominy 244.    Saratoga Chips 171.
Porterhouse Steak 97.
French Griddle Cakes 235.
Brown Bread 216.    Coffee 408.

### Luncheon.
Scrambled Mutton 125.
Welsh Rarebit 198.    Olives.
Hominy Croquettes 244.
Currant Jelly 383.    Molasses Cup Cake 274.
Chocolate 410.

### Dinner.
Oyster Soup 38.
Roast Loin of Pork 128, Apple Sauce 143.
Boiled Sweet Potatoes 175.
Scalloped Onions 177.    Stewed Carrots 189.
Pickled Green Peppers 162.
Royal Sago Pudding 357, Sweet Sauce 375.
Crullers 281.
Fruit.    Cheese.
Coffee 408.

430                  *MENUS.*

## Wednesday.

### Breakfast.
Old-fashioned Apple Sauce 143.
Fried Mush 243.
Pork Tenderloins 129.    Fried Sweet Potatoes 175.
Parker House Rolls 224.    Omelet 208.
Wheat Bread 213.
Coffee 408.

### Luncheon.
Cold Roast Pork 128.    Stewed Codfish 55.
Green Tomato Pickles 161.
Rusks 227.    Strawberry Jam 387.
Tea 410.

### Dinner.
Beef Soup 25.
Roast Fillet of Veal 112, Tomato Sauce 140.
Browned Potatoes 175.
Macaroni a la Creme 193.    Parsnip Fritters 180.
Piccalili 165.
Lemon Pie 292.    Cocoanut Tarts 303.
Cheese.
Coffee 408.

## Thursday.

### Breakfast.
Stewed Peaches.
Corn Meal Mush 243.
Stewed Beef Kidney 109.    Crisp Potatoes 173.
Egg Muffins 229.    Ham Toast 248.
Coffee 408.

### Luncheon.
Veal Croquettes 114.
Sardines.
Cold Slaw 153.    Cheese Toast 247.
Canned Plums 392.    Soft Ginger Cake 272.
Cocoa 411.

### Dinner.
Chicken Cream Soup 27.
Boiled Corned Beef 104.
Boiled Potatoes 104.    Boiled Turnips 104.
Boiled Cabbage 104.    Beets Boiled 186.
Charlotte Russe 320.
Preserved Strawberries 377.
Fruit Jumbles 280.    Fruit.
Coffee 408.

## Friday.

### Breakfast.
Orange Marmalade 386.
Oat Flakes 245.
Codfish Balls 54.    Baked Eggs on Toast 248.
Lyonnaise Potatoes 173.
Sally Lunn 226.    Raised Doughnuts 282.
Coffee 408.

### Luncheon.
Cold Corned Beef 104.
Vegetable Hash 188.    Deviled Lobster 59.
Graham Bread 216.    Peach Butter 393.
Golden Spice Cake 267.
Tea 410.

### Dinner.
Celery Soup 35.
Baked Halibut 49, Hollandaise Sauce 142.
Browned Potatoes 170.
Scalloped Oysters 66.    Stewed Tomatoes 181.
Fried Salsify 186.
Suet Plum Pudding 367, Brandy Sauce 371.
Sponge Drops 277.    Fruit.
Coffee 408.

*Whitehouse Cook Book,* 1887 pg 430

### *The Home Medical Manual Could be Found in Every Cookbook Prior to 1930.*

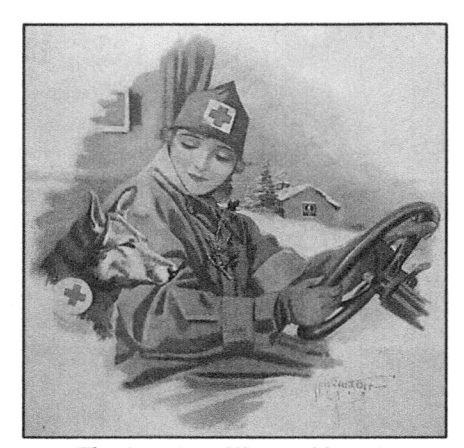

The American Woman Magazine
December 1918, Augusta Main

The Canyonville Historical Society allowed Tammera to travel through the pages of their copy of The *White House Cook Book* from 1905. This sizable cookbook provided over 100 pages of information on fresh ingredients, preparation, care, and nutrition (for the infirm, infant, and healthy), and dedicated several chapters to the *toilet,* health, and medicinal preparations. One section on medicinal recipes caught Tammera's attention in her 1891 edition of the *White House Cook Book* on page 488 for treatment of felons. Even after reading through five recipes, she still had no idea what a felon was. Perhaps a boil or form of infection was all she could think of; so off to the internet, where she learned a felon is an infection inside the fingertip. Generally, the abscess is deep in the palm side of the finger and very painful, usually caused by bacterial infection from *Staphylococcus*. Amazing what you learn from old books, and we seriously doubt the recipes are effective in the modern age of antibiotic resistance. In the 1891 edition of the *White House Cook Book,* Tammera found a chapter on Medicinal Food. Medicinal foods in the 21st century is largely viewed as prescriptive liquids for gastric tube feeding or Ensure® type drinks. Many biomedical or allelopathic providers do not realize they can write prescriptions for *Medical Foods* for clients with failure to thrive (elderly and children). Today's version, however, contains high levels of sugar, and chemicals, bearing little resemblance to the medical foods of the past or in other cultures.

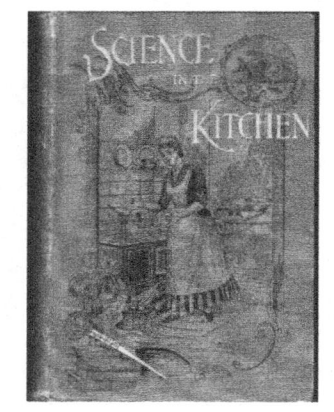

The historical society also shared one of their oldest cookery books, the *Science in the Kitchen* from 1893, a book few know about. This impressive volume was written by Dr. John Harvey Kellogg's wife for patients to use after leaving the famous sanitorium. *The Science of the Kitchen* goes into detail about the value of selecting only the freshest of meats on page 393, which was a surprise to Tammera, considering the bulk of the writing discussed the varied and debased nature associated with meat. The chapter includes information on cooking methods and recipes for mutton, beef, poultry, game, and fish. The dietary views of the Kellogg's can be considered extreme even by today's standards. A friendship developed between Ellen White and the Kellogg's during John Harvey's time as director of the Health Institute, which was associated with the fledgling Seventh Day Adventist church. Ellen White and Dr. Kellogg corresponded for years, which heavily influenced the dietary views of both parties. In *Science in the Kitchen*, Mrs. Kellogg stressed the Victorian value of economy when preparing meals and limiting waste. *The Great 20ᵗʰ Century Cook Book* and *My Mothers Cook Book* from 1902, contain additional chapters for health also.

## Medicinal Foods (1891) [218]

"Spinach has a direct effect upon complaints of the kidneys; the common dandelion, used as a green, is excellent for the same trouble; asparagus purifies the blood; celery acts admirably upon the nervous system, and is a cure for rheumatism and neuralgia; tomatoes act upon the liver; beets and turnips are excellent appetizers; lettuce and cucumbers are cooling in their effects upon the system; beans are a very nutritious and strengthening vegetable; while onions, garlic, leeks, chives and shallots all of which are similar, possess medical virtues of a marked character, stimulating the circulatory system, and the consequent increase of saliva and the gastric juices promoting digestion. Red onions are an excellent diuretic, and white onions are recommended raw as a remedy for insomnia. They are tonic, and nutritious."

"We might go through the list and find each vegetable possessing its special mission of cure, and it will be plain to every housekeeper that a vegetable diet should be partly adopted and will prove of great advantage to the health of the family."

## Mustard Poultice (1891) [219]

*Equal parts of ground mustard and flour made into a paste with warm water and spread between 2 pieces of muslin, form the indispensable mustard plaster.*

Into 1 gill* of boiling water stir 1 tablespoon of Indian meal;** spread the paste thus made upon a cloth, add 1 teaspoon of mustard flour.***
If you wish a mild poultice, use 1 teaspoon of ground mustard as it is prepared for the table, instead of the mustard flour.
*4 oz     **cornmeal     ***ground

## Invalid Cookery (1902) [220]

"For the patient, sick and weary with suffering, food should be prepared with the utmost care and served in the daintiest manner.
Convalescence depends much upon the appetite and proper food.
Fevers require that the patient's strength be kept up; at the same time, everything that quickens circulation should be avoided.

On giving an invalid a drink of water when liquids are restricted, hand him a small glass full. This will satisfy his thirst.

Never leave food standing by the patient with hopes that an appetite may be aroused by its presence. Remove at once and return after an interval in a fresh and attractive manner. "

**Regarding diet for the ill:** The text book of *The Principles and Practice of Nursing,* 1938, Chapter IX pg. 114, contained some insight into standards of nursing and use of nutrition.

**Importance of Food in Health and Disease Prevention** *(verbatim)*: The human body has been compared to a lifeless machine in that both wear out; but both need repair; both do work, and both need fuel. But the human body, unlike the lifeless machine, has an active mind and soul as well as an active body; it has the power to enjoy as well as use food; and given the proper materials and conditions, it has the power *within itself* to grow, to build to adapt, to create, and in life but to make it useful and happy.

The **essential materials** are food and oxygen – the maintenance of life itself is dependent upon them. Amounts and kinds of food required – A diet to maintain health and prevent disease must provide, in both total amount and composition of following:

1. For growth and repair of tissue. 2. For the production of energy – the power to do work and supply heat. 3. For the stimulation and regulation of body processes.

The essentials for growth and repair are 1. Protein. 2. Mineral salts. 3. Water
The essentials for production of energy are 1. Carbohydrates and fats

Conditions which favor digestion and assimilation of food
1. Freedom from painful emotions. 2. Freedom from excessive mental or physical fatigue, strain, or other discomfort. 3. Freedom from hurry, 4. Attractive, pleasant surroundings and a cheerful atmosphere.

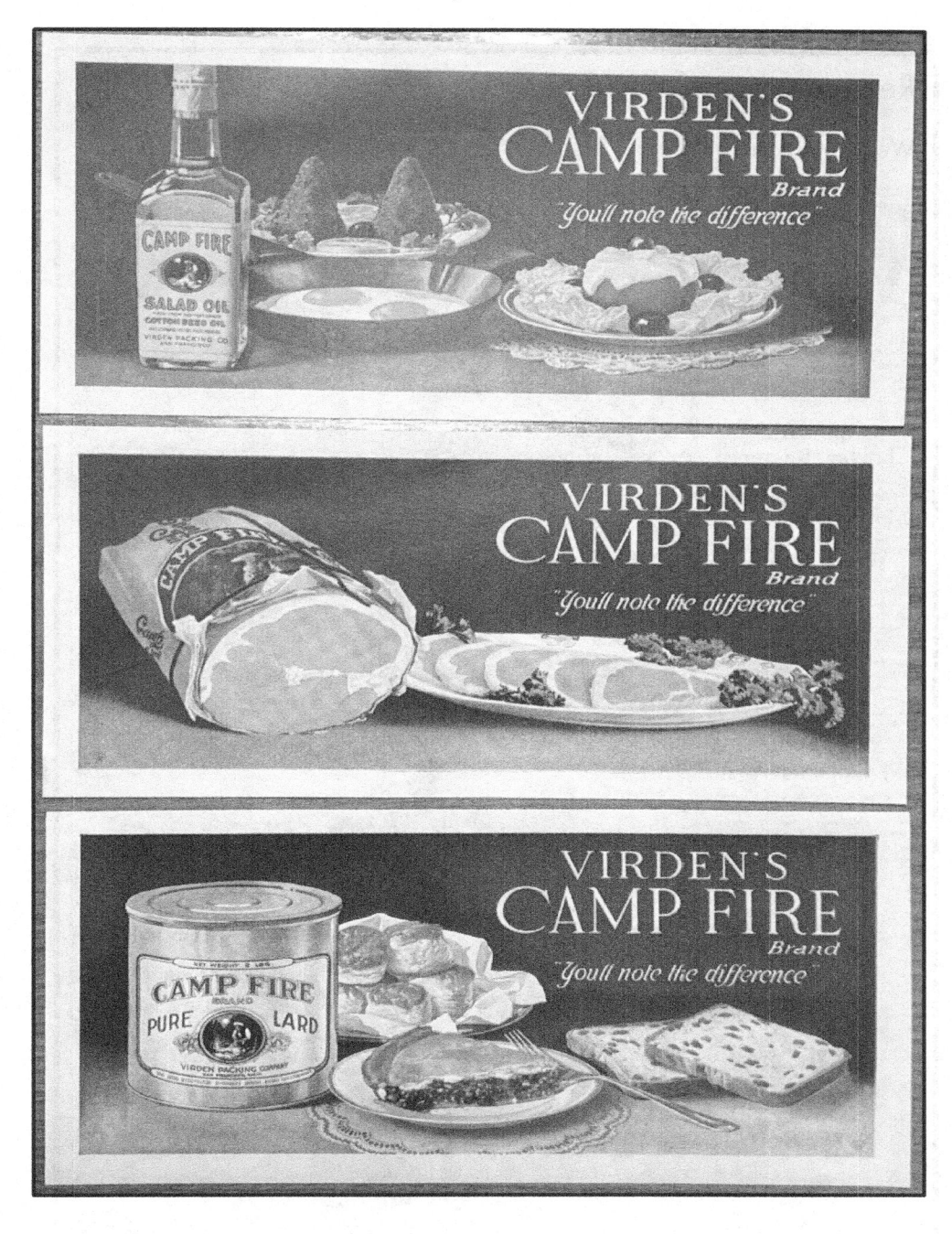

These 1920s postcards were free to customers. Each contains 5 recipes on the back using the Camp fire brand products. The company started out as a meat packer, but expanded in 1919-1922 into the canned fruit business, describing itself as "A New California Packer." Supposedly, peaches were one of its specialties. Both meat and fruit were canned under the Camp fire brand. By 1932, the company had been taken over and absorbed into Del Monte, Armor, and Western Canner and Packer.

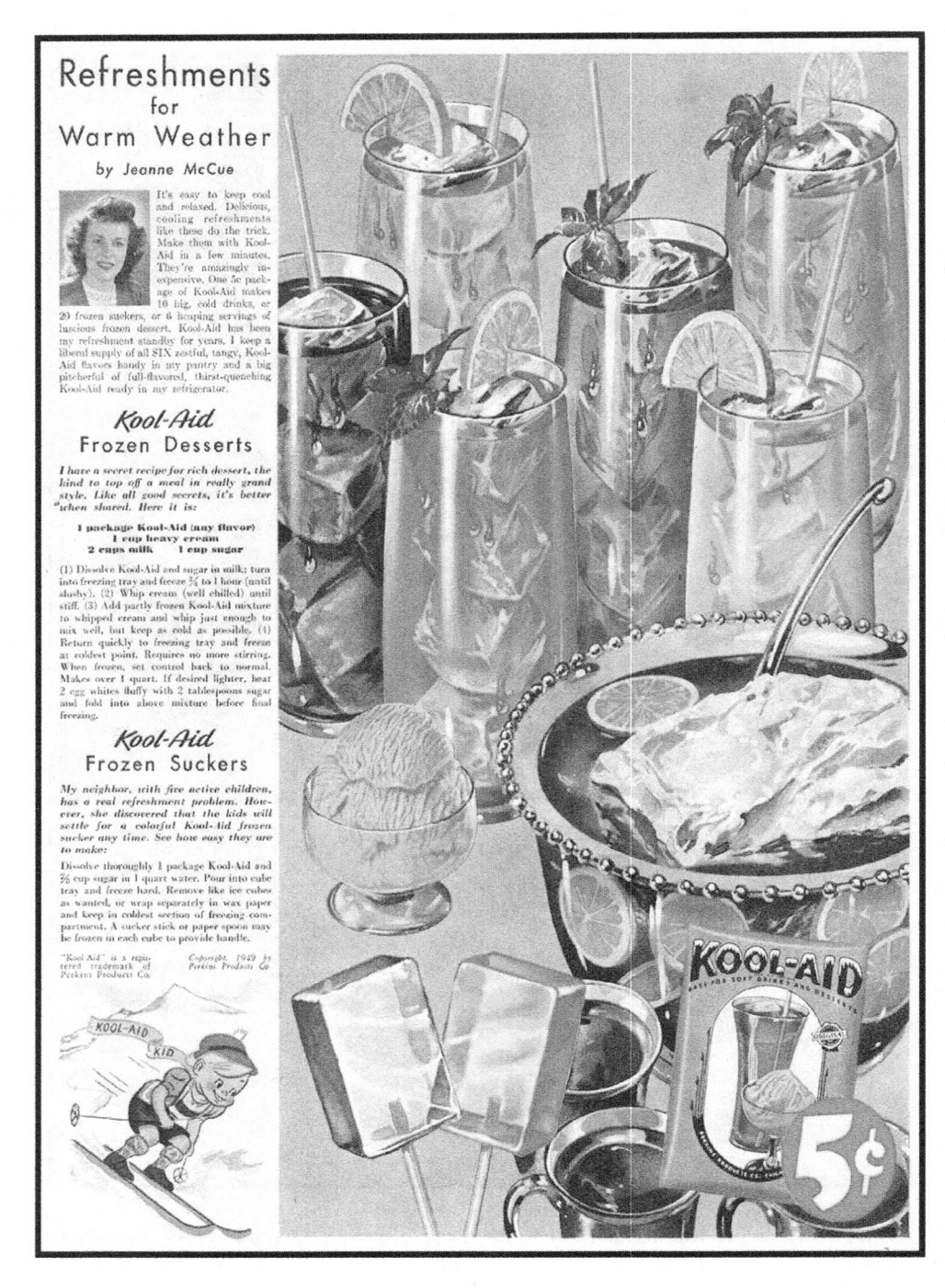

Kool-Aid has been a part of homes since 1927 and was inspired by Jell-O. Pre-sweetened Kool-Aid was developed in 1964 and redeveloped in 1970. This ad appeared in the Ladies' Home Journal in 1949.

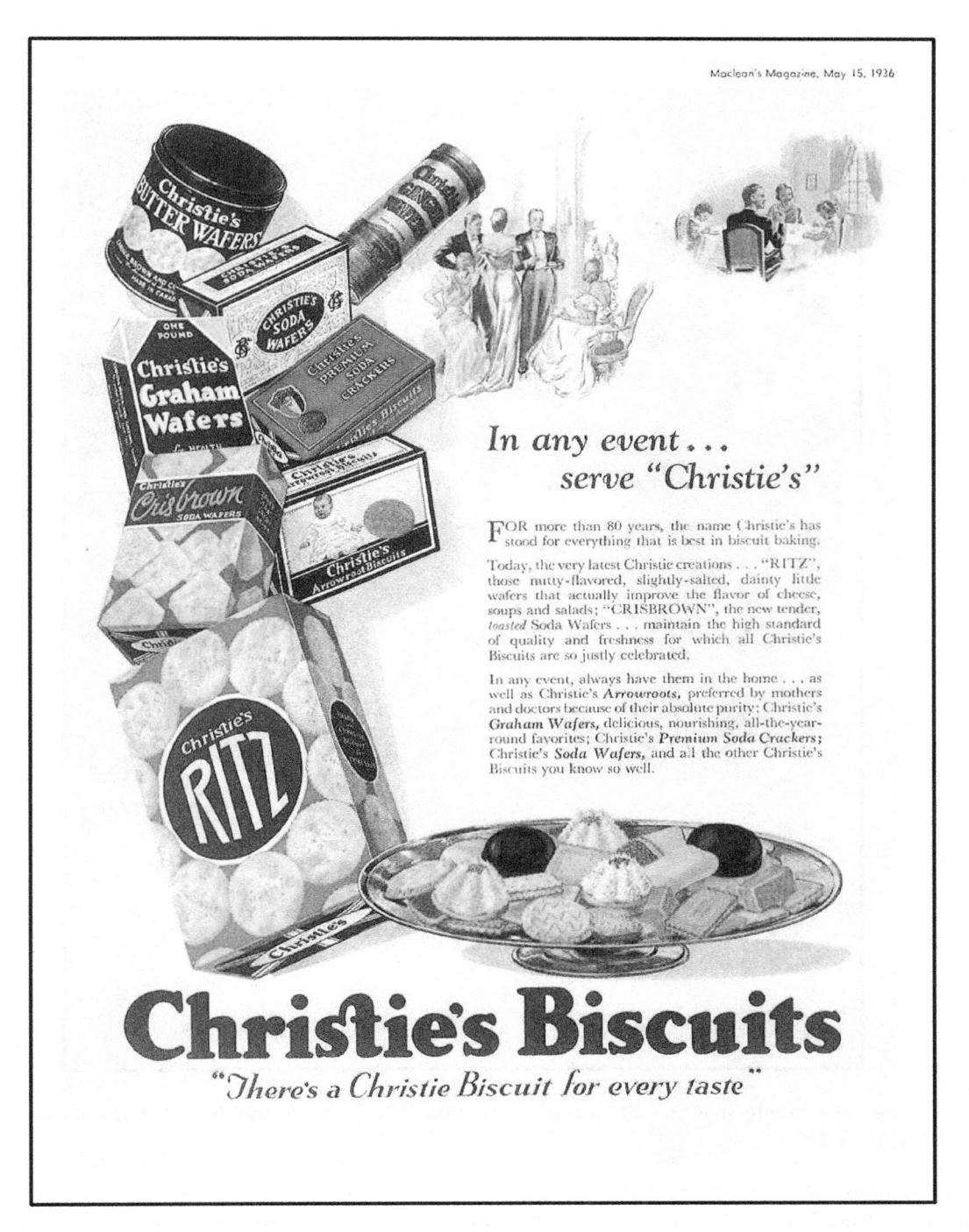

Before Nabisco provided cracker and cookie favorites, there was Christie's, just one of many companies that folded during the 1930s. MacLean's Magazine 1936.

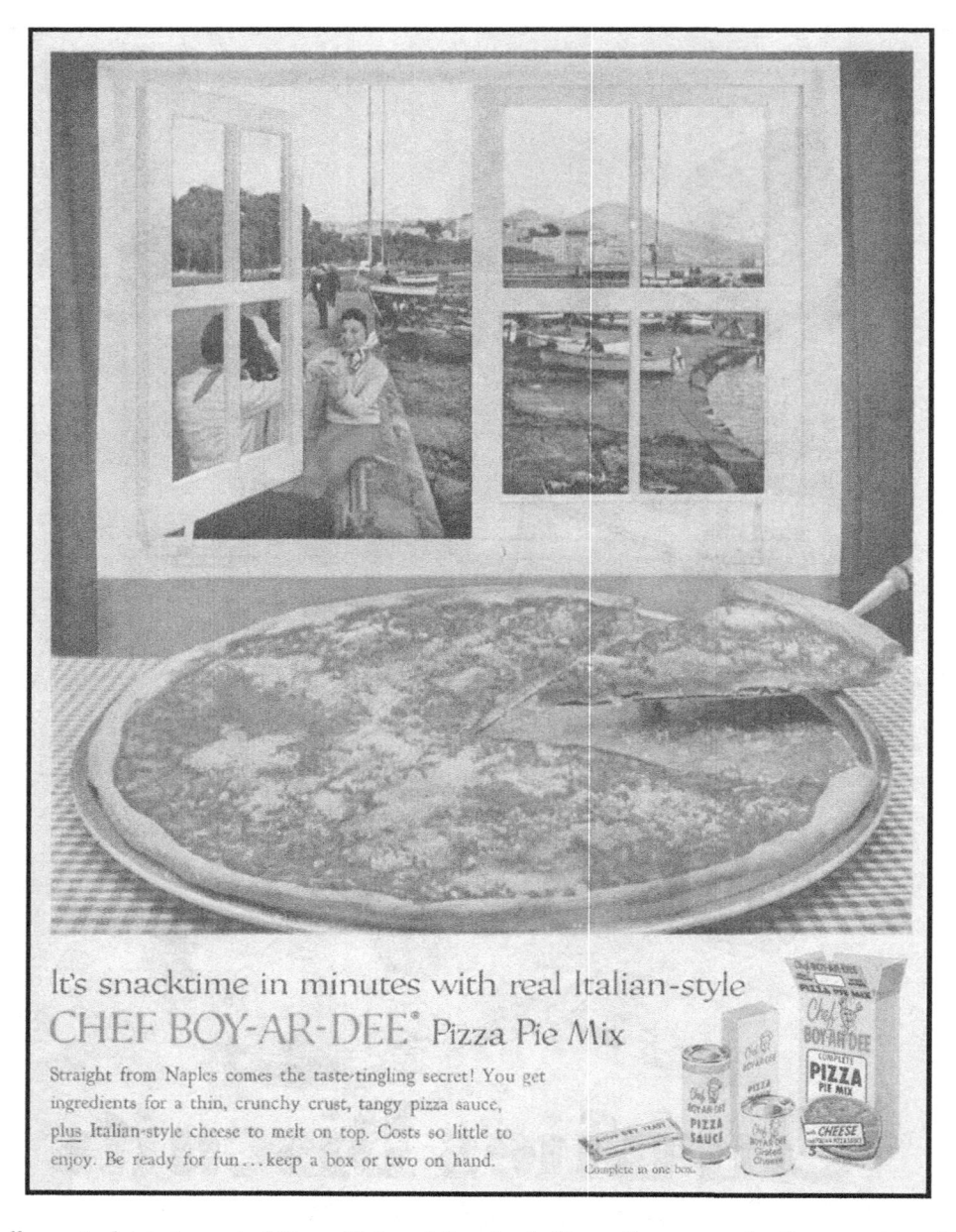

It's snacktime in minutes with real Italian-style
CHEF BOY-AR-DEE® Pizza Pie Mix

Straight from Naples comes the taste-tingling secret! You get ingredients for a thin, crunchy crust, tangy pizza sauce, plus Italian-style cheese to melt on top. Costs so little to enjoy. Be ready for fun...keep a box or two on hand.

Before college students invented Pizza Hut and Domino's Pizza, there was the first meal in a box. Life Magazine 1958

Ettore Boiardi, a classically trained French chef came to America as an Italian immigrant in 1914. He became head chef at New York Plaza Hotel. In 1924, he and his brother opened the first Italian Restaurant outside of little, Italy. Chef Hector's pasta dishes quickly became the talk of the neighborhood, and demand for his food grew. Hector did not trust that individuals would reheat his take-home meal to his satisfaction and came up with the very first boxed meal with a jar of sauce and dried pasta. His invention was soon followed by J. L. Kraft launching the Macaroni and Cheese dinner. [221, 222]

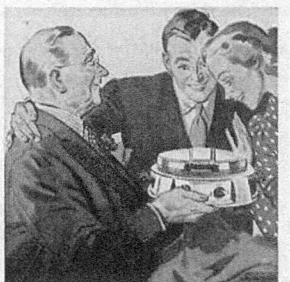

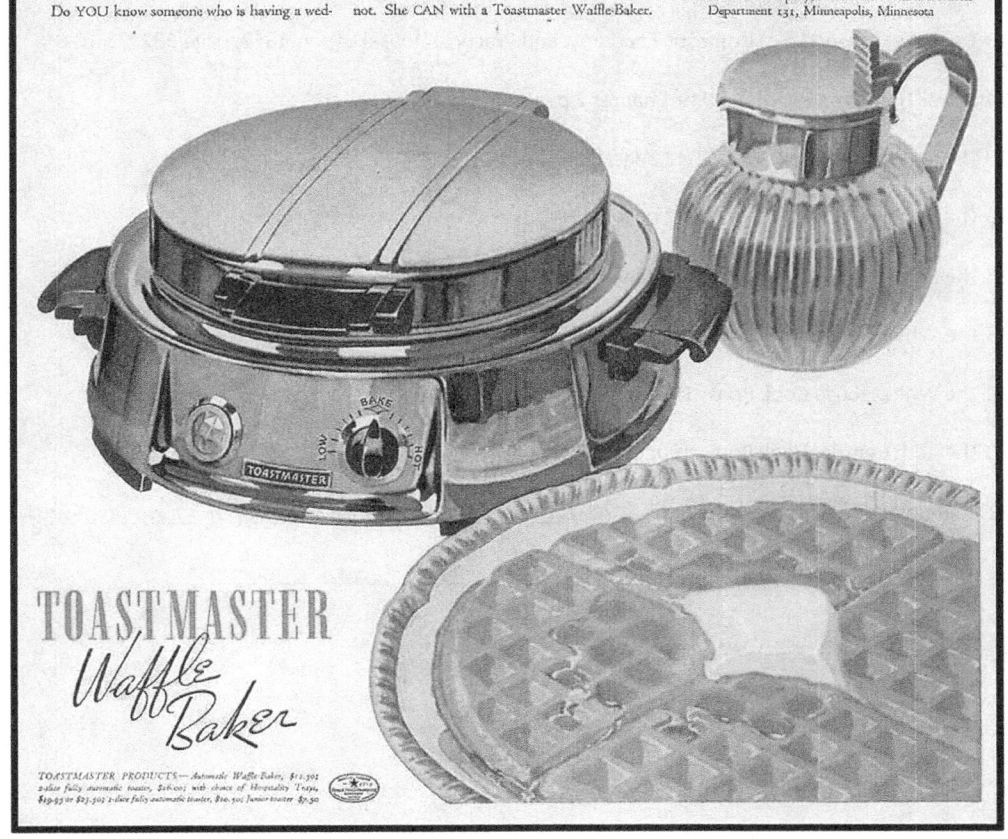

Toastmaster Appliances, Life Magazine 1937

In the 1920s and 1930s waffles became a favorite food for lunch and dinner made at the table with an electric waffle iron. Waffle suppers where a fashionable meal guests would remember, touted the *All about Home Baking* published by General Foods in 1933. Waffles were made with cheese and tomato, pea pulp, cornmeal, peanut butter, coconut, pineapple and more.

207 The Settlement Cook Book, 1942 page I

208 The American Woman's Cook Book, 1947 page 23

209 Meat Tops the Menu – Recipes Menus, Reducing Menus, Compliments of National Live Stock and Meat Board, Chicago, Illinois 1936  Goes with Chapter on Wisdom from the Past

210 Meat Tops the Menu – Recipes Menus, Reducing Menus, Compliments of National Live Stock and Meat Board, Chicago, Illinois 1936

211 The American Woman's Cook Book, 1947 page 24

212 *Household Discoveries and Mrs. Curtis's Cook Book*: Preserving of Meat and Vegetables, 1906 pages 595 , 597, 600, 605

213 The New Cyclopedia of Domestic Economy, and Practical Housekeeper, 1872, page 382

214 Better Homes and garden 1949, chapter 2 page 17

215 The Settlement Cook Book, 1942 page 12

216 The Settlement Cook Book, 1942 page 623

217 The Settlement Cook Book, 1942 page 623

218 The White House Cook Book, 1891 page 496

219 The White House Cook Book, 1891 page 477

220 The 20th Century Cook Book, 1902 page 479

221 Chef Boyardee History, Retrieved July 2022: https://www.wideopeneats.com/chef-boyardee-history/

222  The History of Kraft Foods Inc.: https://web.mit.edu/allanmc/www/kraftfoods.pdf

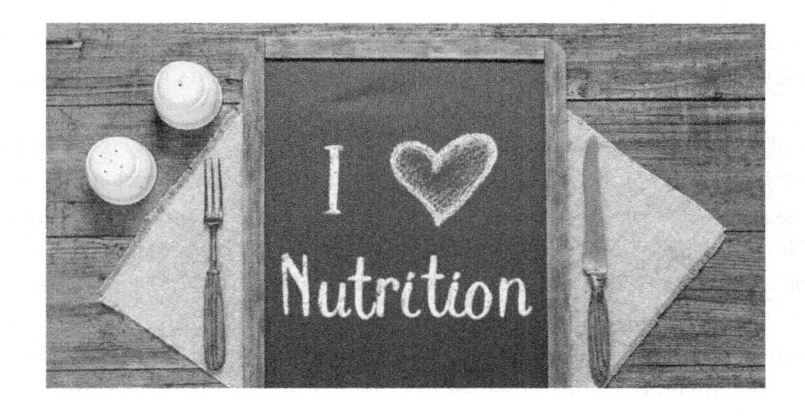

## *Final Thoughts from Chef Christine*

There is nothing more satisfying or more joyful than creating a delicious meal or dish out of nature's offerings. Maybe it's taking the lowly turnip - considered to be the poor man's food in Europe and fed to livestock, and creating a silky soup from it. It's the beauty of distilling the essence of the simple things into the ethereal.

When we sauté garlic and onions, when we braise a piece of meat, we connect ourselves with everyone who has ever braised meat and everyone who will ever braise meat. We share with countless women and men throughout history that same pleasure, amazement, sensory stimulation, and that same sense of mindful gratitude for what Mother Nature provides for us.

The passing down of recipes, the familial and cultural continuum of traditional foods, the nurturing of the preparer and the gratefulness of the receiver is all the collective connectivity we yearn to have.

> *"The nourishment of the body is food,*
> *while the nourishment of the soul is feeding others."*
>
> - Iman Ali

Something so communal as a shared meal can become a battle zone, a polarization of opinions. Instead of this sacred space of collective nourishment, we've turned it into a place of segregation and judgment. In a world that is so divided on so many issues, splitting hairs over how we are to eat, and what only widens the division. Now is time to circle back to the basics, and close the door on food wars.

Delicious, exquisite food is banished by some well-meaning people in the name of certain diet trends. We need to stop labeling food and start embracing it for all its goodness and beauty.

I am reminded of a story that took place about 2,000 years ago. A vision was given to a hungry man who had strict religious taboos about certain foods thought to be unclean. He saw heaven open and a large sheet was let down to earth by its four corners. It contained many different types of food. He was told to nourish himself. He resisted saying he had never eaten anything impure or unclean. He was told not to call anything impure that God has made clean.

A new conversation can take place. A dialogue over the virtues of the variegated colors of our foods and what they mean. We could speak about the energy of our food and the beautiful life-support they provide.

Let us create a new world. A world of harmony and not disenfranchisement, one of nourishment, not the deprivation of body and soul.

> **Principle 30:** *The foods consumed are much more than calories, nutrients, sugars, and fiber. It is medicine, joy, and comfort for all ages. Food connects the world while remaining unique to each person, time, and culture.*

## *List of Principles*

**Principle 1**: Food Knowledge and Culinary Skills must be taught to children and adults in order to improve health outcomes. Pg. 3

**Principle 2**: Our cells carry information on Ancestral Foods. Pg. 5

**Principle 3**: Grow a garden, buy locally, know your farmer and rancher, and converse with the avatar and butcher. Pg. 8

**Principle 4**: An organized and stocked pantry allows for greater food security and dietary flexibility. Pg. 12

**Principle 5**: Make one or two larger meals, so you have leftovers to turn into weekly meals in a hurry. Pg. 13

**Principle 6**: Freezers allow for the seasonal rotation of plants and a complete protein profile of amino acids through the diet for balance, reducing the development of food sensitivities. Pg. 14

**Principle 7**: The How of food preparation and processing is as important if not more so than the What when it comes to health and wellness. Pg. 18

**Principle 8**: While the Industrial Revolution brought about many beneficial changes, it diminished our connection to local food and lore. Pg. 19

**Principle 9**: When it comes to fats and oils, read the label, consider the packaging, and look for the country of origin to determine quality. Pg. 36

**Principle 10**: Quality cooking utensils and cookware last a lifetime and are a measure of safety from unknown chemical contaminants. Pg. 54

**Principle 11**: Lower dependence on plastics by using bees wax coated papers, cotton, and parchment paper bags. Pg 56

**Principle 12**: Reduce lead exposure by verifying the heavy metal content of stoneware, ceramic, and china dishware. Dishware manufacturers utilize heavy metal in the glazing process still. Pg. 60

**Principle 13**: Filter all the water used in drinking and cooking. Filtered water reduces toxic chemicals, solvents, and pathogens from contaminating food. Fermenting requires filtered water. Pg. 63

**Principle 14**: Understanding the healing properties of herbs and their inclusion in cookery is essential to fully grasp the concept of "food as medicine." Pg. 68

**Principle 15**: Herbs, spices & seasonings ~~use~~ are shared and interconnected worldwide. Pg. 77

**Principle 16**: Prepare yourself to cook. Mise en place = putting in place or gather. Read recipes all the way through, and assemble ingredients and tools before beginning. Pg. 82

**Principle 17**: To reduce high lectin and phytic acid content, soak beans and quinoa before cooking under pressure. Pg 120

**Principle 18**: The care and kindness we show others should follow us into the kitchen. Small, meaningful adjustments made in relationships apply to recipes, too. Pg. 132

**Principle 19**: Target exotic edible weed species is guaranteed ethical harvesting. This helps control exotic populations so native species can thrive. Pg. 182

**Principle 20:** Ethical harvesting reduces and assists the species you harvest so they can continue growing successfully. Ensuring future harvests are abundant for foragers, including animals. Pg. 183

**Principle 21:** Consider what aspect of nutrition or medicinal benefits you are harvesting a plant for. Pg. 186

**Principle 22:** Let Go ~ stop trying so hard and allow your generational intuition guide you. The best way to get the flavor of the past is to use your senses versus precision measurements. Pg. 260

**Principle 23:** Home fermenting is an easy and affordable way to preserve food, and add pro and pre biotics to the diet. Pg 270

**Principle 24**: Too much of a good thing can lead to digestive health challenges for some individuals. Not everyone can do fermented foods, due to imbalances in the gut microbiome. Pg. 271

**Principle 25**: Fermentation reduces carbohydrate content and naturally occurring toxins present in plant foods. Pg. 278

**Principle 26**: Traditionally prepared dairy, that is naturally fermented and cared for, can provide valuable nutrition for those not allergic. Pg. 296

**Principle 27:** Condiments act as flavor enhancers and digestive aids when made with clean ingredients and in traditional ways. Pg. 306

**Principle 28:** Special foods are always a part of cultural events. So be kind to yourself and those around you and savor the flavor and connection of traditions. Pg. 350

**Principle 29:** Consider how much money you are saving by cooking yourself! For example, it costs less to buy grass-fed steak for four people than it does to buy a feedlot steak cooked in a mediocre restaurant for one. Pg. 352

**Principle 30:** The foods consumed are much more than calories, nutrients, sugars, and fiber. It is medicine, joy, and comfort for all ages. Food connects the world while remaining unique to each person, time, and culture. Pg 400

# Modern & Historical Cookery Resources

Allen, D. (2005). *Irish Traditional Cooking.* Kyle Books.

Apelian, N. (2021). *The Forager's Guide to Wild Foods: The North American Edition.* Global Brothers SRL.

Archibald, A. (2019). *The Genomic Kitchen.*

Ayrton, E. (1975). *The Cookery of England.* Great Britain: Purnell Book Services.

Beard, J. (1972). *American Cookery.* New York: Little Brown and Company.

Beard, J. (1976). *New Fish Cookery.* New York: Little Brown and Company.

Berolzheimer, R. (1947). *The American Woman's Cook Book.* Chicago: National Binding.

Better Homes and Garden. (1949). *Better Homes and Garden Cook Book.* De Moines: Meredith Publishing Company.

Betty Crocker. (1952). *Betty Crocker's Picture Cook Book.*

Bitterman, M. (2010). *Salted.* New York: Ten Speed Press.

Blackstone, E. M. (1910). *The American Womans' Cook-Book: Approved Hosehold Recipes.* Chicago: Laird & Lee.

Board, N. L. (1936). *Meat Tops the Menue.* Chacago: National Live Stock and Meat Board.

Breed, L. M. (1934). *The Human Machine.* Boston: The Alpine Press.

Buhner, S. H. (1998). *Sacred and Herbal Healing Beers - Secrets of Ancient Ferminutestation.* Boulder: Siris Books.

Capoano, A. (Director). (2022). *True Texas Mexican: Cuisine and Culture* [Motion Picture].

Cernohous, S. (2017). *The Funky Kitchen.* Flagstaff: Living Wellness, LLC.

Civitello, L. (2011). *Cuisine & Culture 3rd edition.* Hoboken: Wiley.

Collester, J. S. (1988). *Old Pioneer Recipes.* Indianapolis: Bear Wallow Books.

Colonial Williamsburg Foundation. (1938). *The Williamsburg Art of Cookery or Accomplifb'd Gentlewoman's Companion.* Williamsburg : Williamsburg Foundation.

Company, M. L. (1922). *The Metropolitan Cook Book.* New York: Metrropolitan Life Insurance Company.

Cooke, M. C. (1902). *The Great 20th Century Cook Book.* Illinois: The Educational Company.

Cordain, L. (2002). *The Paleo Diet.* Hoboken, New Jersy: John Wiley & Sons.

Cortes, M. (n.d.). *A Seacret History of Coffee, Cocca & Cola.* Brooklyn: Akashic Books.

Cressman, L. S. (1961, 1981, 2005). *The Sandle and the Cave - The Indians of Oregon.* Corvallis: Oregon State University Press.

Cruess, W. (1948). *Commercial Fruit and Vegitable Products.* New York, Toranto, Lundon: McGraw-Hill Book Company.

Cuny, J.-M. (1971). *La Cuisine Lorraine*.

De Pay, F. A. (1900). *The New Century Home Book*. New York: Eaton & Mains.

Dods, M. L. (1902). *My Mothers Cook Book: of the South Kentington School of Cookery*. Chicago: Thompson and Thomas.

Dukes, G. H. (2016). *A Short History of Eating*. London: London Press.

Ellet, E. F. (1872). *The New Cyclopaedia of Domestic Housekeeper: adapted to all classes of society*. Norwich: Henry Bill.

Ellet, M. E. (1972). *New Cyclopaedia: Domestic Economy, and Practical Housekeeper*. Norwich, CO: Henry Bill.

Fallon, S. &. (2001). *Nourishing Traditions*. Washington, DC: New Trends.

Farm Journal. (1963). *Freezing and Canning Cookbook*. New York: Doubleday.

Farmer, F. M. (1917). *A New Book of Cookery*. Boston: Little Brown and Company.

Fernandez, A. F. (2002). *Near a Thousand Tables a history of food*. New York: Free- Press.

Fisher, K. A. (1929). *Good Meals and How to Prepare Them*. New York: Good House Keeping Institute.

Fitzgerald, K. N. (2016). *Methylation Diet & Lifestyle*. Medford: www.drkarafitzgerald.com.

Flandrin, J. L. (1996). *FOOD a culinary history from antiquity to the present*. New York: Columbia University Press.

Fraioli, J. O. (2011). *Wild Alaskan Seafood*. Guilford: Lyons Press.

Gaia Original. (1988). *The New Age Herbalist*. New York: Gaia Books Ltd.

Gately, I. (2008). *Drink : A Cultural History of Alcohol*. New York: Gotham Books.

Gilbert, F. C. (1931). *Historic Cookery*. Layton : Gibbs Smith Publisher.

Gillette, H. Z. (1905). *The White House Cook Book*. New York: The Saalfield Publishing Company.

Gillette, M. F. (1891). *The White House Cook Book*. Cinncinati: Central Publishing House.

Ginger, B. H. (1900). *California Mexican-Spanish Cook Book*. VintageCookbooks.com.

Gladstar's, R. (2008). *Herbal Recipes*. North Adams: Strorey Publishing.

Good Housekeeping. (1944). *The Good Housekeeping Cook Book*. New York: Farrar and Rinehart.

Grieve, M. (1971). *A Modern Herbal Vol I & Vol II*. New York: Dover Publications.

Hale, H. H. (1968). *The Horizon Cookbook and Illistrated History of Eating and Drinking through the Ages*. American Heritage Publishing Co.

Hamilton, A. V. (1873). *The Household Cyclopaedia*. Springfield: W.J. Holland & CO.

Harmer, B. (1938). *Text-Book of the Principles and Practice of Nursing*. New York: The MacMillan Company.

Hay, W. H. (1929). *Health via Food*. East Aurora: Sun-Diet Press.

Health Department Cookware Company of America. (1935). *Healthward: Cooking and Eating for Health, Happiness and Success.* Hartford.

Herrick, C. T. (1913). *Consolidated Library of Modern Cooking and Household Recipes.* Akron: The New Werner Company.

Hetzler, R. (2010). *The Mitsitam Cafe Cookbook.* Washington Dc: Smithsonian National Musium of the Amrican Indian.

Hewitt, J. R. (1872). *Coffee: Its History, Cultivation and Uses.* New York: Digital Text Publishing.

Hirsch, D. (2005). *The Moosewood Restaurant Kitchen Garden.* New York: Ten Speed Press.

Hopkins, K. (2009). *99 Drams of Whiskey.* new York: St. Martin Press.

Household Magazine. (1931). *Searchlight Recipe Book.* Topeka: The Household Magazine.

Hutchens, A. R. (1991). *Indian Herbalogy of North America.* Boston: Shabhala.

Issued by the Medical Department of the General Confrence of the Seventh-day Adventists. (1921). *Home Nursing a comprehensive series of lessions on hygiene and the practical care of the sick.* Washington, D.C.: Review and Herald Publishing Association.

Kamps, A. D. (2011). *What's Cooking Uncle Sam?* Washington DC: The Foundation for the National Archives.

Kander, M. S. (1947). *The Settlement Cook Book.* Milwaukee: Settlement Cook Book Co.

Karr, T. (2018). *Our Journey with Food 2nd edition.* Summerland.

Karr, T. a. (2020). *Empty Plate Food Sustainability Minutesdfulness.* Summerland.

Karr, T. J. (2015). *Our Journey with Food.* Bozeman: Summerland.

Katz, S. E. (2016). *Wild Fermentation.* White River Junction: Green Press Initiative.

Keal, B. (2008). *Tupperware Unsealed.* Gainsville FL: University Press.

Keepsake Cuisine Series. (n.d.). *Chuck Wagon Cooking.* Terrell Publishing Co.

Keith, L. (2009). *The Vegitarien Myth.* Cresent City CA: FlashPoint Press.

Kellogg, M. E. (1893). *Science in the Kitchen - Principles of Healthful Cookery.* Chicago: Modern Medicine Publishing Co.

Kerr. (1920). *Kerr Home Canning Book.* Portland: Kerr Glass Manufacturing Corporation.

Kingry, J. (2012). *Ball Complete Book of Home Preserving.* Toronto: Robert Rose Inc.

Kirschmann, J. (2007). *Nutrition Almanac 6th edition.* New York: McGraw Hill.

Kopec, L. N. (2013). *Let's Get Real About Eating.* Bloominutesgton, IN: Balboa Press.

Kurlansky, M. (2009). *The Food of a Younger Land.* New York: Penguin Group.

Kurlansky, M. (2010). *Salt: A world History .* New York: Walker and Comp.

LaBella, L. (2012). *Seasoning CastIron.* Smashwords.

Lassiter, W. L. (1959). *Shaker Recipes for Cooks and Homemakers*. New York: Greenwich Book Publishers.

Lemcke, G. (1906). *European and American Cuisine*. New York: D. Appleton and Company.

Lindlahr, V. H. (1942). *You Are What You Eat*. New York: National Nutrition Society.

Lovegren, S. (2005). *Fashionable Food: Seven Decades of Food Fads*. Chicago: University of Chicago Press.

Lovegren, S. (2005). *Fashionable Foods, Seven Decades of Food Fads*. Chicago: The University of Chicago Press.

Lowell, J. P. (2005). *The Gluten-Free Bible*. New york: Henry Holt and Comp.

Mabey, R. (1988). *The New Age Herbalist*. New York: A Fireside Book.

Marrone, T. (2012). *Cooking with Wild Berries & Fruits*. Cambridge: Adventure Publications.

Martinez, M. (2020). *The Mexican Home Kitchen*. NY: Rage Kindelsperger.

Medical Department of the General Confrence of Seventh-day Adventists. (1927). *Home Nursing*. Washington, DC: Review and Herald Publishing Associasion.

Minutesich, D. (2016). *Whole Detox: 21 Day Personalized Program* . New York: Harper One.

Minutesich, D. P. (2018). *The Rainbow Diet*. Newburyport: Conari Press.

Montanari, M. (1949, 2004). *Food is Culture*. New York: Columbia University Press.

Morales, N. (2020). *The Native Mexican Kitchen: A journey into Cuisine, Culture and Mezcal*. Skyhorse Publishing.

Morse, S. (1908). *Household Discoveries: Encyclopaedia of Practical Recipes and Processes*. NY: The Success Company.

Mueller, J. (2014). *Delicious Probiotic Drinks*. New York: Skyhorse Publishing.

Mueller, T. (2012). *Extra Virginity: The Sublime and Scandalous World of Olive Oil*. New York, London: WW Norton & Comp.

Murphy, J. (1986). *A Little Irish Cookbook*. San Fransico: Chronicle Books.

National Livestock and Meat Board. (1936). *Meat Tops the Menu*. Chicago: National Live stock and Meat Board.

National Presto Industries Inc. (1966). *The Modern Guide to Pressure Canning and Cooking*. Eau Claire: National Presto Industries, Inc.

National Presto Industries Inc. (1955). *National Presto Cooker Recipe Book*. Eau Claire: National Presto Industries Inc.

Neil, M. H. (1917). *Ryson Baking Book*. New York: General Chemical Company - Food Department.

Orey, C. (2010). *The Healing Powers of Chocolate*. New York, New York: Kensington Books.

Pendergrast, M. (2010). *Uncommon Grounds: The History of Coffee and How it Transformed our World*. New York New York: Basic Books.

Phillips, A. L. (1906). *A Bachelors Cupboard*. Vintage Cookbooks.com.

Pollan, M. (2001). *The Botany of Desire - Plants Eye View of the World*. New York New York: Random House.

Quelus, A. L. (2011). *The Natural history of Chocolate.* Five Star Publishing.

Reavis, C. G. (1981). *Home Sausage Making* . North Adams: Storey Publishing.

Richards, Mary Anne, Staff Home Economist. (1965). *Favorite Recipes of America - Vegitables.* Louisville: Favorite Recipies Press Inc.

Robinson, J. (2013). *Eating on the Wild Side - the Missing Link to Optimum Health.* New York: Bantom Books.

Rombaur, I. S. (1942). *The Joy of Cooking* . Indianapolis: The Bob-Merrill Company.

Ronald, M. (1897). *The Century Cook Book.* NY: The Century CO.

Rore, S. (1886). *Mrs. Rorer's Philadelphia Cook Book: A Manual of Home Economies.* Philadelphia: George H Buchanan and Company.

Rorer, S. T. (1914). *Mrs Rorer's Diet for the Sick.* Philadelphia: Arnold and Company.

Schatzker, M. (2011). *Steak.* New York: Penguin Books.

Schindler, B. (2021). *Eat Like a Human.* Little Brown Spark.

Sharol Tilgner, N. (1999). *Herbal Formulas.* Creswell: Wise Acres Publishing.

Sherman, S. (2017). *The Sioux Chef's Indigenous Kitchen.* Minutesneapolis: University of Minutesnesota Press.

Shimer, P. (2004). *Healing Secrets of the Native Americans.* New York: Black Dog.

Shulman, M. R. (2007). *Mediterranean Harvest.* New York: Rodale.

Sitz, K. (2008). *Basque Heritage Cookbook.* Burns: Self Published.

Sloan, E. S. (1901). *Sloan's Handy Hints and Up-To-Date Cookbook.* Boston: Dr. Earl, S Sloan.

Snodgrass, M. E. (2004). *Encyclopedia of Kitchen History.* New York: Fitzroy Dearborn.

Sonnenfeld, A. (1999). *Food A Culinary History from Antiquity to the Present.* Columbia University Press.

Spice Islands Home Economics Staff. (1961). *The Spice Islands Cook Book.* Menlo Park: Lane Book Company.

SRM - Society for Range Managment. (1990). *Trail Boss Cowboy Cookbook.* Blackwell: SRM - Society for Range Managment.

Standage, T. (2009). *A Edible History of Humanity.* New York: Walker & Company.

Strawbridge, D. a. (2012). *Curing and Smoking Made at Home.* Richmond Hill: Firefly Books Ltd.

Strehlow, W. P. (1988). *Hildegard of Bingen's Medicine.* Rochester: Bear and Company.

Tannerhill, R. (1988). *Food in History.* New York: Three Rivers Press.

Tason, M. (2011). *A Guide to History of Chocolate.* www.enjoyablebooks.com.

Thayer, S. (2015). *The Forager's Harvest; A guide to Identifying, Harvesting and Preparing Edible Wild Plants.* Bruce, WI: Forager's Harvest.

The W.T. Rawleigh Company. (1942 & 1943). *Rawleigh's Good Health Guide: Almanac, Cook Book*. The W.T. Rawleigh Company.

Throop, P. (1998). *Physica - Hildegard von Bingen's*. Rochester VT: Healing Arts Press.

Tilgner, N. S. (1999). *Herbal Formulas*. Creswell: Wise Acres Publishing.

Tilgner, S. (1999). *Herbal Medicine from the Heart of the Earth*. Creswell: Wise Acres Press.

Trader Vic's. (1968). *Trader Vic's Pacific Island Cookbook*. New York: Doubleday.

US Department of Agriculture. (1928). *Pork on the Farm, Killing, Curing, and Canning*. Washington, DC: US Department of Agriculture.

Wahls, T. M. (2017). *The Wahls Protocol Cooking for Life*. New York, New York: Penguin Group LLC.

Wang, Y. a. (2010). *Ancient Wisdom, Modern Kitchen*. Life Long.

Weaver, L. B. (1917). *A Thousand Ways To Please A Husband*. New York: A. L. Burt Company.

Webster, M. J. (1914). *The Apsley Cookery Book*. London: J & A Churchi;;.

Williams, M. E. (1912). *Elements of the Theory and Practice of Cookery*. MacMillan Company.

Williamson, D. (1993). *Basque Cooking and Lore*. Caldwell: Craxton Printers, Ltd.

Wilson, B. (2012). *Consider the Fork*. New York: Basic Books.

Wilson, B. (2019). *The Way We Eat Now*. New York: Basic Books.

Wise Books. (1948). *The Wise Encyclopedia of Cookery*. NY: Wm Wise & Co. Inc.

Woman's Home Companion. (1942). *Woman's Home Companion Cook Book*. New York: P.F. Collier and Son Corporation.

Wrought Iron Range Co. (1923). *Home Comfort Cook Book*. St. Louis: Wrought Iron Range Co.

# Index

18th Century Apricot Ice Cream, 343
5 Minute Guilt Free YUMM-OHH pudding, 341
845- To Melt Lard, 380
A Note on Fish Broth, 267
Alaskan Summer, 256
Almandrongila Euskalduna Moduda, 215
Alubias de Tolosa Stew, 123
Amaranth Pilaf, 165
American Indian Health and Diet Project, 192
Apple Crumble, 323
Apricot Silk, 325
Apricot Tansy, 346
Arroz con Leche, 337
Ashure, 338
Asparagus and Roasted Red Peppers and Garlic, 86
Asparagus Leek Soup, 85
Aunt Pari's Picnic Cutlets, 245
Avocado Cream Sauce, 312
Avocado Dip, 308
Aymara Spoke with the Stars, 150
Bacalao Con Tomates Y Pimiento, 260
Bacalo A La Vizcaina, 259
Baked Apples with Blackberries, 321
Baked Pheasant, 206
Baked Turnips, 117
Banana Crunch Muffins YUMM, 332

Basil Pesto, 309
Basque Apple Compote, 320
Basque Beans and Chorizo, 123
Basque Beef Tongue, 218
Basque Chorizo, 227
Basque Cod with Tomatoes and Peppers, 260
Basque Cuisine, 259
Basque Pasta, 262
Basque Rabbit Stew, 207
Basque Roast Leg of Lamb, 222
Basque shellfish and rice, 260
Basque Tenderloin with Peppers, 212
Basque Tomatoes Stuffed with Foie Gras, Duck Confit, and Chanterelles, 173
Basque Tuna and Potato Soup, 261
Beans & Grains, 22
Bear Fat Pie Crust, 210
Beef Heart Jerky, 355
Beef Tongue, 218
Beetroot Raita, 113
Ben's Barbecue Sauce, 308
Berry Lemonade, 362
Berry Vinaigrette Salad Dressing or Glaze, 310
Best Ever Broccoli Soup, 88
Bitterroot Pudding, 184
Black Bean Chili, 122

Blackberries & Peaches, 321
Blackberry Liqueur, 360
Blackberry Sorbet, 321
Bleaching Lard, 381
Blitva, 99
Blueberry Tea, 360
Bobotie, 216
Braciole, 212
Broad-Leaf Maple Flower Fritters, 183
Broccoli and Chickpea Curry, 128
Broccoli and Red Onions, 87
Brotchan Foltchep, 153
Broths/Bouillon/Stocks, 221
Brown Kale with Chestnuts, 133
Brussels Sprout-Potato Hash, 87
Buckwheat Grits, 162
Buckwheat Naan Bread, 162
Buckwheat Rye Bread, 163
Buckwheat Waffles, 161
Buffalo Berry Jelly, 188
Buffalo Steak in Red wine, 209
Bull Kelp Pickles, 84
Burrito in Turmeric Buttermilk, 236
Buttered Cabbage, 94
Camp Coffee, 365
Camp Cookery, 386
Carbohydrates, 27
Cast Iron, 64, 65

Cattail Pollen Dumplings in Sweet Onion soup, 197
Cattails on the Cob, 197
Cauliflower Kuku, 95
Champ, 107
Championak Salsa Berden, 315
Chard & Potatoes, 99
Chat Masala, 131
Chicken Kabob, 244
Chicken Liver Sautéed, 251
Chicken Livers and Mushrooms, 249
Chicken Pie, 246
Chicken with Purple Cabbage and Chard, 236
Chickweed Salad, 197
Chinese Bright Eyes Soup, 320
Chokecherry Jelly Recipe, 187
Chokecherry Syrup, 187
Citrus Poached White Fish, 268
Clarified butter or Ghee, 34
Coconut Milk Ice-Cream, 343
Coconut Milk Yogurt, 276
Conejo Guisado, 207
Cookies That Bring Joy, 333
Cookware, 56
Corn Griddle Cakes, 145
Corn Silk Tea, 368
Crabapple Jelly, 326
Crabapplejack, 364
Cranberry Spritzer, 362
Creamy Basque Dressing, 315
Creamy Cabbage-Potato & Pork Soup, 229
Creamy Mushroom Soup, 174
Cucumber Catsup, 308
Cucumber Sauce, 310
Culinary Spices, 75
Custard Cream, 348
Dads Bacon Curls, 231
Dads No-Bake Cheese Cake, 349
Dandelion and Hibiscus Kombucha, 274
Dandelion Greens, 190
Dandelion Greens (1902), 190
Dandelion Jelly, 189
Dandelion Risotto soup, 190
Dandelion Wine, 188
Dressing for Dandelion Greens, 189
Drop Biscuits or Dumplings, 159
Duck Liver Pâté, 203
Duck, Date, and Rutabaga Pot Pie, 242
Dulse and Yellowman, 82
Dulse Slaw, 83
Easy Chicken Parmesan, 251
Easy Cream Cheese Made at Home, 302
**Easy Fermented Kraut and Veggies, 292**
Easy Sourdough Starter, 282
Eggs, 238
Eggs and Sausage, 240
Egyptian Tigernut Sweets, 151
Elderberries and Rosehips Syrup, 184
Elderberry Infused Honey, 185
Elderberry Jelly, 185
Elevation Adjustments, 44
Elk in Wine, 208
English Muffins, 284
Ezekiel Bread, 153
Fall Foods Breakfast Sausage, 228
Fats & Oils, 33
Feel Better Italian Soup, 121
Fennel and Delicate Squash Soup, 96
Fermented Cranberry Apple Relish, 275
Fermented Foods to Brine Ratio, 293
Fermented Fruits, 291
Fermented Potato Chips, 278
Filets' Con Pimentos, 212
Finnish Sima Spring Mead, 274
Fire Cider, 361
Fish With Green Peppers and Clams, 265
Flan, 332
Flaxseed Lemonade, 365
Flaxseed Tea, 365
Flummery, 323
Food for the God's Chocolate Mousse, 345
Food Placement in Refrigerator, 385
French Dressing, 313
French lentils Stew, 124
French Onion Soup, 96
Fricase De Pollo, 246
Fried Cornmeal Mush, 144
Fried Dandelion Blossoms, 189
Fried Sweeting, 324
Fruit French Dressing, 314

Fruits & Vegetables, 32
Game Meat & Offal, 199
Garam Masala, 130
Garlic Soup, 89
Garlic, Onions, Shallots, & Chives, 74
German Caraway Bread, 164
German Lentil-Sausage Soup, 128
German Potato Salad, 106
Ginger, 80, 327
Ginger Beer, 363
Ginger Molasses Cookies, 335
GingerPoached Peaches with Goat cheese and Blueberries, 326
Going Greek, 222
Goji Berries, 320
Grain-Free Granola, 165
Grandmothers Family Spring Bitters, 366
Granola - Gluten free, 354
Greek Greens and Rice Salad, 152
Green Beans and Chanterelle's, 176
Green Corn Griddle Cakes, 143
Green Tea Ginger Moscow Mule, 367
Grilled Steak with Spicy Argentinian Sauce, 213
Grits Waffles, 160
Gumbo File, 264
Halibut with Green Beans and Quinoa, 256
Harvey's Sauce, 314
Hebridean Broth, 83
Heritage Grains and Native Preservation, 137
History of Sourdough Bread, 155

Hoe-Cake, 143
Home Food Preserving Resources, 22
Homemade Dairy Yogurt Instructions for Pasteurized Milk, 276
Homemade Ketchup, 307
Hominy, 140
Hominy Balls, 140
Hominy Griddle, 141
Hominy Pudding, 140
Horchata made from Chura, 368
Hot Toddy, 364
How to Care for Fats, 380
How to Clarify Fat, 379
How to Clean Cast-Iron, 58
How to Make Nixtamal, 139
How to Try Out or Render Fat, 379
Huitlacoche Tacos, 142
Hungarian Farina Dumpling Soup, 213
Hungarian Fried Cabbage and Noodles, 89
Hungarian Goulash, 214
Hungarian Mushroom Soup, 172
Hungarian Walnut Cookies, 339
Hunters Stew, 204
Injera - Ethiopian Flatbread, 288
Instant Turmeric Golden Milk, 365
Invalid Cookery, 391
Irish Moss Lemonade, 194
Irish Soda Bread, 157
Italian Salad Dressing, 311
Italian White Bean Soup, 126

Kale Sauté with Garlic and Lemon, 93
Karen's Awesome Banana Nut Muffins, 328
Karr, Tammera, 416
Kidney, 200
Kitchen Appliances, 61
Kohlrabi, 93
Kombucha, 272
Korean Five Grain Rice, 134
Kunun Aya Refresher, 151
Kuru Fasulye, 120
Lamb and Potatoes, 223
Lamb Gravy, 316
Latkes, 104
Lemon Bliss Bars, 329
Lemon Ginger Water Kefir, 273
Lemonade Syrup, 317
Lengua, 218
Lenten Borscht with Beans, 113
Lentil and Chorizo Casserole, 129
Lentil and Lemon Soup, 124
Libby's Buttermilk Baking Mix, 158
Libby's Mayonnaise, 311
Liver and Onions, 219
Mac & Cheese, 301
Macaroni Pie, 300
Mango Chutney, 306
Marmitako, 261
Marrow Bones, 220
Matsutake Cracker Hors d'oeuvre, 176
Meat Balls Basque Style, 215
Meat Tops the Menu, 381
Medicinal Foods, 391
Meghli, 148
Mexican Coffee, 369

Migas, 239
Mincedmeat, 344
MinceMeat, 199
Mint Sauce, 316
Mock Apple Fritter, 346
Moms Cornbread, 145
Moms Peach Cobbler, 322
Moose Steak, 208
Mugolio: Pine Cone Syrup, 195
Mushroom Medley-Miso Soup, 177
Mushroom Stir Fry, 176
Mushrooms Sautéed, 174
Mushrooms with Parsley Sauce, 315
Mussels in White Wine, 266
Mustard Poultice, 391
Mutter Paneer, 130
Natillas, 348
National Center for Home Food Preservation, 47
Nettle Broth, 194
New Mexico Green Chile Sauce, 313
Nixtamalization, 138
No-Bake Cranberry Nut Energy Bites, 336
Nona's Pasta e Fagioli Soup, 126
Nona's Salmon Spread, 316
Norms Buckwheat Pancakes, 162
Norwegian Rye Bread, 164
Nuts and Seeds, 29
Oatmeal Muffins, 153
Ogokbap, 134
Old Fashioned Irish Watercress Soup, 193
Old Fashioned Tomato Sauce, 312

Onions, 19
Orangeade, 366
Oregon Grape, 185
Oxalate, 30
Oxtail Casserole, 220
Paella, 260
Pakora plate, 90
Paleo Eggnog Recipe, 369
Pancake Mix, 159
Parmesan Polenta with Bacon and Greens, 289
Parsnip Cakes with Crispy Bacon, 115
Parsnips with Ham and Basil, 115
Persian Basmati Rice, 150
Pierna De Cordero Asada, 222
Pizzelles, 333
Plain Waffles, 160
Polenta, 143
Pone, 144
Pork & Fennel, 228
Pork Loin with Fruit, 230
Pork Steak Grill with Spicy Sauce, 230
Pork with Mulberry Chutney, 230
Porru Sada: Leek Soup, 90
Potato Cheese, 112
Potato Cheesecake, 112
Potato Pancakes, 116
Poultry Stock, 250
Pre-Biotic Onion Bread, 277
Proteins, 32
Pumpkin Kibbeh, 91
Purple Potato Salad, 107
Quinoa and Watercress Salad, 149
Quinoa Salad, 149
Rabbit and Gravy, 207
Radishes with Butter and Parsley, 116

Rainbow Chard and Pecans, 100
Raised Hominy Muffins, 141
Raisin Sauce, 317
Rajma Masala, 132
Raw Lemon Cheesecake Bars, 340
Red Cabbage and Apples, 94
Refried beans, 126
Restorative Pâté, 249
Rhubarb-Berry Spoon Cake, 341
Rice Waffles, 160
Ricotta Pie, 345
Roast Wild Goose, 206
Roasted Cauliflower and Cabbage with Lamb Burger, 223
Roasted Cauliflower with Pomegranate Glaze, 95
Roasted Chanterelle Mushrooms with Caramelized Fennel, 175
Roasted Squashes Moroccan Style, 97
Rocky Mountain Oysters, 201
Rose Hip Jelly, 188
Rose Oyster Mushroom with Epazote & Chipotle Soup, 178
Rustic Potato Pie, 105
Rutabagas, 117
Salmon Kabobs, 258
Salt Rising (Risen) Bread, 155
Salted Caramel Pecan Pie, 347
Sandwich Fillings, 383
Sarvisberry Pie, 186
Sauces and Stuffing, 314

## Index

Sausage & Brussels Sprouts Soup, 232
Sausage and Wild Grains, 240
Sausage Spezzatino, 231
Sautéed Broccoli and Fresh Basil, 88
Sautéed Brussels Sprouts with Chestnuts, 86
Savory Creamy Root Soup, 111
Scotch Oat Cake, 165
Scottish Haggis, 219
Scrambled Eggs with Shaved Oregon White Truffle, 177
Sea Vegetables, 82
Sea Vegetables & Seaweeds, 30
Seared Salmon with Mushrooms and Spinach, 258
Seasonings, 78
Self-Brining Vegetables, 292
Semolina Dumplings, 146
Shaved Apple, Fennel and Celery Salad, 85
Sherry's Easy Baked Figs, 327
Sherry's Tigernut Pancakes, 152
Shortening, 379
Shredded Spicy Chicken, 247
Shrimp & Broccoli, 262
Sicilian Olive Oil, Almond Flour Cake, 342
Silver-Wrapped Fish with Tangerine Peel, 267
Size of Cans, 41
Slippery-Elm Tea, 368
Smoke point, 35
Smoked Sausage, 229

Sopa De Ajo, Sopa De Borracho, 89
Sorrel for the Holidays, 363
Sourdough Apple Oat Muffins, 285
Sourdough Bread Adjustments, 45
Sourdough Pizza Crust, 286
Sourdough Starter, 282
Southern Rockefeller, 263
Southern Way of Cooking Rice, 265
Spiced Brown Rice Bowl, 148
Spiced Cider, 370
Spiced Truffles, 348
Spicy Green Soup Starter, 100
Spicy Meat bars, 200
Spicy Sweet Potato Fries, 108
Split Pea Soup with Dulse, 125
Sprouted and Cultured Spelt Pancakes, 287
Sprouting Seeds & Supplies, 30
Steamed Purslane, 193
Stinging Nettle Sauté, 194
Strawberry Mango Salsa, 309
Stuffed Delicata Squash with Sausage, Greens, & Garlic, 233
Stuffed Heart, 205
Substitutions, 40
Swede Turnip, 117
Sweet Coconut Brown Rice, 147
Sweet Potato "Noodle" Pad Thai, 110

Sweet Potato Noodles with Garlic & Kale, 109
Sweet Potato Pudding, 108
Sweetbreads, 201
Sweetened Condensed Milk, 41
Sweeteners, 38
Switchel, 270
Taco Spice Mix, 216
Tahini Sauce, 313
Tammera's Whole Chicken Routine, 235
Tams Anytime Tortillas, 241
Terms Used in Cooking, 378
The Noble Way To Hunt, 210
The Piperade, 112
Thick Pickle with Pearl Barley & Beef Ribs, 221
Timpsila, 192
To Build A Camp Fire, 386
To Preserve, 381
Toasted Squash Seeds, 91
Tomates Farcies, 173
Tomato Basil and Shrimp Soup, 262
Tomato Soup, 98
Tongue, 201
Traditional Irish Soda Bread, 158
Traditional Salsa, 310
Traditional South African Potjiekos – Cape Malay Chicken Curry Potjie, 247
Trail Mix in Minutes, 353
Tripe, 225
Triple Berry Bars, 324
Triple Mushroom Mélange, 179
Trying Out and Storing Lard, 380

Turkey and Fermented Quinoa Patties, 290
Turkey Stir Fry, 252
Turkish dessert, 338
Types of Flour, 25
Types of Yeast, 27
Vegetables, 85
Venison or Elk Bresaola, 202
Venison with Cranberry Apples Sauce, 209
Waffles, 160, 161
Warm Salmon and Asparagus Salad, 257
Wassail Recipe, 370
Water Filters, 62
Water Kefir, 271
Watercress Dressing, 192
Welsh Cookies, 334
West African Plantain and Okra Stew, 92
What is in that Lunch Box?, 382
White Beans with Olive Oil & Parsley, 128
White Chicken Chili, 241
Whole Grains, 24
Wienerschnitzel, 226
Wild Berry Flummery, 323
Wild Greens Pie, 197
Wild Huckleberry Bars, 186
Wild Rice Salad, 196
Wolfberry fruits, 320
Wrought Iron Range Company, 318
Yam and Ham Soup, 117
Yellow Split Pea Dhal, 127
Zing'n Hot Sauce, 253
Zing's Hot and Saucy Turkey Meat Balls, 252
Zucchini Soup, 98

## Your Authors

TAMMERA J. KARR, Ph.D., BCHN®, CGP, CNW, is an author, educator, researcher, and clinician. She has served as a nutrition advisor to wellness programs and presented at local, regional, and national conferences. She writes blogs, reviews and contributes to national board exams.

Passionate about nutrition as the key to stopping many modern illnesses, Tammera authored *Our Journey with Food* and *Our Journey with Food Cookery Book* adds to the story filling in many gaps in our modern food knowledge for health. Believing "Traditional Foods" are all about community, Tammera invited colleagues, students, friends, and family to contribute to this work.

A native of Oregon, Tammera has over 50 years experience with whole foods and the HOWs for preparing them. She currently resides with her family in rural central-southern Oregon.

CHEF BENJAMIN QUALLS, moved into the world of professional cooking following an active U.S.A. Army career, where he learned first hand about global cuisine. A self-proclaimed chef with over 35 years of experience as head cook for retirement communities and restaurants, Ben provides a practical and varied approach to food for individuals.

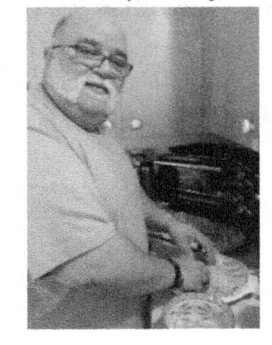

Reminding us that *not everyone has a Whole Foods in their backyard.* Bens passion is developing recipes and menus while revitalizing historical dishes that remind residents of younger days. Ben enjoys experimenting with multicultural and global cuisine.

Chef Ben serves as the Holistic Nutrition for the Whole You culinary advisor. Ben and his family, live along the majestic Columbia River in north-central Oregon.

CHRISTINE WOKOWSKY, CN, CGP, was born in Strasburg, France. She learned cooking from her mother and father, which later formed the foundation for over 30 years in the professional kitchen.

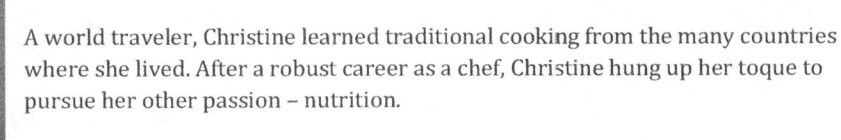

A world traveler, Christine learned traditional cooking from the many countries where she lived. After a robust career as a chef, Christine hung up her toque to pursue her other passion – nutrition.

A graduate of Huntington College of Nutrition, Christine is a Certified Gluten Practitioner and the author of RADIANT DETOX- Your 21-Day Gateway to Vitality. Christine lives in NW Washington state, where she is working with clients.

# It's not about WHAT we eat, but HOW we eat it.

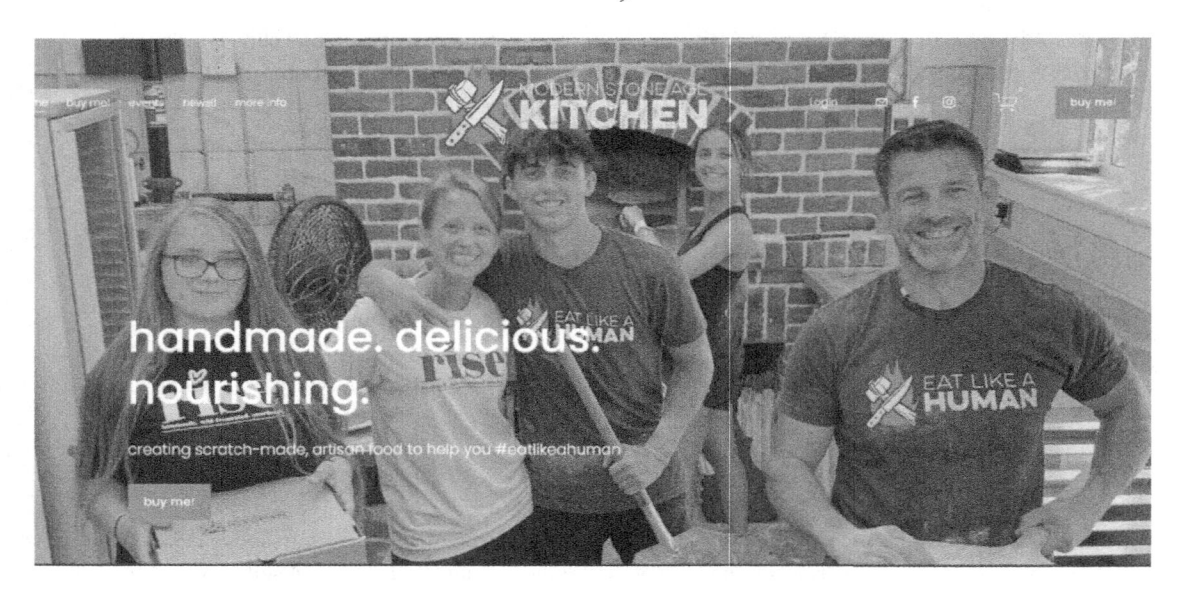

https://modernstoneagekitchen.com/

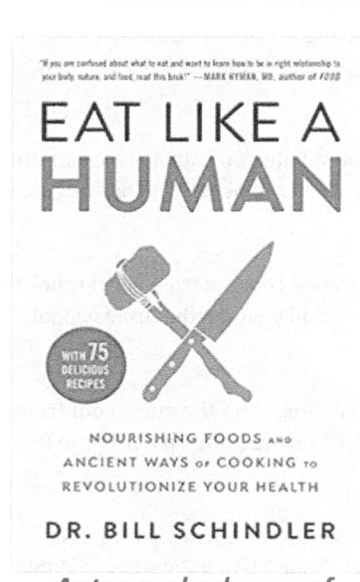

**EASTERN SHORE FOOD LAB**
Informed by the past ~ inspired by the future
innovative classes & events

Learn how to nourish your family
&
EAT LIKE A HUMAN

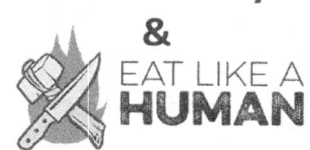

Check our Bills Blog @
https://eatlikeahuman.com/category/blog/

*Autographed copy of
Eat Like a Human
$28.00*

# Books by Tammera Karr

## Available through YourWholeNutrition.com and Amazon.com

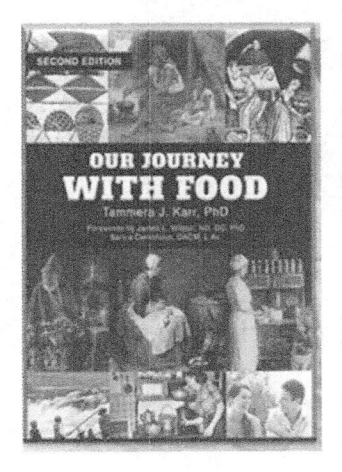

The majority of our population has moved from rural America to the cities and has radically changed their diet from farmed fresh food to corporate prepared food. Our Journey with Food, by Tammera Karr, is a fascinating account of our history of food that explains this process.

Tammera captures this information and, with interest and relevant examples, provides the reader with insights into health and disease. This second edition has included important information on medical cannabis and plasticity of the brain as it is related to the aging process. This book is such an important resource on nutrition that it has been implemented into our required reading for the curriculum at Hawthorn University. We are pleased to be able to provide our students this perspective into nutrition and health.

~Janet Ludwig, Ph.D.
Dean of Integrative Health and Nutrition
American College of Healthcare Sciences

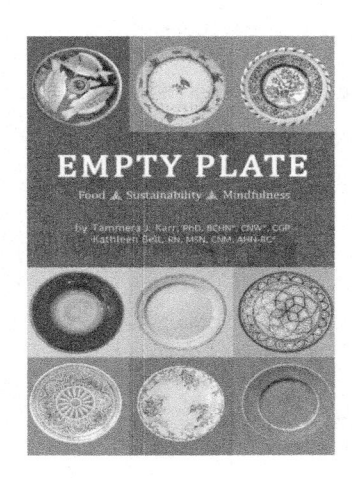

"Empty Plate is a refreshingly original and insightful approach to true "Holistic" health. An enjoyable, thought-provoking blend of history, tradition, and science .... A must read for those with a serious interest in integrative approaches to health."

~Terry Wahls, MD
researcher, educator, and author of the Wahls Protocol

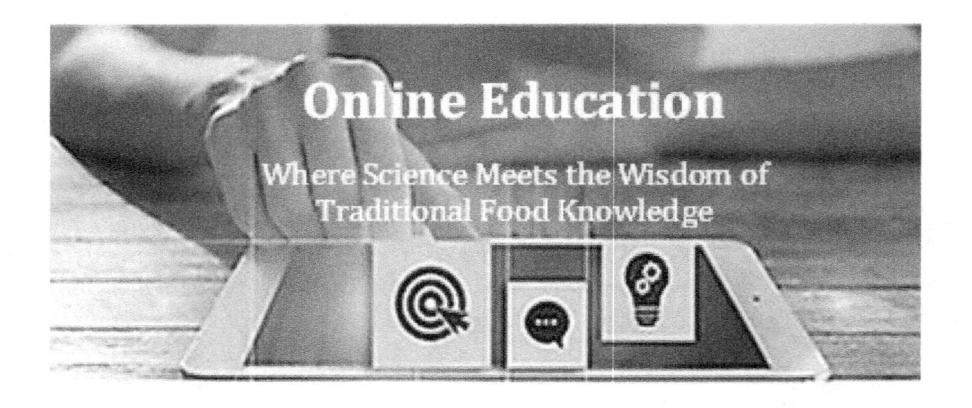

## HN4U Our Journey with Food @ Yourwholenutrition.com

**Who is this program for?**

This course, while initially created for nurses eager to use food as medicine, is also suitable for anyone motivated to learn how to create delicious meals with health-promoting qualities.

**Evidence-Based**

**Why You Want to Take This Program**

**Food and Health**

> "Cutting edge science, practical application for clinicians and clients, history to add context and more... Incredible Value"
> ~Mary Hagood, FNP-C

There is a growing body of science supporting traditional food choices for sustainable health.

- Self-Paced Course with Instructor Access
- 12 Evidence-Based Presentations
- Over 20 Videos with Downloadable Tools
- 3 Exams to Test Knowledge
- Scientific and Historical Citations
- Group Interaction, Recommended Reading, Activities, Support, Tips, and Tools
- 25 credit-hour Approved Certificate of Completion for Nurses.
- 10 credit-hour Certificate for NANP Members
- CEs approved by the American Naturopathic Certification Board

**This Course Will Cover:**

- Nutrition Foundations
- Sustainability in Food Choices for Health
- Mindfulness in Food Selection and Lifestyle

Made in the USA
Monee, IL
05 January 2025